THE WELLNESS BOOK

Also by Herbert Benson, M.D.

The Relaxation Response
(*with Miriam Z. Klipper*)

The Mind/Body Effect

Beyond the Relaxation Response
(*with William Proctor*)

Your Maximum Mind
(*with William Proctor*)

Also by Eileen M. Stuart, R.N., M.S.

Together Toward a Healthier Heart
(*Editor and major contributor*)

THE WELLNESS BOOK

The Comprehensive Guide to Maintaining Health and Treating Stress-Related Illness

Herbert Benson, M.D.
Eileen M. Stuart, R.N., M.S.
and Associates at the Mind/Body Medical Institute
of the New England Deaconess Hospital and Harvard Medical School

Illustrations and graphics by Michael P. Goldberg

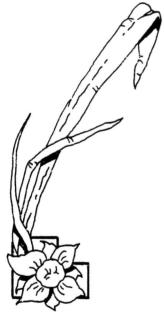

Birch Lane Press
Published by Carol Publishing Group

A Birch Lane Press Book
Published by Carol Publishing Group
Birch Lane Press is a registered trademark of Carol Communications, Inc.

Editorial Offices: 600 Madison Avenue, New York, N.Y. 10022
Sales & Distribution Offices: 120 Enterprise Avenue, Secaucus, N.J. 07094
In Canada: Canadian Manda Group, P.O. Box 920, Station U, Toronto, Ontario M8Z 5P9

Queries regarding rights and permissions should be addressed to Carol Publishing Group, 120 Enterprise Avenue, Secaucus, N.J. 07094

Carol Publishing Group books are available at special discounts for bulk purchases, for sales promotions, fund raising, or educational purposes. Special editions can be created to specifications. For details contact: Special Sales Department, Carol Publishing Group, 120 Enterprise Avenue, Secaucus, N.J. 07094. Proceeds of *The Wellness Book* will be donated to the Mind/Body Medical Institute, Boston.

Lyrics on page 354 from the recording "Wherever You Go"
© 1972, the Benedictine Foundation of the State of Vermont, Inc., Weston, Vt. 05161; composer: Gregory Norbet, O.S.B.

Manufactured in the United States of America

10 9 8 7 6 5 4 3 2 1

Library of Congress Cataloging-in-Publication Data

The Wellness book : the comprehensive guide to maintaining health and treating stress-related illness / by Herbert Benson, Eileen M. Stuart, and the staff of the Mind/Body Medical Institute of New England, Deaconess Hospital, Harvard Medical School.
        p.   cm.
    "A Birch Lane Press book."
    Includes index.
    ISBN 1–55972-092-1
    1. Stress management.   2. Medicine, Psychosomatic.   3. Relaxation.
I. Benson, Herbert, 1935–   . II. Stuart, Eileen M.   III. New
England Deaconess Hospital.
RA785.W45   1992
613—dc20   91–28808
                                                              CIP

Dedicated to:

Our patients who have taught us so very much.

Our colleagues in Medicine, Nursing, Psychology, Dietetics, Physical Therapy, Social Work, Allied Health, and the Clergy who recognize the completeness of their patients and continue to contribute to furthering this understanding.

Marilyn, Jennifer, Gregory, and Steven, with love.   HB

My family: my parents who taught me to believe in myself, and Michael, Josh, and Katie who make all things possible for me.   EMS

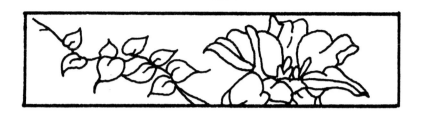

CONTENTS

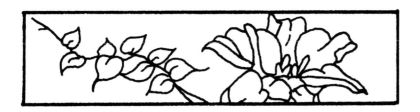

FOREWORD

The Wellness Book combines the best of what you can do to enhance your health and well-being with the marvels of modern scientific health care. It is the result of more than twenty-five years of our scientific research and clinical practice at the Harvard Medical School and three of its five major teaching hospitals. At the time that our research and clinical programs were evolving, they were contributing in a significant fashion to the emerging field of Behavioral Medicine. This *Wellness Book* is a guide to our successful Behavioral Medicine clinics at the New England Deaconess Hospital in Boston. Through it we hope to make our experience available to those not able to attend our clinics.

Behavioral Medicine is a field that combines the many different disciplines related to the integration of mind and body as it relates to health and illness. It applies this model of health to prevention, diagnosis, treatment, and rehabilitation. This approach to health-care recognizes and respects the contribution of individuals to their own health and well-being.

Our clinical programs at the New England Deaconess Hospital had their beginnings after Herbert Benson, M.D., completed his fellowship training in cardiology at the Thorndike Memorial Laboratory in 1967. He then spent two years in the Department of Physiology at Harvard Medical School under the supervision of Dr. A. Clifford Barger. It was there that the remarkable physiological alterations of the relaxation response were discovered. At the same time, Drs. Robert Keith Wallace and Archie F. Wilson were making similar physiologic measurements of meditation in California. Both research teams found that it was possible for you, by simply changing the content of your thoughts (that is, by thinking in a fashion called meditation), to significantly decrease your bodily metabolism, heart rate, rate of breathing, and blood pressure. Your brainwaves would change to distinct slower patterns called alpha, theta, and delta waves, patterns usually associated with deep rest. Benson labeled these physiologic changes the relaxation response and later wrote about it in *The Relaxation Response.*

From 1969 to 1974, our research continued at the Thorndike Memorial Laboratory and from 1974 to 1987 at Boston's Beth Israel Hospital. Since 1987, both the research and clinical programs have been based at the New England Deaconess Hospital. Through this research we came to understand that the relaxation response is successful in reducing symptoms to the extent that any disease or disorder is caused or made worse by stress. The addition of Joan Z. Borysenko, Ph.D., Margaret A. Caudill, M.D., Ph.D., Richard Friedman, Ph.D., Ilan Kutz, M.D., and Eileen M. Stuart, R.N., M.S. to the clinical and research team in the years 1979–1982 brought other Behavioral-Medicine strategies such as cognitive restructuring, multiple risk factor reduction, exercise and nutrition to our programs. Accordingly, we developed and currently offer programs for hypertension, chronic pain, general stress-related symptoms, cancer, HIV + disease, infertility, cardiovascular disease, insomnia, pre-surgery symptoms, and menopause.

This brief history illustrates the development of our programs within the context of medicine based on traditional science. The approaches are designed to interact and work hand in glove with modern medicine. They are not an alternative. If you are considering following this book as adjunct treatment for any chronic symptom or disease, do so under the advice and supervision of a physician or other qualified health-care professional.

In October 1988, the Mind/Body Medical Institute was founded at the New England Deaconess Hospital and Harvard Medical School. It is a non-profit scientific and educational organization dedicated to advancing research, teaching, and training in Behavioral Medicine. The publication of this book is a project of the Mind/Body Medical Institute. All revenues accrued from *The Wellness Book* will be used to help support the work of the Institute.

Each of the chapters of *The Wellness Book* was written by the health professionals who specialize in that area within our clinical programs at the Deaconess Hospital. This book contains short histories of real patients. In all cases, their names and nonessential circumstances have been altered to ensure anonymity. All writings have been directed, coordinated, and edited by Eileen M. Stuart and Herbert Benson.

Important advances in modern medicine are often not glamorous and frequently go unheralded. For example, public health initiatives that saved many lives in the nineteenth and twentieth centuries included sanitation, immunization, and provisions to ensure clean, healthy food. If you consider the advances that make news, such as heart transplantation, you find that they are often necessary because of an illness which could have been prevented and was the result of a lifetime of unhealthy behaviors. Current priorities in health care are shifting because we recognize the implications of the unhealthy lifestyle behaviors which are so common in our country. The challenge for the twenty-first century is to help individuals to change these longstanding, detrimental lifestyle behaviors. This is one challenge the Mind/Body Medical Institute is working to meet.

The Wellness Book is in concert with the goals of the U.S. government initiative Healthy People 2000. By using it, you are on the cutting edge of health care. You have recognized the need to get involved in your health care and make positive changes in your life. You may have recognized that health is not simply the absence of illness, or you may be looking for a way to maximize your ability to control the symptoms of an illness. Whatever your personal goals, we are delighted that you have chosen *The Wellness Book* to guide you on this journey, and hope its teachings will enhance your health and well-being. We wish you the very best of health.

Herbert Benson, M.D.
Eileen M. Stuart, R.N., M.S.
Boston, Massachusetts
January 1992

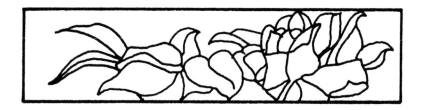

ACKNOWLEDGMENTS

Aspects of *The Wellness Book*, including those meant to ensure an aesthetically pleasing design, were made possible by a grant from Amyas Ames. We are most grateful.

For their excellent editorial coordination we are deeply indebted to Carolyn J. Conte, B.S.; Patricia C. Zuttermeister, M.A.; and Maureen Shirley, B.A. We thank Carol Shookhoff for her editing expertise, superb attention to detail, and good humor. For his help in the writing of an early draft of our clinic workbook we are grateful to Christopher Tilghman, B.A.

We thank the members of our administrative staff who have supported the writing of this book as well as our clinical programs throughout this long process: Patricia Melnick, B.S.; Joyce Rich, M.S.W.; Nancy E. MacKinnon; Kristin Medich, B.S.; and Kim Heath, B.A.

The Wellness Book grew out of the workbooks and manuals developed over the years by the providers in our clinical programs. We gratefully acknowledge the contributions of our many colleagues who have helped shape our clinical programs and contributed to the evolution of this book through their clinical and research work. We thank: Joan Borysenko, Ph.D.; Ilan Kutz, M.D.; Steve Maurer, M.A.; Elizabeth Florentino, R.N., M.S.; Jane Alter, M.S.W.; Carol Mandle, R.N., Ph.D.; Jared Kass, Ph.D.; Richard Parker, M.D.; David Eisenberg, M.D.; David Arond, M.D.; E. Duff Bailey, M.D.; Basil Barr, M.D.; Robert Bengston, M.S., P.T.; Sue Cummings, R.D., M.S.; Christine Doherty, R.N.; Joan Drevins, M.S., P.T.; David Farrar, M.D.; Irene Goodale, Ph.D.; Carol Ginandes, Ph.D.; Harrison Hoblitzelle, Ph.D.; Janice Brazeau-Knuuttunen, P.T.; Margot McCool, R.D., M.S.; Elizabeth Nation, R.N., M.S.; Lou Natividad, R.D.; Patricia Paine, R.N.; Matthew Winer, M.D.; and Carolyn Schwartz, Ph.D.

We would also like to acknowledge our past administrative staff without whose support our programs would never have grown to their current level: Cathy Ball, M.S., P.T.; Debra Corison, R.N., M.S.; Sheila Cusak, M.A.; Roxanne Daleo, M.A.; Claudia Dorrington, B.S.; Anne Jacobs, M.A.; Dianne Katz, M.A.; Norah Mulveney, M.A.; Sandra Pevey; Jennifer Sargent; and Margaret Sweet, B.A.

We are deeply indebted to the many volunteers—students and work-study students—who have contributed their time and expertise to our clinical programs. Unfortunately, too numerous to identify each one by name, their personal contributions have influenced the richness of our programs, and they are very much appreciated and valued by the clinical staff.

We thank Ellen Smith, M.A., and Marilyn Wilcher, B.A., of the Mind/Body Medical Institute executive staff, who have given so freely of themselves to promote the research and teaching programs of the Institute.

Support for the research and clinical programs also came from the Advanced Medical Research Foundation, the American Cancer Society, Mr. and Mrs. Melvin Cohen, Mr. and Mrs. David A. Colker, the Adolph Coors Foundation, William K. Coors, Norman Cousins, Lois Stiles Edgerly, the Nathan Cummings Foundation, Amey A. DeFriez, the Paul P. Dosberg Foundation, Inc., the Fetzer Institute, David Firestone, Hannah Greenbaum, the Harold Grinspoon Charitable Foundation, Eileen Growald, Graham Gund, T. George Harris, Mr. and Mrs. William B. Hood, Jr., Richard M. Hunt, Ph.D., the Hunt Foundation, George Johnson, the Charles F. Kettering Foundation, Arthur Kornhaber, M.D., David B. Kriser, Mr. and Mrs. A. Dix Leeson, Masco Corporation Charitable Foundation, Francis X. Meaney, Esq., the National Institutes of Health, the National Institutes of Mental Health, Laura C. Negley, Domenic C. Pepe, Ann R. Roberts, Laurance S. Rockefeller, the Honorable David M. Roseman, Arman Simone, Ruth Stricker (the Wood-Rill Foundation), Lucy R. Waletzky, M.D., George S. Warburg, John P. Weitzel, Mr. and Mrs. Abrasha Wilcher, Marilyn Wilcher, the Rev. Robert and Kathryn Windsor, and Katharine Winthrop.

PART 1

THE MIND/BODY CONNECTION

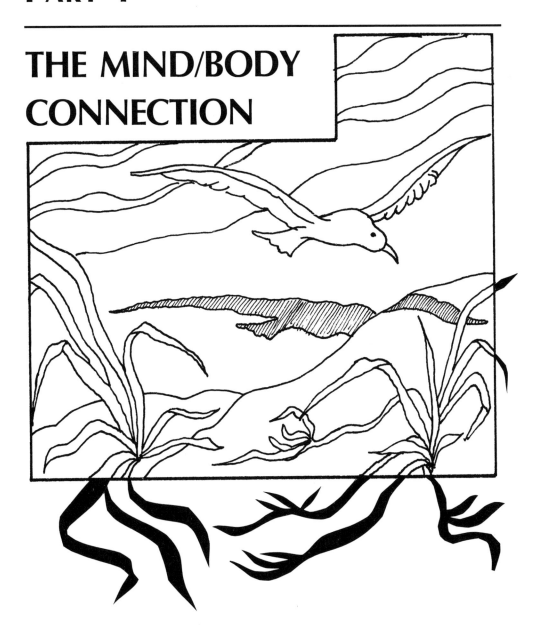

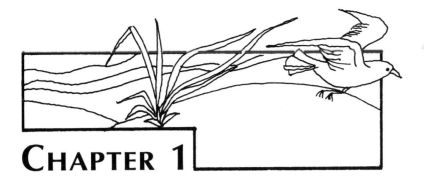

CHAPTER 1

THE BEGINNING

A tree as great as a man's embrace springs from a small shoot.
A terrace nine stories high begins with a pile of earth.
A journey of a thousand miles starts with the first step.

Lao-Tsu, *Tao Te Ching*

In this chapter you will explore

- what this book is about, how to use it, and what to expect in future chapters
- your role in implementing the suggestions in this book

Welcome to *The Wellness Book*. This book is written in a self-help format, designed to provide you with basic information and valuable skills to help you make health-enhancing changes in your life. What you get out of it depends on your motivation as well as your individual health needs and goals. We recognize that you as an individual are unique. Therefore, we have developed exercises to help you clearly identify these needs. Your active participation will enable you to address your needs and learn strategies to achieve your goals. Some of you may want to prevent disease or improve general well-being. Some of you are looking for ways to increase your coping ability or sense of control over a chronic or life-threatening disease. Yet others want to reduce anxiety or stress and related symptoms. Just as participants in our behavioral medicine clinics have various symptoms and motives for enrolling, people have diverse reasons for reading this book. Are any of these reasons yours?

- I want to know how to use my mind and body to help me lead a healthier life.

- I want to sleep better.
- My doctor says I need to lower my blood pressure.
- I have premenstrual syndrome (PMS) and heard that this approach can alleviate my symptoms.
- I've tried everything else for my migraines; this can't hurt.
- I want to understand more about stress so I can manage it.
- I have chronic lower-back pain, and a friend told me this approach helped her.
- I want to exercise more, but I have heart disease (or diabetes or both).
- I want to decrease the stress of having cancer and get on with my life.
- I've had a heart attack and need to reduce my risk for another one.
- I want to do whatever I can to cope with having AIDS.

If so, this book will provide you with a basic outline for healthy lifestyle habits and teach you specific ways to cope with the symptoms of illness.

 Take a Moment To . . .

Identify your motivation for reading this book.

_____

_____

_____

_____

_____

Keep in mind that the approach and specific techniques you will learn here are supplements, not alternatives, to your regular medical care. We expect that you will maintain a close relationship with your physician and other relevant health-care providers for routine medical care and monitoring of your condition. We also expect that you will become more active in promoting your own health and well-being. We give you specific techniques to accomplish this.

Behavioral medicine unites modern scientific medicine, psychology, nursing, nutrition, and exercise physiology to enhance the natural healing capacities of your body and mind. Behavioral medicine strategies have helped many thousands of men and women reduce the stress that contributes to such conditions as joint pain, hypertension, diabetes, cardiac disorders, gastrointestinal disorders, infertility, migraine headaches, and chronic pain. These techniques are also useful in reducing stress, promoting positive attitudes, and improving the quality of life for those with life-threatening diseases. Furthermore, behavioral medicine approaches can prevent disease, such as cardiovascular disease for those at high risk, by encouraging and helping them to change adverse lifestyles.

Behavioral medicine, or mind/body approaches, work because they address not only the physical symptoms of your condition, but also the framework of attitudes and behaviors that surround the condition. They deal with the cycle of stress, anxiety, physical tension, symptoms, and disease. Mind/body approaches teach you to break old, harmful patterns and to develop positive attitudes and behaviors. And, as this book shows, these changes can bring about a sense of well-being which can affect your health and your daily life.

THIS BOOK IS FOR YOU IF . . .

This book is for you if you want to learn more about mind/body interactions and how to use them to improve your health or sense of well-being. This book is for you if you notice that lifestyle and stress can or does affect your health. This book is for you if you have any illness or symptoms which may be caused or made worse by stress. It has been reported that between 60 and 90 percent of those seen in a primary-care physician's office have symptoms or illnesses which can be attributed to stress and lifestyle habits.

> Of the ten leading causes of illness and death in the U.S., seven
> could be greatly reduced if the following lifestyle habits were
> modified—alcohol abuse, lack of exercise, poor diet, smoking, and
> unhealthy maladaptive responses to stress and tension.
> Former U.S. Surgeon General Julius B. Richmond, M.D.

Do you see in yourself any of the risk factors outlined by the Surgeon General? By recognizing the relationship between lifestyle, stress, and your health, you have a foundation for understanding the mind/body connection and the importance of establishing an active role in your health care.

Knowledge is a necessary first step toward initiating change, but it is not sufficient in and of itself. If knowledge alone were enough, no nurse would smoke, no physician would be obese, no psychologist would be burned out by stress, and each health-care professional would exercise. Once you have identified an adverse lifestyle behavior, the next step is to work toward changing it. *The Wellness Book* provides a structure to help you identify what changes are important and how to make these changes successfully.

HOW THIS BOOK IS ORGANIZED

Each chapter of *The Wellness Book* focuses on a specific aspect of the mind/body approach, which includes the relaxation response, nutrition, exercise and body awareness, cognitive restructuring, stress management, coping, problem-solving, and humor. Basic information provided on each topic will help you develop the skills and attitudes necessary to begin to make healthy changes.

Although each chapter may be read alone, we recommend that you first read through the entire book. In that way, what you learn about yourself and the techniques and attitudes you develop in one chapter can be reinforced and built upon in later chapters.

HOW TO USE THIS BOOK

The popular saying "Today is the first day of the rest of your life" imparts a sense of hope and renewal, and it contains simple wisdom. A new beginning is what *The Wellness Book* offers you, a chance to change for the better your behaviors, attitudes, or ways of thinking that may be aggravating your symptoms, interfering with your healing process, or hindering self-improvement. This new beginning includes an invitation to take a more active role in your health. We will present a variety of techniques and approaches that will help you let go of old habits and behaviors that serve you badly and replace them with new habits that serve you well.

The Wellness Book is based on the philosophy that you can enhance the process of healing or staying well by first understanding how the mind and body work together and then by practicing your new skills daily. Read it with pencil, pen, crayons, and paper handy—it asks for a good deal of your own input as you read and work toward change. Plan to reflect and to practice the new skills you will be learning. Discuss your plans for using this book with your health-care professional so that your efforts are coordinated with the care you are already receiving.

The chapters in *The Wellness Book* were written by clinical experts in the Mind/Body Medical Institute who share a common belief in the mind/body model of health and illness. All the chapters have a similar format, designed to help you apply specific knowledge, skills, and awareness to your situation or condition. This format includes:

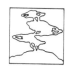

In this chapter you will explore
the objectives of the chapters.

Case Histories
stories describing the experience of patients who have completed our program, to help you see how one person applied what is taught in the clinic.

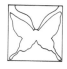

Take a Moment to . . .
series of questions, exercises, or reflections designed to help you apply what you are learning. This may involve writing, taking a deep breath, or paying attention to your thoughts.

The illustrations, diagrams, photographs, charts, and quotes found throughout these pages may help you see your situation differently or reinforce new ideas. You may find it helpful to photocopy some of them to use as reminders. References for each chapter are at the end of the book; we encourage you to turn to these works to explore further any aspect of what you are learning or experiencing.

Although we understand that making health-enhancing changes in your life may seem like an overwhelming task at this point, we expect you to succeed. Thousands of people have successfully completed our clinical programs and have found them both helpful and enjoyable. Now it's your turn.

> Look to this day!
> For it is life, the very life of life.
> In its brief course
> Lie all the verities and realities of your existence:
>   The bliss of growth;
>   The glory of action;
>   The splendor of achievement;
> For yesterday is but a dream,
> And tomorrow is only a vision;
> But today, well lived, makes every yesterday
>   a dream of happiness,
> And every tomorrow a vision of hope.
> *Look well, therefore, to this day!*
>
> "Kalidasa," ancient Sanskrit poem

Sue C. Jacobs, Ph.D.
Cynthia Medich, R.N., M.S.

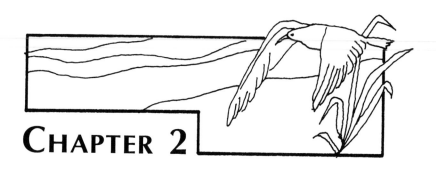

CHAPTER 2

THE MIND/BODY MODEL OF HEALTH AND ILLNESS

Then deem it not an idle thing,
  A pleasant word to speak;
The face you wear—the thoughts you bring—
  The heart may heal or break.

> Daniel Clement Colesworthy
> "A Little Word"

In this chapter you will explore

- how the mind and body interact
- the mind/body model of health and illness

The term *mind/body* is used frequently in *The Wellness Book* to describe the many complicated interactions that take place between your thoughts, your body, and the outside world. According to this mind/body model, your general health depends on a multitude of factors. It depends, for example, not only on your genetics or such measures as your cholesterol and blood-pressure levels, but also on such factors as your health habits and lifestyle, your emotional state, social support, and environment. Within this model, you can potentially achieve health benefits from positive changes in any of the biological, psychological, or social areas.

The awareness that mind and body interact has important implications for the way we view illness and treat disease. According to the mind/body model, the treatment of illness will be most effective if attention is paid to the mind and body as well as to their interaction with the outside world. For example, taking prescribed blood-pressure medication helps lower high blood pressure and reduce the risk of heart disease, but smoking, social isolation, and high cholesterol should also be taken into account as important risk factors for developing heart disease. The mind/body relationship implies that if you address only one of these factors you may not be able to achieve the best possible results.

BECOMING AN ACTIVE PARTICIPANT IN YOUR HEALTH CARE

The mind/body model emphasizes that beliefs influence health and well-being. For example, your beliefs affect how you comply with medical treatments; if you do not believe your medications are helpful, there is a strong possibility you will not take them. Furthermore, even if you do take them, you may not benefit as much as you would if you believed they were worthwhile. Believing in your treatment may bring you additional benefit through the placebo effect. The placebo effect has three components: (1) the beliefs of the patient; (2) the beliefs of the health practitioner; and (3) the relationship between patient and health practitioner. When these are positive, a placebo has a 37 percent chance of working as well as an active medicine. If you believe in your surgeon and in the surgery you will have better results than if you believe in neither. Believing in the benefits of your treatment and in your health practitioner is important because belief enhances the effectiveness of the treatment.

One dramatic example of the power of belief and the placebo effect came from Dr. Stewart Wolf while he was at New York Hospital in 1950. Patients suffering from the nausea and vomiting of pregnancy were told they were to be given a drug that would alleviate their problem. In truth, they were given Ipecac, a drug used to induce vomiting. The patients' nausea and vomiting disappeared after taking the Ipecac—their *belief* in the drug's powers actually counteracted the biologic actions of the drug.

A more recent example of the importance of belief came from a study by Dr. R. Horowitz and his colleagues reported in the *Lancet* in 1990. They analyzed data from a large, multicenter study called the Beta Blocker Heart Attack Trial. This study compared the rates of death among patients who did or did not take their medication (a beta blocker) as prescribed. Those patients who *did not* take their medication as prescribed were 2.6 times more likely to die than those who did take their medication. The pills, taken as prescribed, appeared to have a protective effect. The astonishing finding, however, was that similar results occurred with the placebo group as well! That is, patients who *did not* take their "medication" as prescribed had an increased rate of death whether they were prescribed the beta blocker *or* the placebo. These results were independent of psychological characteristics, smoking, or family history—all of which could have influenced the results.

Believing in your ability to control your health has other important implications. Your success in making changes in your lifestyle, such as losing weight or stopping smoking, is directly related to your belief that you can make those changes and that they will positively affect your health and well-being.

The mind/body approach to health requires your active participation. Your decision to use *The Wellness Book* may be part of a history of multiple doctor visits, medications, and therapies. Or it may be the start of a new partnership that includes you in your heath care. Regardless of the reason, your belief in mind/body medicine will help you help yourself.

Joan's Experience

Joan, thirty-six and working as a computer programmer, consulted a primary-care physician because she was bothered by headaches. During the brief history and physical exam, the physician found Joan's blood pressure to be quite high (150/100 mm Hg). She was twenty pounds overweight, and blood tests revealed that her cholesterol was high (280 mg/dl). She admitted to smoking one pack of cigarettes a day.

The physician prescribed medication to treat her blood pressure and elevated cholesterol. She told Joan to lose weight and stop smoking, and she scheduled a follow-up appointment in two months.

When Joan returned, she complained that her headaches had not improved. Her blood pressure was still high (160/102 mm Hg), she had lost no weight, and she had not been able to quit smoking. When the doctor asked why she had not followed through on her recommendations, she began to cry. She was feeling overwhelmed; she was new to the area and had no support to help her. She could not afford the medications because they cost ninety dollars a month. Her husband had recently left her after a stormy marriage, and she was having difficulty supporting their two children. She had taken a second job as a waitress on the weekends. This left her little time for her children or herself, and she was feeling guilty about this. She felt overwhelmed, tired, and depressed. She was not sleeping well, her headaches were occurring daily, and she wondered how she could take time to exercise and eat properly at a time like this. To attempt to quit smoking now seemed impossible to her.

Her physician realized that to treat Joan's headaches and blood pressure successfully, she would need to consider much more than the physiology of these conditions. She reiterated the importance of the medications she had prescribed but she also spent time listening to Joan, allowing her to give vent to her countless difficulties. She referred Joan to a social worker to see if she qualified for financial assistance and for guidance regarding social support. Her physician also referred her to the

Behaviorai Medicine Hypertension Clinic at the New England Deaconess Hospital for help in understanding mind/body interactions as well as learning specific interventions to decrease the frequency of her headaches and lower her blood pressure and cholesterol. The physician assured her that she could get her symptoms and blood pressure under control and that Joan could cope with her current crisis. She also encouraged Joan to begin to address her lifestyle changes, emphasizing how important this was for her.

Joan left the office feeling much better (her blood pressure on repeat measure that day was 140/95 mm Hg). She felt someone had finally listened to her, and so she felt less helpless and hopeless. Joan subsequently met with the social worker and was evaluated for participation in the Hypertension Clinic. Within six weeks, her headaches were gone. She was sleeping normally and, although still under great stress, was less anxious. Furthermore, her blood pressure and cholesterol were now normal.

Joan's case illustrates just how integrally connected the mind and body are. In the mind/body model, your health depends on a multitude of factors. Physical symptoms are influenced by thoughts, feelings, and behaviors. And conversely, thoughts, feelings, and behaviors are influenced by physical symptoms. Social factors are also fundamentally important. By attending to Joan's immediate need for financial help, social support, and reassurance, her physician acknowledged the multiple factors that influenced her blood pressure and her symptoms. Her physician also engendered belief, her belief that Joan could succeed, and her belief that changing her lifestyle was important to Joan's health. Further, she treated the physical dimension of high blood pressure with medication.

CHANGING PERSPECTIVES

For decades Western medicine has searched scientifically for specific causes of diseases and treatment for the symptoms. This proved to be a successful approach to diseases such as tuberculosis and smallpox; patients were cured if the specific cause was eliminated. This method, however, is not always effective. For example, blocked arteries can be bypassed with heart surgery. But if the patient continues to smoke, has a high cholesterol intake, or does not take his blood-pressure medication, the heart vessels can become blocked again. In this instance, the disease is likely to progress if underlying habits, lifestyles, and compliance with treatment are not addressed.

Besides incorporating the most sophisticated discoveries and treatments of modern medicine, the mind/body model recognizes that your thoughts, your emotions, and your behaviors directly influence your health, and therefore takes a more comprehensive approach to health care. The mind/body connection is based on a well-documented series of research studies conducted over several decades (Engel, Goldman, Pennebaker, Ornstein). The results of these studies lead to two firm conclusions:

1. *Specific behaviors contribute to illness.* Our behaviors with respect to food, alcohol, tobacco, exercise, and drugs profoundly affect the development of and recovery from disease. We also know that systematic, formal approaches to modifying behavior can be more successful than unsystematic, informal approaches. Throughout *The Wellness Book*, you will be given carefully planned and integrated exercises intended to help bring about changes which have been proven to enhance well-being.

2. *Psychological and emotional reactions directly affect physiological function.* The way you react to your environment, both psychologically and emotionally, determines, in part, your physiological state. These so-called psychophysiological interactions are an important component of living. When we have calm peaceful thoughts, we tend to have a comparable emotional reaction and similar physiological reaction as well. When we have angry or fearful thoughts, we tend to be emotionally aroused, and consequently our physiological reactions are more dramatic.

    We now know that stress-induced physiological reactions, if repeated or prolonged, can contribute to illness. Hence, the thoughts and emotional reactions which give rise to these physiological reactions must be addressed. You will learn the mechanisms by which stress causes physiological change, and you will also be given specific strategies to manage stress and thereby reduce problematic physiological reactions. Learning to manage stress, using the techniques described in this book, will not only make you more comfortable psychologically, but will also help you stay healthy by reducing the by-product of psychological stress–physiological arousal.

In 1979, Julius B. Richmond, M.D., then Surgeon General, issued *Healthy People: The Surgeon General's Report on Health Promotion and Disease Prevention.* As noted earlier, this report stated that as many as half the premature deaths in the United States may be due to unhealthy behaviors or lifestyles. It further suggested that of the ten leading causes of premature death, at least seven could be substantially reduced if Americans altered their bad habits. These included poor diet, smoking, lack of exercise, alcohol abuse, and unhealthy responses to tension and stress. This document began to shift the focus of our thinking about health and illness away from identifying and treating one specific cause of disease to a much broader understanding of disease prevention and treatment.

Another important study contributing to the shift away from one specific cause of disease is the research on cardiovascular disease conducted in Framingham, Massachusetts. This study, spanning four decades, clearly identified smoking, sedentary lifestyle, stress, and obesity—in addition to elevated blood pressure and cholesterol—as important factors in predicting heart disease. (In fact, poor diet, lack of exercise, smoking, and alcohol abuse can be identified as contributing to many diseases.)

The mechanisms by which personal beliefs, psychosocial factors, and stress affect the development of disease are not as well understood. What we do know, however, is that the mind and body communicate constantly with each other. What the minds thinks, perceives, and experiences is transmitted from our brain to the rest of our bodies. It also works the other way: our bodies send messages to our brain.

Take a Moment To . . .

Clench your fists and jaw. Close your eyes, and wrinkle your eyebrows for thirty seconds.
Did you hold your breath? Did you feel tense?
Pay attention to what thoughts go through your mind.
Did you have angry thoughts?

The *physical* action of clenching your fists and jaw or wrinkling your eyebrows induces the emotions and thoughts that usually lead to feelings of anger. Your thoughts, your emotions, and your physical actions tend to act together in this way. It is possible for thoughts (*I can't stand this! How dare that car cut me off!*) and emotions (anger, frustration) to be associated with physical changes (increased blood pressure, increased muscle tension) that can be potentially harmful.

Take a Moment To . . .

Hold a pen in your mouth tightly with your lips; about one-third of the pen will be in your mouth and the remainder will extend straight out of your mouth, pointing in the same direction as your nose. Do not let your teeth touch the pen. Hold the pen with your lips only, pursing your lips around it. Hold this position for a few moments. Besides feeling "foolish" or "silly," how would you describe your physical and emotional feelings within this facial expression?

_____

_____

Now hold the pen gently between your front teeth without touching it with your lips. Hold this position for a few moments. Does this feel physically or emotionally different from the above experience? Note any differences.

_____

_____

In the first position you were using muscles that typically inhibit smiling. In the second position you were using muscles that typically facilitate smiling. Recent psychological research has shown that these simple physical differences alter mood. Many of us believe our mood results from external situations, but this is not necessarily true. How we choose to respond or act has as much if not more impact on our mood than events that occur outside ourselves. This simple demonstration illustrates how inextricably linked the mind and body are and how you can use this interaction to influence your health positively.

By learning how to use your mind to alter your lifestyle and minimize the mind's negative effects, you will assume more control over your own health. You will also learn what is beyond your control and when you should adopt a more accepting attitude. This is the beginning of the beginning!

Margaret Caudill-Slosberg, M.D., Ph.D.
Richard Friedman, Ph.D.

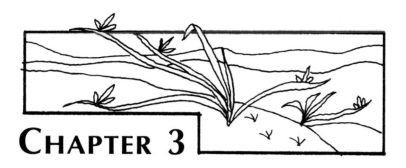

CHAPTER 3

GETTING STARTED

Are you in earnest? Seize this very minute—
What you can do, or dream you can, begin it,
Boldness has genius, power, and magic in it.
Only engage, and then the mind grows heated—
Begin it, and the work will be completed!

Goethe, *Faust, Part I*

In this chapter you will explore

- where you are in relation to your health
- how to identify long-term goals
- how to develop strategies to achieve long-term goals
- how to make an initial Health Commitment
- how to see change as a challenge, rather than a threat

In chapter 1 you contemplated *why* you are reading *The Wellness Book*. You have made a choice to read this book, recognizing that your health status can profoundly affect your lifestyle, and that your lifestyle may be affecting your health. They are inseparable. You may have decided to adopt a new pattern of behaviors to reduce certain risk factors or symptoms in order to improve your overall health and well-being. Our goal is to guide you toward that decision with an adequate level of awareness and help you take action toward better health.

Each person learns and approaches change in their own unique way. This chapter addresses the change process, including getting started and being successful. While some people find that they would prefer to learn the principles of how to change first, others would prefer to read content first, then come back to this chapter. In our clinical programs we have found that it is helpful to look at the how-tos of change and set goals early in the program. Whether you read this chapter now or later, take the time to consider carefully and participate in its many exercises.

Developing an awareness of yourself and your behavior will enable you to take increased responsibility for your choices. Your current level of motivation as well as your ability to identify and think about feelings, strengths, and personal assets all influence the choices you make and your degree of success. As a first step in developing self-awareness, we are going to ask you to stop and take a moment to complete the following exercise.

Take a Moment To . . .

Look back to chapter 1 where you identified why you are reading this book. Imagine how you would like to be different, what would change if you reached your goals? Can you put it in words? Can you draw it or visualize it? Express it some other way—in song or movement?

Use This Space to Write/Draw In . . .	
ME NOW	ME AS I WANT TO BE

Was this exercise difficult for you? It was for Kate. Let's look at her experience with change.

Kate's Experience

Kate, a fifty-one-year-old elementary school teacher, entered one of our clinical programs to stop smoking, reduce the symptoms of bronchitis, and reduce her anxiety and fears. She came because she was afraid of what would happen if she continued smoking. She worried about developing heart disease and lung cancer; she already had chronic bronchitis. She had wanted to stop smoking by the age of fifty and had tried to quit three times before. At the beginning of her program she was able to imagine herself not smoking, but she could not imagine feeling calm and relaxed. During the course of the clinical program she learned to elicit the relaxation response and other behavioral techniques to help her become more calm and stop smoking. She began to exercise. She enlisted the support of her family and the help of a health-care professional.

Slowly, Kate's image of herself changed. She saw herself not only as a nonsmoker, but as a more vibrant, healthy woman possessing increased self-confidence and self-respect. Kate's is a success story. She was able not only to quit smoking, but also to improve her breathing problems, and she felt calmer. In addition, she decreased her blood pressure, a goal she had not originally sought to achieve.

Changing a particular lifestyle behavior is usually not easy. It is not a single event or a one-time decision, but a dynamic process of self-reflection, gathering information, making choices, developing skills, constantly readjusting a plan, and having important personal needs met along the way. It means developing a sense of humor so that you can be free to see those unwanted behaviors in a way that is nonjudging. It means adopting the attitude that although you may want to change certain behaviors, parts of you are excellent.

Throughout *The Wellness Book* you will be asked first to identify and then to evaluate and reevaluate your goals, plans, and progress. We will give you specific tools and strategies to succeed in this process. But before we begin, let us be certain that these goals are consistent with what is important, meaningful, or valuable to you.

CLARIFYING WHAT IS IMPORTANT / MEANINGFUL / VALUABLE TO YOU

One technique to help you get in touch with what you value and ultimately, to help you identify your long-term goals is the "Ten Loves" exercise. Developed by Dr. Sidney B. Simon, a pioneer in the field of values-clarification and humanistic education, this exercise asks you, "Am I getting what I really want out of life?"

First, read how this exercise helped Kate, and then try it yourself. When she completed her list of loves, it included such things as going on adventure tours and cruises, taking walks in the park, ballroom dancing with her husband, and playing with her new grandchild. By listing her "Ten Loves," Kate realized she was taking fewer tours, not walking, and not dancing because she tired easily and became short of breath. She knew she would have more energy and breathe better if she stopped smoking. The exercise raised her awareness of the limitations that cigarette smoking was imposing on those things which were important to her. It gave her the reason and increased her motivation to set smoking cessation as a goal, and to go about the hard work of successfully making this change.

Take a Moment To . . .

Complete this "Ten Loves" exercise by using the following format. List ten things you love to do. To the right of each love, answer these questions:

a. The date when you last did this.
b. Do your prefer doing this alone (A) or with other people (P)?
c. Would the person closest to you approve of this?
d. Did you like to do this five, ten years ago?
e. Do you expect to do this five, ten years from now or when you retire?
f. Does it involve risk, either physical or emotional?
g. Is your health status interfering with doing this?
h. Put a star by the five you love best.

To help you, we show part of Kate's list.

Ten Loves

	Date	Alone?	Approve?	Past?	Future?	Risk?	Health
1. Dancing	2 yrs	P	Yes	Yes	Yes	No	Yes
2. Walks	6 Mo	A	Yes	Yes	Yes	No	Yes

Your list:

Ten Loves

	Date	Alone?	Approve?	Past?	Future?	Risk?	Health
1.							
2.							
3.							
4.							
5.							
6.							
7.							
8.							
9.							
10.							

What did you learn from this exercise? Are there things you love to do that you no longer do? Are you not doing things because of your health? How balanced is your time between leisure and work? Write down at least three things you discovered or rediscovered about yourself.

What do you want to change in your life? What would bring you fulfillment or balance? What is it you want to do?

This process you have just completed will be important as you think about specific behaviors you want to change and goals you want to accomplish. It is important that these goals be personally relevant and consistent with those life values you just identified. Thinking about your long-range goals will force you to consider important life values, detect inconsistencies between your ideal values and actual living habits, and establish a working plan for fulfilling them.

DETERMINING YOUR LONG-TERM GOAL OR GOALS

Let us first briefly define some terms we will use frequently.

- *Long-term goal:* A goal which you plan to achieve within three, six, twelve months or longer.
- *Short-term goal:* Specific strategies or actions to assist you in achieving your long-term goal.
- *Stage of change:* The place from which you are beginning the process of achieving your goal. Different stages of change require different strategies to reach the same goal.

The first step in changing behavior is to identify your long-term goals. They can be described as your destination. They should be measurable, realistic, positive, and attainable. They should be viewed as a challenge rather than a threat. To help you identify your long-term goals:

- Decide what areas in your life are important. In which of these do you need or want to make changes? What is it you want to do?
- Think of your long-term goals as your destination. How will you know when you get there, when you have made the changes you want?
- Make sure your goals are realistic and attainable. Examples of long-term goals might include: "I will have stopped smoking in six months," "I will lose twenty pounds," "I will not get stressed when someone cuts me off in traffic," or perhaps "I will become aware of the physical sensations I experience when I am stressed."

Take a Moment To . . .

List your long-term health goals. You may have identified these goals earlier as you completed the values-clarification exercise, or you may have been clear on these goals when you bought this book. In addition to these initial long-term goals, as you continue to read *The Wellness Book*, you will undoubtedly add new goals to your list. This is exactly what should occur with this dynamic, evolving process.

My Long-Term Goals

1. _____
   _____

2. _____
   _____

3. _____
   _____

4. _____
   _____

5. _____
   _____

THE HEALTH COMMITMENT—
A WAY TO ACHIEVE YOUR LONG-TERM GOALS

Writing out specific plans for reaching goals can help you make continued progress toward them. We have developed the Health Commitment form, a formal contract with yourself, as a tool to guide your progress through the stages of successful behavior change. (See the blank Health Commitment form for your own use, page 31.) As you proceed through *The Wellness Book* and learn more about the mind/body model for health, the relaxation response, nutrition, exercise, and stress management, you may well be inspired to create additional long-term goals or identify more specific strategies (short-term goals). Therefore we have included additional copies of the Health Commitment form at the end of every chapter. We recommend using one form for each long-term goal.

Let's get started writing *your* Health Commitment. There are five main steps.

Step 1.   Choose one long-term goal

Choose one long-term goal from the list that you just identified in the previous exercise.

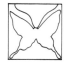

Take a Moment To . . .

Turn now to the blank Health Commitment form at the end of this chapter and begin to create your own contract. Write down the *one* long-term goal you have just chosen from your list on page 20. (Repeat this process for each of your long-term goals.)

Ask yourself the following:

- Have I stated what I want in a positive way?
- Is my long-term goal realistic and attainable?
- How will I know when I've reached my destination, achieved my goal?
- Do the benefits of achieving the goal outweigh the costs? If the answer is no, give this more thought and consider a more realistic goal. Unrealistic goals are frustrating and the biggest contributors to lack of success.
- What other kinds of barriers may get in the way of reaching my goal?
- Should I revise my goals to be more realistic and attainable if the benefits do not outweigh the cost?
- When do I expect to reach my goal?
- What is my time frame?

To illustrate, we will construct a sample Health Commitment using Kate's experience. One of her goals was to stop smoking (see opposite).

As you identify your long-term goal, it is important to think of it as your destination. How will you know when you get there? Kate stated her destination in a positive way. She would know she had reached her goal when she no longer smoked cigarettes and when she had the energy to do the things she liked; she would be living her image of herself as a nonsmoker. She gave herself three months to quit smoking.

Consider your readiness to change

Drs. James O. Prochaska and Carlo DiClemente, behavioral scientists known for their research in behavior change, have shown that if you understand your readiness to change, you are better able to identify what you need to do to achieve and maintain specific changes. We have adapted their model as follows.

Ask yourself which of the following best describes your readiness to change in relation to each long-term goal you have chosen:

> Never considered change; need information
> Considered change, but not yet committed
> Desire change; need motivation
> Attempting change; need structure, support, and skills
> Change made; need reinforcement
> Change made; slipping back into bad habits (relapse); need renewed
> motivation and support

Understanding your readiness to change becomes useful as you go on to select strategies (short-term goals) to achieve your goal, because different stages of change require different strategies to reach the same goal.

Step 2. Choose short-term goals

One of the most important, but often most difficult, parts of writing a Health Commitment is determining your short-term goals. Short-term goals are *strategies* to achieve your long-term goal. They are specific, realistic, measurable, and behavior-oriented. Stating that you will walk one mile today is more effective than stating you will walk a hundred miles over the next six months. You have more control over what is happening today than at some distant point in the future. If your long-range goal is to lose twenty pounds over twelve weeks, it is helpful to say that you will lose one-and-a-half pounds this week, but even more effective to say that you will have fruit instead of ice cream for dessert today.

The following goal-setting model, with examples from Kate's experience, should help you write your short-term goals.

EXAMPLE
KATE'S HEALTH COMMITMENT

Long-Term Goal:

Become a nonsmoker

Signature

Witness

Expected Date of Reaching Goal: _____ 3 months _____

Readiness to Change	Short-Term Goals	Comments (supports, rewards, etc.)
Attempting change; need structure, support, and skills.	a) Purchase only one package of cigarettes at a time. b) Switch brands with each package. c) Buy only low-tar, low-nicotine brand. d) Purchase cigarettes at only one store and must walk to the store each time. e) Limit my coffee intake to two cups per day. f) Elicit the relaxation response every day.	Supports—Walk with dog to store; she needs to be walked anyway. Also, walk with daughter, which will give us some quality time together. Walking to store will also increase my resolve to quit smoking if I am short of breath.

Take a Moment To . . .

- Compile a list of all the positive actions you are currently taking that will help you achieve your long-term goal.

    Kate's example: I now only purchase one package of cigarettes at a time. I switch brands with each package I buy. I buy only low-tar, low-nicotine brands.

    Your list of positive activities:

    _____

    _____

    _____

    _____

- Now compile a list of behaviors you would like to change or eliminate because they interfere with your ability to reach your long-term goal.

    Kate's example: I smoke with each cup of coffee I drink. I drive to the store to get cigarettes, making it as easy as possible to get them.

    Your list of behaviors to change:

    _____

    _____

    _____

    _____

- Select one behavior from this list of behaviors to change.

    Kate's example: I will walk to the store to get cigarettes.

    Your behavior to target for change:

    _____

    _____

    _____

    _____

- Now list all the positive effects of changing that behavior.

Kate's example: Walking to the store to purchase cigarettes makes it a more difficult task, increases my awareness of what I am doing, and improves my breathing. All of these reinforce my goal to quit.

Your list of positive effects of change:

_____

_____

_____

_____

- List all the negative effects of not changing.

  Kate's example: Continuing to smoke will increase my respiratory problem and my risk for developing coronary artery disease.

Your list of negative effects of not changing:

_____

_____

_____

_____

- Consider the obstacles to changing this behavior.

  Kate's example: The store was a mile away, and since she was not used to walking, this seemed almost too far for her.

Your obstacles to change:

_____

_____

_____

_____

- Consider some of your supports for change that can help you overcome obstacles. Supports can be the social support of people who cheer you on or engage in an activity with you. Supports can be within you, such as feeling good about yourself. Or supports can be rewards, things you find pleasant or desirable. It may be something you have not done in a while. It can be a social reward: have lunch with a friend, talk on the phone, play with children or animals, help someone in need, ask someone for a hug—or give one. A reward can be giving yourself "alone time," going to a ball game, working on a hobby, reading a good book, going fishing, or simply watching the stars. Or a reward can be taking the time to take a walk, play a game of tennis, or go dancing. A reward can be enjoying a fresh, crisp apple, treating yourself to the shirt you have been eyeing, smelling a summer rose, feeling the softness of a puppy's fur, or watching a sunset.

> *Kate's experience*: Kate found support for walking to the store by taking the dog with her and inviting her daughter along. She bought new exercise clothes which made her look healthy and fit, and she treated herself with fruit to eat on the walk home.

Your supports for change:

_____

_____

_____

_____

Take a Moment To . . .

Set short-term goals you can *live* with.

Now that you have carefully considered and written your long-term goal, a date to achieve that goal, your readiness to change, and the benefits, barriers, and supports for change, it is time to write your short-term goals. Refer to Kate's example on page 23 if this will be helpful.

Turn to the Health Commitment form at the end of the chapter and write your short-term goals. Emphasize performance and outcome. Use action-oriented statements. Some verbs helpful in writing your goals include *recognize, prepare, practice, plan, choose, decide, participate in,* and *complete.* Take time with this portion of the process. It is worth the effort.

Step 3.   Sign the commitment

Now is the time to maximize your commitment by signing your list of goals in front of a witness. This is a good way to involve a friend or family member. Involving other people is a way of letting them know what you are doing and asking for their encouragement and support. Let them know that smiles, hugs, and praise are helpful. Perhaps people you are close to are also interested in improving their diet or stopping smoking or starting an exercise program. Working together can provide additional incentive for all of you.

Take a Moment To . . .

Sign your Health Commitment and choose someone close to you to witness this.

Step 4.   Evaluate your Health Commitment

Your Health Commitment will need to be updated on a regular basis. Look at it frequently to evaluate your progress. The following guidelines and questions will help you assess your progress as you work through *The Wellness Book*:

- Evaluate your progress daily or weekly. Did you reach your short-term goals? If not, should you try again or back up a step? Is your goal still appropriate? Slipping up once or twice is okay. Do not throw out the whole plan if it is still reasonable. If you continue to slip, reevaluate your plan. It may not be reasonable. You may need to change your plan or establish your short-term goals in smaller, more attainable increments. Try incorporating more rewards.
- Use your Health Commitment throughout the process. Describe your experience with your short-term goals in the Comments column. Emphasize your accomplishments. It helps to say aloud to yourself what you accomplished—affirm that you can do it. For example, write "I smoked one less cigarette today" or "I practiced the relaxation response for twenty minutes." Reward yourself for reaching short-term goals. Visualize yourself meeting your next short-term goal. At least once a day imagine what life will be like once you accomplish your goal. Take a few minutes to reflect on what you learned about yourself, regardless of whether you achieved the day's goal or not.
- As you progress, reassess readiness to change and modify your short-term goals to reflect your changing needs. Enter any new short-term goals on your Health Commitment.

MOVING TO THE NEXT STEP

> Habit is habit, and not to be flung out of the window by any man, but coaxed downstairs a step at a time.
>
> Mark Twain, *Pudd'nhead Wilson*

By completing the exercises, you have already started to gain some of the skills you need to achieve your goals. Keep in mind that change is a complex process best accomplished by a series of small steps and a workable plan such as the one you have begun to map out with your Health Commitment. You have passed through the starting gates. The task now is to concentrate on one step at a time.

You must also *be patient*. Slow and steady wins the race. Also, slow and steady can be interesting and fun.

Before going on to the next chapter, take a break and look at yourself in a mirror. Note what is beautiful about you, inside and out. Imagine how much more attractive you will find yourself as you achieve each of your goals. Try making a face. Laugh if you like. It is important that we take ourselves seriously enough to not always be serious!

Sue C. Jacobs, Ph.D.
Cynthia Medich, R.N., M.S.

SAMPLE
SMOKING CESSATION
HEALTH COMMITMENT

Long-Term Goal:

Become a nonsmoker

_____

_____
Signature

_____
Witness

Expected Date of Reaching Goal: _____ 3 months _____

Readiness to Change	Short-Term Goals	Comments (supports, rewards, etc.)
Never considered change; need information.	1. Contact American Cancer Society for information on health hazards of smoking and for information on strategies for quitting. 2. Have a complete phsyical examination.	
Considered change, but not yet committed.	1. List reasons why becoming a nonsmoker is important for me. 2. Talk with others who have become nonsmokers to determine cost/benefit of not smoking.	
Desire change; need motivation.	1. Attend a stop-smoking program. 2. Talk with others about how they quit smoking and if those strategies allowed for long-term cessation.	

(continued)

Readiness to Change	Short-Term Goals	Comments (supports, rewards, etc.)
Attempting change; need structure, support, and skills.	1. Purchase only one package of low-tar, low-nicotine brand cigarettes at a time, and switch brands with each package. 2. Each time I get the urge to smoke, I will Stop, Take a Breath, then decide if I really need/want the cigarette.	
Change made; need reinforcement.	1. List all the positive effects I am now experiencing by not smoking. 2. Play a game with my children after dinner instead of lingering with coffee and a cigarette.	
Change made; slipping back into bad habits, need renewed motivation and support.	1. Elicit the relaxation response whenever a strong urge to smoke comes. Watch the urge come and go. 2. Affirm that "I am a nonsmoker" each morning in front of the mirror and each time I overcome the urge.	

HEALTH COMMITMENT

Long-Term Goal: _____

_____
Signature

_____
Witness

Expected Date of Reaching Goal: _____

Short-Term Goals	Comments (supports, rewards, etc.)

HEALTH COMMITMENT

Long-Term Goal:

_____

_____

Signature

_____

Witness

Expected Date of Reaching Goal: _____

Short-Term Goals	Comments (supports, rewards, etc.)

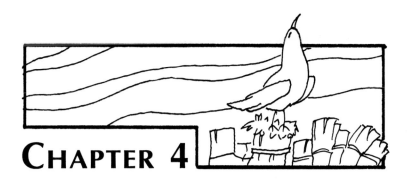

CHAPTER 4

THE RELAXATION RESPONSE

In this chapter you will explore

- the fight-or-flight response
- the relaxation response
- the relationship of the relaxation response to breathing
- different types of breathing

The mind/body model of health suggests that our modern world—with its stresses, strains, and incessant changes—causes or aggravates many of our symptoms. You cannot always change your environment, and in many cases may not want to. But what can you do about the stresses of modern life? One answer lies within you. By learning to use your awareness and your mind, you can begin to control your physical reactions to stress. You can cultivate the ability to turn within to give yourself a respite—a chance to slow down, relieve tension and anxiety, and renew yourself. First let us examine the physiology of stress.

THE FIGHT-OR-FLIGHT RESPONSE

The *fight-or-flight response,* also called the stress response, was first identified by Dr. Walter B. Cannon of the Harvard Medical School early in this century. It is a profound set of involuntary physiological changes that occur whenever we are faced with a stressful or threatening situation. This response, critical to the survival of primitive humankind, prepares the body for a physical reaction to a real threat—to fight or flee. Today, however, we do not often face the life-threatening situations that primitive people responded to frequently, and the fight-or-flight response cannot distinguish between a serious threat and the everyday stresses of modern life. In fact, simply recalling a threatening or frightening situation is often enough to trigger the fight-or-flight response.

Take a Moment To . . .

Recall a frightening event in your life . . . or think of a scary movie you have seen recently. Remember how you felt as a passenger on a plane that lurched violently, or during a near accident on the highway. Picture the situation as vividly as possible. Now become aware of your body. What has happened to your heartbeat? How has your breathing changed?

The fight-or-flight response is an integrated reaction controlled by the hypothalamus, an area of the brain. Confronted by a threat—physical or emotional, real or imagined—the hypothalamus causes the sympathetic nervous system to release epinephrine and norepinephrine (also called adrenaline and noradrenaline) and other related hormones. When rapidly released into the body, these powerful messengers propel you into a state of arousal.
Here is what happens:

Physiological Changes of the Fight-or-Flight Response	
Metabolism	Increases
Heart rate	Increases
Blood pressure	Increases
Breathing rate	Increases
Muscle tension	Increases

Recently, researchers studying the long-term effects of the fight-or-flight response have concluded that it may lead to permanent, harmful physiological changes. The fight-or-flight response is useful and, in fact, necessary in times of emergency. But the stressors of modern living elicit it at times when it is inappropriate for us to run or fight. We must find ways to control the harmful aspects of this primitive physiological response and so neutralize the negative effects of modern stress on our health and well-being. The relaxation response can do just that.

Paul's Experience

Paul, a forty-five-year-old artist, came to the Mind/Body Clinic for relief from frequent headaches. Fairly early he noted the correlation between the incidence of his headaches and times of work stress. After learning to elicit the relaxation response, he wrote on his weekly diary card:

> I have learned daily use of the relaxation response and pay constant attention to keeping my body well balanced. I have found the key to wellness for me. Now I need to relax into it until my practice is part of my nature.

THE RELAXATION RESPONSE

An anecdote from Herbert Benson

> In the late 1960s, my colleagues and I were conducting research on the causes and effects of hypertension. We were using biofeedback techniques to train squirrel monkeys—with a system of rewards and punishments—to control their blood pressure.
>
> One day, several practitioners of transcendental meditation came to my office and told me they believed they could lower their blood pressure through the practice of meditation. They invited me to conduct research on them to validate this claim. It was 1968, and it was the Harvard Medical School; I was having difficulties even trying to convince my colleagues that stress might be related to hypertension. Not wanting to get involved with anything so out of the mainstream, I politely showed them the door.
>
> Persistent in their claims, the practitioners returned repeatedly until I agreed to measure key physiological responses. At the same time, at the University of California-Irvine, Drs. Robert Keith Wallace and Archie F. Wilson were conducting similar studies. We all found that several major physiological systems responded to the simple act of sitting quietly and giving the mind a focus: the metabolism decreased, the heart rate slowed, respiratory rate decreased, and there were distinctive brain waves. Maybe, I thought, these people had a point. Later, Dr. Wallace joined me at Harvard, and we continued our work together.
>
> The evidence we gathered had compelling implications about the control you can exert over physiological functions. It suggested strongly that you could use your mind to change your physiology in a beneficial way, improve health, and perhaps reduce your need for medications. I subsequently coined the term *relaxation response* to describe this natural restorative phenomenon that is common to all of us.

As demonstrated by researchers around the world and suggested by age-old wisdom, there is a *counterbalancing mechanism* to the fight-or-flight response. Just as stimulating an area of the hypothalamus can cause the stress response, so reducing the stimulation results in relaxation. The relaxation response is an inborn set of physiological changes that offset those of the fight-or-flight response. These changes are coordinated; they occur together in an integrated fashion.

Compare the changes of the relaxation response to those of the fight-or-flight response:

Physiological Changes of the Fight-or-Flight Response	
Metabolism	Increases
Heart rate	Increases
Blood pressure	Increases
Breathing rate	Increases
Muscle tension	Increases

Physiological Changes of the Relaxation Response	
Metabolism	Decreases
Heart rate	Decreases
Blood pressure	Decreases
Breathing rate	Decreases
Muscle tension	Decreases

If the stresses of modern life cause the fight-or-flight response, the relaxation response can be used to counteract the harmful effects of stress. Just as the heart begins to beat rapidly when you imagine a frightening situation, your mind can be used to slow your heart rate.

There is one other significant difference between the fight-or-flight response and the relaxation response: the fight-or-flight response usually occurs involuntarily, whereas conscious elicitation of the relaxation response most often needs to be practiced.

LEARNING TO ELICIT THE RELAXATION RESPONSE

The relaxation response is a state of profound rest that can have lasting effects throughout the day if you practice it regularly.

What is relaxation? Many of us use the image of "letting go." Physically, we mean releasing muscles from habitual, unconscious tension. We try to breathe more slowly and regularly, letting go of tension with each outbreath. Emotionally, we mean cultivating an attitude of greater equanimity. Mentally, we mean observing and letting go of troubling, worrisome thoughts. All of us can experience an enhanced ability to relax as we practice these different approaches to letting go.

A classic teaching story illustrates the themes of holding on and letting go. In a country where the monkeys wreak havoc by stealing newly ripened fruit, the farmers devised a clever trick to stop the monkeys' mischief. They hollow out a coconut, drill a hole just the size of a monkey's outstretched paw, and place a piece of tempting fruit inside. After the greedy monkey grabs the fruit inside the coconut, it cannot withdraw its paw while still clutching the fruit. Since the monkey will not let go of the fruit, it is caught in a trap of its own making. Like the monkey, we need to learn to let go of tensions that may be contributing to troublesome physical symptoms and behavioral patterns.

Many people have difficulty relaxing their bodies: you may think you are relaxed, when, in fact, your neck muscles are still tense. Cultivating a state of quiet acceptance in a world that demands so much is a new experience for many of us. To use an automotive image, shifting down from overdrive can be difficult for those accustomed to the fast lane. Yet, to restore a healthy balance, your body and mind need exactly such a change in pace.

Margaret's Experience

Margaret, a fifty-seven-year-old housewife who is the sole caretaker for her severely disabled husband, came to the Mind/Body Clinic because of increasing fatigue. On her exit evaluation she wrote:

> It's a life-long struggle to take care of yourself and know what's right for you . . . The message I got from the Mind/Body Group was "be good to yourself. You're doing the best you can. The best you can is going to get you there, so just try and keep doing it. When you fail, you'll still learn something." Just this kind of "be gentle with yourself" attitude is very important—that has been valuable for me.

To elicit the physiological state called the relaxation response, you need to develop techniques that help you "let go" more deeply than most of us can without such help. Remember that the relaxation response is a physiological response inborn to everyone, and it can occur at times when you are not even aware of it. Bring to mind, for example, a time when you were lying on the beach on a warm summer day or moments at night when you drift into sleep. In both instances, the relaxation response is believed to account for the pleasant state and its measurable physiological changes. You can develop your innate ability to use these techniques in the most beneficial ways possible.

The relaxation response can be elicited by a number of techniques that involve mental focusing. The techniques commonly used in the programs of our behavioral medicine clinics include:

Techniques Which Elicit the Relaxation Response	
Diaphragmatic breathing	Repetitive prayer
Meditation	Progressive muscle relaxation
Body scan	Yoga stretching
Mindfulness	Imagery
Repetitive exercise	

All these techniques have two basic components: the first is the *repetition* of a word, sound, phrase, prayer, image, or physical activity; the second is the *passive disregard of everyday thoughts* when they occur during relaxation.

As you try the different methods of eliciting the relaxation response described in this and the next chapter, you may find that one method works better than others or that one or two of the techniques prove to be the most helpful. Or you may choose to make a combination of all the techniques part of your personal health regimen. We will introduce you to each of these techniques and help you find your own balance. Bear in mind that the goals of eliciting the relaxation response are straightforward, practical, and potentially transformative. The participants in our clinic programs commonly report these kinds of changes:

- decrease in stress-related physical symptoms
- decrease in anxiety
- freedom from compulsive worrying, self-criticism, and negative thoughts
- increase in concentration and awareness
- improved sleep
- greater self-acceptance
- enhanced performance and efficiency

Research studies confirm that such changes can occur with regular elicitation of the relaxation response. In addition, a recent study of the relationship between spirituality and health conducted by Jared Kass, Ph.D., and colleagues at Boston's Deaconess Hospital, found that a significant number of those who regularly elicit the relaxation response, regardless of method, reported an increase in positive attitudes associated with spirituality. Spirituality in this study was linked to increased life purpose and satisfaction. They also found that increases in positive attitudes contributed to improvements in health. Regular elicitation of the relaxation response cultivated health-promoting attitudes which decreased the frequency of medical symptoms.

As our patients practice regularly, they generally begin to describe themselves as more peaceful, energetic, self-accepting, happier, and so forth. Less preoccupied with past and future, they learn to enjoy the present moment more fully. In short, whatever their cultural or spiritual tradition, people can enjoy the benefits of the relaxation response in whatever way is most appropriate for them.

Nancy's Experience

As a first-year law student, Nancy was seized by anxiety and terror whenever called upon in class. She suddenly realized that she needed to find a permanent solution to the performance anxiety she experienced in class and in her former career as a singer and conductor. She couldn't continue her legal studies or become a lawyer when paralyzed like this.

On her weekly diary card she noted the following:

I came to the Mind/Body Clinic and the relaxation response helped me to solve what I believed was an insurmountable crisis. I learned that I could control situations. Now I can stop my mind from creating the horrible physical and psychological symptoms associated with performance anxiety. Now my clinic group has ended and with the skills I've learned, I am performing admirably in class, get called on often, and even raise my hand! My classmates have noticed the difference and as they sit in fear, waiting for their names to ring out, they ask me, "How did you do it?" "Relax and breathe," I say. "It's all in your mind."

THE RELAXATION RESPONSE AND BREATHING

> Life is in the breath. He who half breathes, half lives.
>
> Proverb

You may be surprised to learn that there is more than one way to breathe or that focusing on how you breathe can help relieve stress and elicit the relaxation response. But awareness of and conscious control over your breath is an important factor in all methods of eliciting the relaxation response.

Cultural norms can adversely affect the natural breathing process: flattening your abdomen (belly) or thrusting out your chest both interfere with more natural, deeper breaths. Over time, the patterns of breathing that develop as we strive for a flat belly may contribute to physical symptoms. Furthermore, the physical tension and shallow breathing that accompany anxiety can both inhibit the breathing process. An awareness of your breathing pattern is a first step in altering the physical, emotional, and mental effects of stress on your body.

Take a Moment To . . .

Notice your breathing now. Can you describe the way you breathe? Are your breaths long or short? Are your inbreath and outbreath balanced, or is one longer than the other? Do you feel you are not getting enough air? What parts of your chest and stomach are moving as you breathe?

UNDERSTANDING BREATHING

With each breath, we nourish the body with oxygen, which is transferred from the lungs to the bloodstream and then transported to every part of the body. Through the process of cellular respiration, the oxygen is used to produce energy. The carbon-dioxide wastes produced in this process are carried back to the lungs through the bloodstream and exhaled on each outbreath. We are not usually consciously aware of this process on which life depends. Breathing, of course, occurs whether we pay attention or not, but it is also one physiological function over which we can have conscious control.

There are two basic ways of breathing: the first is diaphragmatic, or abdominal breathing; the second is chest, or thoracic breathing. Normally, breathing is a combination of the two. However, you may benefit from shifting toward more diaphragmatic breathing. Compare the following descriptions of two kinds of breathing:

Chest or thoracic breathing.   Chest breathing is relatively shallow. The chest expands and the shoulders rise as the lungs take in air. Under stress, we all have a tendency to breathe shallowly. Breathing can become irregular, involving both holding your breath and exhaling incompletely. Because of this pattern, your breathing may feel constricted, creating uncomfortable or even

Chest Breathing

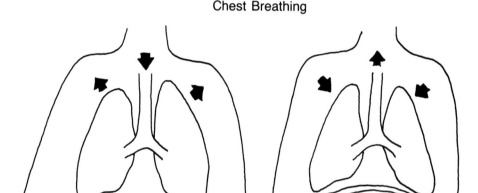

Inhalation   Exhalation

anxious sensations of not getting enough air. Breathing thoracically can cause symptoms such as shortness of breath and tightness in your chest. Culture has taught many of us to breath this way exclusively.

Diaphragmatic breathing.   The diaphragm is a large, domelike sheet of muscle that stretches over the bottom portion of your lungs, separating the lungs from your abdominal organs. As you inhale, this muscle contracts and

Diaphragmatic Breathing

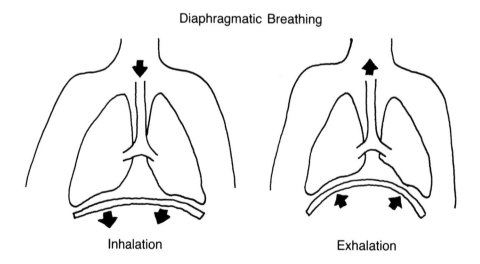

Inhalation   Exhalation

moves down, drawing air into your lungs. When you exhale, the diaphragm relaxes and moves upward. Air is then moved out of your lungs. By shifting to more emphasis on diaphragmatic breathing, you can alter the restricted breathing patterns of chest breathing.

Though deceptively simple and subtle, the act of breathing diaphragmatically can offer control over some of the anxieties and tensions that contribute to stress-related physical symptoms. How remarkable that one of the important stress-management tools is as close as your own breath!

Donald's Experience

Donald is a thirty-year-old business executive who came to the Mind/Body Clinic seeking relief from panic attacks. He found diaphragmatic breathing to be a great help:

> Whenever I felt as though I was choking (from the panic attacks), I would just sit back and breathe to my stomach and it would go away. It was like instant relief . . . It gave me something to do that I felt was helping me. It wasn't like I was ignoring my illness; I felt like I was addressing my illness. If I didn't get anything else out of this whole program besides learning how to breathe to my stomach, that was worth it. That's something you could share with people. You'd be surprised how many people I've told.

Many Eastern disciplines place great emphasis on diaphragmatic breathing as a way to bring balance to both mind and body. In the words of Thich Nhat Hanh, a Vietnamese Zen master and internationally known teacher of mindfulness meditation:

> Learn to practice breathing in order to regain control of body and mind,
> to practice mindfulness, and to develop concentration and wisdom.

People are often dismayed when they start paying attention to how they breathe. Suddenly a lifelong, unconscious process becomes new and foreign. "I'm not sure I know how to breathe!" patients have exclaimed, frustrated by the awkwardness. This reaction is very common, but with patience and practice, you can relearn the ease and positive benefits that come with deep, rhythmic breathing.

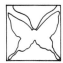

Take a Moment To . . .

Lie on your back in a comfortable position to become aware of your breathing. Close your eyes and place one hand on your belly just below the navel (belly button). Because of the movement of the diaphragm with each breath, as you inhale your hand will rise slightly. As you exhale, your hand will fall. Focus your attention on the rising and falling of your hand. This is diaphragmatic breathing. An ideal time to practice this is just before going to sleep. You can also practice during the day while standing or sitting.

You may wonder how diaphragmatic breathing helps you, but consider what happens when you experience intense emotions like anger, fear, or sadness. Do you sometimes notice yourself gasping or "catching your breath," or even struggling to get enough breath? Strong emotions tend to disrupt diaphragmatic breathing and trigger more shallow breathing patterns. By consciously shifting to diaphragmatic breathing, you can reduce the intensity of your emotional response and approach the situation more effectively. Try the old maxim "Take ten deep breaths before you get angry." Sometimes you can do just that and find you don't become angry!

You may also want to reflect on the important link between awareness of breathing and the handling of pain. For example, breathing techniques are one major tool used for natural childbirth. Breathing awareness is a powerful tool for handling other types of pain as well. Through breathing techniques, you can actually learn to uncouple the sensations of pain from the emotional reactions, tensions, and fears that tend to accentuate pain. By focusing on the experience of your breathing, the sensations of pain may begin to change, shift, or recede into the background.

But it takes a little time to learn how to experience the subtleties of breathing and to bring about its benefits. Be patient. You will be rewarded. In our program evaluations we have asked patients what part of the program proved most useful to them; awareness of their breath was a common answer. Breathing, then, can become an indispensable ally in your healing process.

Mary's Experience

Mary, a forty-year-old graphic designer with diabetes, came to the Cardiovascular Program to get her life in better balance and to control the symptoms of her diabetes. As she began to elicit the relaxation response, she noted:

> I'm more in control as I make these behavioral changes. I deep-breathe and it helps quiet my mind so I can get a perspective on what's happening. I have more good feelings that last longer, and a stronger sense of self is breaking through. I know I can be who I once was and I'm very happy with that thought.

Becoming more aware of your breathing

Besides noticing the rising and falling of your abdomen, another place to focus awareness on breathing is at the nostrils. You may be able to observe how the air is slightly cooler as it enters your nose and somewhat warmer as it leaves. As your breathing becomes quieter and more regular, you may notice a very subtle pause when the inhalation ends and before the exhalation begins, and vice versa. Some people find this kind of focusing on the breath helps them to concentrate, and the subtle pause offers moments of stillness.

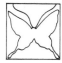

Take a Moment To . . .

Try a focused-breathing exercise now. First, sit comfortably in a chair or lie on the floor, and close your eyes. Take several deep diaphragmatic breaths. As you continue to breath diaphragmatically, begin to count down on each outbreath, starting with *ten* and proceeding down to *one*. As you exhale, imagine the tension draining out of your body from head to toe. And allow your state of letting go to deepen gradually with each outbreath.

As diaphragmatic breathing becomes more natural, you can begin to incorporate an awareness of your breath into everyday activities. For example, try taking three deep diaphragmatic breaths

when the phone rings . . .
when you leave your house or apartment . . .
when stuck in traffic . . .
before eating . . .
before you start a new project at work . . .
before you go to sleep and as you awaken . . .

Although awareness of breathing appears to be a simple technique, it can help you become aware of tensions in your body so you can begin to release them. Furthermore, any time you bring awareness to breathing, you can refocus your attention and come more fully into the present moment. It is a centering device that allows both your body and your mind to become calm.

> If you would foster a calm spirit, first regulate your breathing; for when that is under control, the heart will be at peace; but when breathing is spasmodic, then it will be troubled. Therefore, before attempting anything, first regulate your breathing on which your temper will be softened, your spirit calmed.
>
> Kariba Ekken, seventeenth-century Sufi

Matt's Experience

Matt was forty and nearly incapacitated by severe panic attacks when he was referred to our program by his physician. His work was suffering, his family was worried, and he was incredulous that his several trips to the emergency room could be explained by something as intangible as anxiety. He believed he had a heart problem and that any one of these episodes might kill him. In our clinic, he learned how to focus on his breathing and how to elicit the relaxation response. A year later he said:

> The whole thing is amazing. A year ago my anxiety was so high I couldn't function at all. I was having these terrible panic attacks with severe palpitations, dizziness, sweating, the whole thing. I was one hell of a mess. I've progressed every month. I guess my symptoms are over ninety percent gone. I can get rid of the dizziness and disorientation completely, and I haven't taken any medication for four to five months.

Now, Matt has developed a conscious awareness of his breathing patterns and elicits the relaxation response once or twice daily. He says that any time he feels anxiety returning, he simply stops and does a breathing exercise.

Rich's Experience

Rich, a businessman who had been diagnosed with esophageal spasm and reflux, was referred to our program by his physician. He had been suffering chest pains and palpitations for six years and had become increasingly distressed by the problem. He had been hospitalized for chest pain; he was taking heart medication and using large amounts of antacids.

Frankly skeptical at first, he began to notice that the diaphragmatic breathing was helping to reduce his symptoms. He reported that the combination of anxiety about his health and his shallow, irregular breathing pattern had caused great rigidity in his upper body. He slowly resumed regular exercise, incorporating yoga stretches that helped to release tight muscle groups. With his own doctor's approval he slowly eliminated the heart medication and began to reduce his intake of antacids.

In his post-program evaluation, he wrote that the most useful part of the program was "understanding the fundamental simplicity of proper breathing and relaxation."

Olivia Ames Hoblitzelle, M.A.
Herbert Benson, M.D.

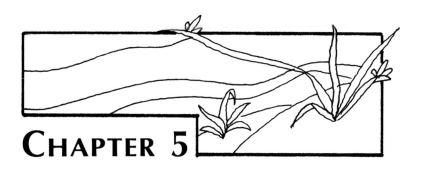

CHAPTER 5

ELICITING THE RELAXATION RESPONSE

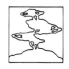

In this chapter you will explore

- how to elicit the relaxation response using meditation
- how to use "minis"
- how to use mindfulness
- how to use imagery

In this chapter, we will describe different ways to elicit the relaxation response. Experiment and discover which methods are best for you. Remember to maintain an attitude of openness and acceptance. To learn any new skill requires patience and perseverance.

Two basic components are involved in eliciting the relaxation response:

1. *A mental focusing device,* such as watching your breath; or repeating a word, phrase, prayer, sound; or using repetitive muscular activity to help you shift your mind from everyday thoughts and worries.
2. *A passive attitude toward distracting thoughts,* which means not worrying about how well you are doing, but gently directing your mind back to your mental or exercise focus when you notice yourself caught up in a train of thought.

The basic steps necessary to elicit the relaxation response are:

Step 1: Pick a focus word, phrase, image, or prayer. It can be rooted in your personal belief system. For example, a Christian might choose the opening of Psalm 23, *The Lord is my shepherd;* a Jew, *shalom;* a Muslim, *Allah.* Or you may prefer a neutral word or phrase like *one* or *peace* or *love.* You may also choose to focus on your breathing.

Step 2: Sit quietly in a comfortable position.

Step 3: Close your eyes.

Step 4: Relax your muscles.

Step 5: Breathe slowly and naturally, and as you do, repeat your focus word or phrase as you exhale.

Step 6: Assume a passive attitude. Do not worry about how well you are doing. When other thoughts come to mind, simply say to yourself, "Oh well," and gently return to the repetition.

Step 7: Continue for ten to twenty minutes.

Step 8: Practice the technique once or twice daily.

Adapted from Herbert Benson, *Your Maximum Mind*

Now, let us explore specific methods in more detail.

MEDITATION

Meditation is one of the techniques for eliciting the relaxation response. In the broadest sense of the word, it is natural and familiar to everyone—it is simply a process of focusing the mind on an object or activity, something you do most of the time. When you use meditation to elicit the relaxation response, you turn your attention inward, concentrating on a repetitive focus such as breathing or a word or a prayer. Your body and your mind begin to quiet down. A state of physiological and mental rest ensues. But, as we all know too well, the mind is usually very active and difficult to focus.

Take a Moment To . . .

Sit up straight and try to release physical tension. Place your hands comfortably in your lap. Close your eyes for a minute or two and notice what happens to your thoughts. Where did your mind go? Did it drift back into the past or move ahead into the future? What kind of thoughts arose? Were they "afflicting" thoughts—the kind that create anxiety and tension? Or were they "nonafflicting" thoughts that allowed you to remain relaxed?

In the process of meditation, you are aware that your mind is active, but you practice several essential methods to reduce reactivity to your thoughts. You take the position of observer or "witness" as thoughts, feelings, or sensations arise and pass. When you become distracted, you choose to bring your mind back to your focus word or phrase or to your breath. You develop an attitude of acceptance toward whatever happens during the relaxation-response process.

Gradually you will develop a conscious, intentional approach to your mind's activity in which you choose your thinking process. You will learn to witness your own thoughts.

Maureen's Experience

Maureen, a young designer in the Cancer Program, found that the relaxation response made her more aware of what was going on in her mind.

> It's the most valuable idea, this idea of the witness, the self. Since I'm having these physical losses, I never want to let go of the idea that you possess this immutable quality, this immutable part of yourself that's unchanging, that's—even perfect, for lack of a better word; that was a revelation to me—the idea that this resource is there and I'm always going to have it.

The observing self, or the witness

When you go to the movies, you may get so emotionally involved that feelings like fear, anger, and sadness arise as powerfully as if the events were actually happening to you. In reality, the movie is only images projected onto a screen. You can choose to pull back from your emotional involvement in the movie, take a deep breath, and say, "Relax, it's just a movie."

In daily life, you may react to events by creating imagined scenarios as if they were actually taking place. These scenarios are frequently distorted and negative and appear automatically. For example, you may instantly react to a loved one being late by reflexively leaping to the conclusion that something dire has occurred. You may feel your heart pounding and may even experience nausea. Some have described these negative, automatic thoughts as "movies of the mind."

With the practice of meditation, you can learn to observe your troubling thoughts and determine which are real and which are simply imagined consequences. One quick method of learning to interrupt this cycle of automatic negative thoughts is to say "stop" to yourself and take several diaphragmatic breaths. Then you can label the troublesome thoughts as "thinking, thinking." As you then take a few more breaths and shift toward witnessing the thoughts, you can begin to let go of these troublesome imaginings.

Take worrying, for example. As soon as you notice that you are experiencing afflicting thoughts, such as worrying or "awfulizing," you can label the mind's activity "worrying, worrying" and shift your awareness to your breathing or your focus word or prayer. With these simple yet effective techniques, you begin to retrain your busy mind. You learn to be aware of anxiety and physical tension without getting caught up in them.

The witness, or nonjudgmental part of your mind, can help break the cycle of negative automatic thoughts and feelings that can adversely affect your body. The witness is one way of describing the ability to adopt a passive attitude by allowing you first to observe and then "let go" of your afflicting thoughts.

Another example may help illustrate this subtle inner skill. Imagine a parade. Standing at the side of the street, you watch the procession pass by, but you do not move from your position—you simply observe all the activity going by. Similarly, you can learn to observe the parade of thoughts that moves endlessly through your mind. And to help steady and focus your mind, you can resume the repetition of your focus.

Jennifer's Experience

Jennifer, a thirty-year-old writer who participated in the Mind/Body Program, found that mindfully watching her thoughts gave her many clues to her emotions, behaviors, and physical symptoms:

> The *truth*—ah-ha! There is a truth—that all these thoughts have been having a heyday—a battle royal—and I'm learning how to observe them without a need to take sides.
>   Choices will come later. In fact, the fact that I'm observing is a choice. And the fact that I'm not fighting and struggling is a major choice and—most importantly, a beginning point. A point of noninvolvement and nonjudgment—a point of detaching from the anxiety of dis-ease that is provoked by the war of words, ideas, thoughts, and feelings.

As you practice eliciting the relaxation response with meditation, you will have moments of entering quieter states quite removed from the stressful levels of activity that make up most of your daily life. In these moments of profound rest, you may experience greater awareness, enhanced self-esteem, and a deepening of your commitment to your health.

GENERAL GUIDELINES ABOUT ELICITING THE RELAXATION RESPONSE

When: For many people the best time is before breakfast because you can set a positive tone for the rest of the day. If you live with others, early-morning practice can become a treasured moment. If this is too difficult to arrange, try before lunch or dinner. If you miss a session during the day, you can also practice as you are going to sleep.

If your regular time for the relaxation response is not the morning, we recommend that you take five minutes then anyway, just to create a foundation of awareness for the rest of the day. The ideal is to develop a routine, a time to bring forth the relaxation response that becomes as much a part of the day as brushing your teeth. Reflect on a maxim attributed to Mohandas Gandhi:

Meditation is the key to the morning and the latch of the evening.

Where: If possible, practice in a relatively quiet place where you will not be disturbed by the telephone (unplug it, if necessary) or by people coming in and out. Choose a place that is attractive and feels safe. Some people enjoy making a special corner for themselves with a few selected objects, like a beautiful plant or picture, that remind them of peaceful moments in their life.

To have a sacred place . . . is an absolute necessity for anybody today. You must have a room, or a certain hour or so a day, where . . . you can simply experience and bring forth what you are and what you might be. This is a place of creative incubation. At first you may find that nothing happens there. But if you have a sacred place and use it, something eventually will happen.

Joseph Campbell, *The Power of Myth*

Position: Any comfortable posture is appropriate for using meditation to elicit the relaxation response. Generally it is preferable to meditate sitting up, in a fairly straight-backed chair that provides good support. If you find sitting uncomfortable, experiment with a reclining chair or lie on your back. You can also sit or even kneel on the floor, with a firm cushion or pillow for support.

How long to practice: Ideally, you would set aside ten to twenty minutes once or twice a day to elicit the relaxation response. Remember that it is a central part of your treatment plan—your prescription, if you will—and that its benefits will be linked to how faithfully you incorporate the relaxation response into your daily schedule. But setting aside the time is also one of the most challenging changes you are being invited to make. Experiment with different approaches to see what works best for you.

How to focus your mind: As you begin to practice eliciting the relaxation response with meditation, you may be startled, even dismayed, at how difficult it is to keep your mind focused. You may observe thoughts either darting from topic to topic, or relentlessly returning to a single area that is worrying you. Many people get discouraged because they seem unable to control their thoughts for more than a few seconds at a time. Fortunately, there are a number of different ways to focus your mind. Awareness of your breath is involved in almost all of them.

Breathing:

Our breath is the bridge from our body to our mind. . . . Breath
is aligned to both body and mind, and it alone is the tool which
can bring them both together, illuminating both and bringing both
peace and calm.

Thich Nhat Hanh, *The Miracle of Mindfulness*

As explained in the previous chapter, diaphragmatic breathing in itself
brings about a state of gentle relaxation. Quite simply, breathing is one of the
keys to meditation and the relaxation response. As you begin to practice, take a
few deep breaths to help turn your attention inward, then allow your breathing to follow its own natural rhythm.

If you experience any tension or anxiety about breathing, it may be
helpful to slow down your outbreath. Breathing tends to become slower and
lighter as the relaxation response takes over. Sometimes your breathing may
even seem to be momentarily suspended. That too is fine. As you will come to
appreciate, awareness of your breathing becomes a companion, not only
during meditation, but during other activities as well, and thereby helps you to
remain calm and balanced.

You may wish to review the previous chapter for various methods of
breath-awareness which can be used as your focus for meditation.

Choosing your focus word or phrase: The most universal methods of focusing
your mind are linked to breathing, either by concentrating on your breath
itself or using it in conjunction with a focus word. Your focus word or *mantra*
can be a word, phrase, or short prayer. "Mantra," in fact, means "the word that
protects." When your mind is focused, you cannot dwell on negative, anxious
thoughts. A mantra has been a part of meditation in both Eastern and
Western cultures for thousands of years; it is an anchor for meditation and
helps you to quiet the chatter or self-talk of your mind as you begin to
meditate.

Choosing your focus word is an important personal step. In our clinic
programs, we have found that tailoring your focus to your personal beliefs is
often the best way to get maximum benefit from the relaxation response. If
your focus has special meaning, it will not only be more effective in meditation,
but most likely you will become more deeply involved in practicing the relaxation response. We call the combination of the relaxation response with a
personal belief system "the faith factor." Some, however, prefer their focus
word to have no connection to a belief system and choose a more neutral word
or phrase. In either case, your focus is a key to meditation and eliciting the
relaxation response.

Keep the word or phrase short enough to coordinate easily with your
breath. The list below, more extensive than those suggested earlier, offers a
range of focus words or phrases from which to choose.

Common Focus Words or Phrases

General

One	*Ocean*
Peace	*Oh well*
Calm	*Let it be*
Let go	*My time*
Relax	*Love*

Christian

Come, Lord	*Lord Jesus Christ, have mercy on me*
Lord, have mercy	*Hail Mary*
Our Father	*The Lord is my shepherd*
Our Father, *who art in heaven*	

Jewish

Sh'ma Yisroel ("Hear, o Israel")	*Shalom* ("Peace")
Echod ("One")	*Hashem* ("The Name")

Eastern

Om (the universal sound)	*Shantih* ("Peace")

Aramaic

Maranatha ("Come, Lord")	*Abba* ("Father")

Islamic

Allah

Henry's Experience

Henry, an elderly gentleman with hypertension, attended the Hypertension Program. Since his wife had died, several months earlier, his blood pressure had been out of control. He found the relaxation response very helpful and chose a focus word that was important to him:

> The first word that came into my mind was *peace*, because I guess that's what I was trying to do within my own body—to bring it to peace; bring my mind and my body into a peaceful state where it was just so much of an uproar before . . . When doing the relaxation techniques, I do just get the feeling that this is great, this is wonderful. I just feel that I could face anything after I've become so relaxed, and I get a better night's sleep for it, and I'm better off all around."

How to use your focus word or phrase: As you experiment with using your mental focus, simply repeat the word or phrase silently to yourself at a relaxed pace, synchronizing the repetition with your breath. A single word, or two, is usually repeated on the outbreath. If using several words, you may want to try different ways of coordinating the words with both inbreaths and outbreaths.

One of our patients uses the word *Ocean:* on his inbreath he thinks *o*, on his outbreath *shunnnn . . .* ; he claims the rhythm is also a reminder of ocean waves.

As your mind begins to quiet down a bit, you may forget to use the word or phrase. But whenever you notice yourself drifting back to "mind-chatter," simply say to yourself, "Oh well," and take that opportunity to return to your breathing and your focus word or prayer. At the same time, remember that it is natural to lose your mental focus. Everyone does. One of the wonders of the mind is its unceasing activity!

Meditation leads to an attitude of awareness of your experience during the process. As you develop this skill, you will find that the same qualities of awareness help you handle the daily challenges of life more easily.

Take a Moment To . . .

1. Repeat the focus thought, word, phrase, or prayer silently to yourself, coordinating it with your breathing or in whatever way is most comfortable for you.
2. When thoughts intrude, as they invariably do, gently keep returning to your breathing and focus.
3. When you lose awareness of both thoughts and the focus, you may be experiencing a more profound stillness of mind. Enjoy it! There is no need to bring back the focus until your mind resumes its activity.

There is no such thing as a "typical" meditation, or a "good" or "bad" meditation. Even those who have practiced meditation for many years recognize that every time is different. Some meditations are more relaxing than others; sometimes your mind is relatively quiet, sometimes it wanders frequently to distracting thoughts. For most of us, the salient element is bringing the mind back from its wanderings into a more focused state. When your mind wanders, instead of getting caught up in thoughts, feelings, or sensations, let them go and once again move gently back to your focus without criticizing yourself for the lapse. You will gradually develop confidence in your ability to observe the restless and sometimes unruly tendencies of your own mind, and with that skill may come both freedom from anxiety and an increased sense of control. As Sujata, a student of meditation, humorously remarked: "My mind has a mind of its own. Where do *I* fit in!"

Sally's Experience

Sally, twenty-five, was anxious, depressed, and felt out of control because of her inability to conceive. After attending the Mind/Body program for infertility, she explained her choice of mantra in a post-program interview:

> To address my need for control, I use three different mantras: *Hamsah* to focus; *Peace in—tension out,* and *Precious Lord, I submit to Your loving grace.* I don't know whether this is correct, but it seems to be working for me. Focusing has meant setting new boundaries and future needs. I think this view has come from the process of meditation, setting up time for myself, explaining my needs to friends, and imagining new ways to heal.

A reminder of the importance of attitude: As you learn to elicit the relaxation response with meditation, try to maintain an attitude of acceptance toward yourself.

- Hard as it is, don't compare one meditation with another.
- Put aside your tendency to judge; remember, the only "bad" meditation is the one you didn't do.
- Even a meditation dominated by busy thoughts can give you reduced physical tension, some personal insights, and an enhanced sense of control.

"MINIS"

Once you habitually elicit the relaxation response, you will feel less anxious and stressed during those ten-to-twenty-minute sessions. You may also find yourself calmer for some time afterward, a wonderful contribution to an increased sense of well-being throughout the day. What, however, can you do when the irritations and stresses of everyday life occur:

- being stopped by five red lights in a row
- being called to the dentist's chair from the waiting room
- everyone's coming in late for dinner
- your boss saying, "Just come into my office for a minute"
- your spouse's not paying attention to what you are saying
- preparing to make an important phone call
- walking into a crowded room
- waiting in line
- paying the bills

A mini-relaxation response—anything from a few conscious breaths to several minutes of sitting quietly—is very useful in dealing with these hassles. Participants in our programs often discover that this simple practice is one of the most effective ways to extend the benefits of the relaxation response into their day. "Mini-meditations" can be remarkably refreshing and powerful; you will be delighted at the effect they have on your ability to concentrate, on how you feel, even on your ability to relate more easily with others.

There are many ways to do a "mini." Here are several:

Mini 1 • Take a deep breath and hold it for several seconds. Then, as you very slowly let your breath out, repeat your focus word or phrase or prayer.

Mini 2 • Put your right hand just under your navel (belly button). Focus on breathing down into your stomach, not breathing up into your chest. Your hand should rise as you breathe in, and fall as you breathe out. Now, as you inhale, say the number *ten* to yourself. Exhale. With the next breath, say *nine*, then breath out. Do this until you reach *zero*.

Mini 3 • Put your hand just under your navel as you did for Mini 2. As you breathe in, count very slowly up to four. As you exhale, count very slowly to yourself back down to one. So, as you breathe in, you count *one, two, three, four*. Then, as you exhale, *four, three, two, one*.

Mini 4 • Breathe in through your nose and then breathe out through your mouth. Do this ten times. Notice how cool the air feels as you inhale, in contrast to how warm it feels when you exhale.

In medical settings, minis are an excellent way to reduce pain and anxiety, helping you feel better physically and psychologically. Many people feel anxious about seeing a dentist. We have found that relaxation-response techniques can help reduce this anxiety. Try doing minis in the waiting room. When the dentist is actually working on your teeth, focus on your breath: count breaths, watch your stomach rise and fall, or count as you inhale and exhale. If injections make you nervous, focus on your breath for thirty seconds before receiving the injection; then, as the needle enters, count your breaths very slowly, from ten to zero.

Physician's examinations upset many people. If you are anxious, do a mini for thirty to sixty seconds or longer while waiting in the exam room. This can help you relax, which will make the examination more comfortable.

Muriel's Experience

Muriel, a forty-year-old participant in the Mind/Body Infertility Program, needed nightly injections at a specified hour. The doctor had trained her husband in the procedure, but every evening both the patient and her husband were so anxious that the sterile needles were dropped on the floor or medicine spilled; by the time both were ready, the injection was too late. Both husband and wife were then trained to do minis. Now, before they even start, they count together down from ten. If either becomes nervous, they both stop and focus on their breathing. Just before the injection, both inhale and exhale very slowly. Result: injections go smoothly, there is less pain, and they are on time.

MINDFULNESS: ANOTHER TECHNIQUE FOR FOCUSING

Janet's Experience

Janet, an unemployed financial analyst, suffered from migraine head-aches since she had been laid off. She learned to elicit the relaxation response and slowly began to notice its effects.

> Even though I had read about mindfulness, it was through this group that I really understand what it is. It has changed my life! It is difficult for someone who worries a lot to be mindful or do one thing at a time because of preoccupation with every other concern. I plan to work very hard at using this in my life.

How often during the day do you find yourself distracted, fragmented, or hurried? Do you sometimes feel as though your mind is going in five directions at once?

Mindfulness is focusing attention on what you are experiencing from moment to moment. You do not allow your mind to become fragmented, drifting into the past or future; rather, you remain fully alert to the thoughts and experiences of the present moment. The practice of mindfulness can be particularly useful to people learning to elicit the relaxation response because it allows them to extend the benefits into more areas of their daily lives.

When using mindfulness to elicit the relaxation response, your breath remains the primary focus. But, in addition, you become mindful of—fully attentive to—the sensations of your body. You remain mindful also of any emotions that arise, exploring their impact on your body. You also remain mindful of your own thinking process. In short, instead of being distracted or fragmented, you are fully aware of your moment-to-moment experiences.

As a meditative relaxation-response technique, you can use mindfulness when sitting quietly or engaged in various activities. It involves a combination of slowing yourself down, doing one activity at a time, and bringing full awareness to whatever you are experiencing.

Alex's Experience

Alex, a thirty-five-year-old legal assistant, found that anxiety and attacks of hyperventilation were interfering with her work and her health. She began to elicit the relaxation response regularly and noticed an immediate improvement in her symptoms.

> Ah-ha! Being mindful! I work very hard on that. Planning is a big part of my work and my mind used to be much more in the future or past. Now I talk to myself. "Stay in the present. Wait until the time comes; then you can deal with that client's project." I notice this mindfulness most when I work with my clients.

Mindfulness effectively helps alleviate pain. By exploring the changing sensations of pain, it is possible for you to separate your physical sensations from emotional reactions, which tend to worsen pain. For example, when you injure yourself, an instantaneous reaction is often aggravated by anxiety. Proficiency at mindfulness can allow awareness of anxiety and reduce your perception of pain. Rather than feeling "I am in pain," you come to think "There is pain." The process of distancing yourself from pain lessens its impact and teaches you that something inside you can separate you from the pain.

> Mindfulness is the miracle by which we can call back in a flash our dispersed mind and restore it to wholeness so that we can live each minute of life.
>
> Thich Nhat Hanh, *The Miracle of Mindfulness*

Using mindfulness to reduce stress during the workday

- As you awaken in the morning, bring your attention to your breathing. Instead of letting your mind spin off into yesterday or today, take mindful breaths. Focus on your breathing, and sense the effects of breathing throughout your body.
- Instead of hurrying to your usual routine, slow down and enjoy something special about the morning: a flower that bloomed, the sound of birds, the wind in the trees.
- On your way to work, attend to how you walk or drive or ride the transit. Take some mindful breaths, relaxing throughout your body.
- When stopped at a traffic light, check your body for signs of physical tension. Drop your shoulders, release your hands on the wheel, soften your facial muscles. Can you break the cycle of running yellow lights and passing cars?
- When stopped at a red light, pay attention to your breathing and enjoy the landscape around you.
- When you arrive at your workplace or begin a project, take a few moments to orient yourself, breathe consciously and calmly, and relax your body; then begin.
- When sitting at your desk or keyboard, become aware of the sub-

tle signs of physical tension. Take some mindful breaths to relax
and release tension.

- Use the repetitive events of the day—the ringing telephone, a
  knock on the door, walking down the hall—as cues for a mini-
  relaxation.
- Walk mindfully to your car or bus. Can you see and appreciate
  something new in the environment? Can you enjoy walking without rushing?
- As you return home, can you consciously make the transition
  from work to home? If possible, after greeting your family or
  housemates, give yourself a few minutes alone to ease the transition.
- As you go to sleep, let go of today and tomorrow, and take some
  slow, mindful breaths.

Take a Moment To . . .

Choose one daily activity that you do alone, such as brushing your teeth,
showering, washing the dishes, walking the dog. Engage in this activity
with mindfulness by combining awareness of your breath with focusing.
Experience every moment as fully as possible. Take a moment now and
try the following exercise using an orange.

- Take a few deep breaths and relax your body.
- Do a mini-relaxation response exercise.
- Let go of the past and the future, and bring your attention to the
  present moment.
- Let your attitude be open and receptive.
- Take a moment to appreciate where the orange came from; look
  carefully at its color, texture, shape.
- Notice the wonderful smell as you begin to peel it.
- See, as if for the first time, how the orange is formed into sec-
  tions and then gently break it apart.
- Eat one section at a time, very slowly, as if you had never tasted
  this fruit before.
- How do you chew? On one side of your mouth, the other, or
  both? How many times do you chew before swallowing? Slow
  down if you start to hurry.
- Whenever you notice any distraction from the moment-to-moment
  experience of eating, stop with your mouth empty, take a deep
  breath, and then continue.
- Allow feelings of enjoyment to arise as you experience the pleasure of eating mindfully.

THE USE OF IMAGERY

> Imagination is a good horse to carry you over the ground, not a
> magic carpet to take you away from the world of possibilities.
>
> Robertson Davies, *The Manticore*

The ancient technique of imagery as a form of meditation appears in many cultures and can be used in numerous ways. In our program, we use imagery to (1) facilitate eliciting the relaxation response and (2) affect attitudes and behaviors.

You use your imagination and create mental images all the time—sometimes for good, sometimes for ill. Imagery, as we use it, is another way to harness the extraordinary power of your mind. You can learn to use the power of your mind not only to deepen meditation, but also to create positive states of mind.

All thoughts and images created by the mind affect the body. When you dream that you are being chased or assaulted or that you are falling, for example, your heartbeat quickens, you tremble, you may even perspire. While the dream is not a reality, but only a series of mental images, the physiological response is real and measurable. The challenge is to use imagery to promote health and well-being.

Because each of us is unique in how we experience the world, so our experiences with imagery will vary widely. Some people may not "see" mental images but may "sense" being part of a scene. Some image in color, others in black and white. Others may enrich their imagery with sounds or smells or imagined physical sensations.

Take a Moment To . . .

Close your eyes and imagine each of the following sensations in turn. Which seem most evocative to you?

> The smell of fresh-cut grass
> The feeling of a swim on a hot day
> The sound of sea gulls
> The taste of your favorite dessert
> The taste of a lemon
> The sight of a beautiful garden or the ocean or a mountain scene

Example: Using imagery can break negative mental cycles and replace them with positive thoughts and feelings. First elicit the relaxation response. Then, in your mind, begin to imagine a "safe place"—a favorite location from childhood, a scene with a beautiful view, a place of protected solitude. The more fully you re-create the scene in imagination, the more likely you are to experience feelings similar to when you were actually there—contentment, calm, peace.

Once you recognize imagery's power to soothe and heal, you can use it as a regular part of your practice of the relaxation response. The two interact naturally: the state of calm helps to evoke images, and imagery helps to further calmness. If you choose to use the imagery of a safe place, you may discover an inner refuge free from physical pain and emotional distress. For some people, this practice effectively reduces pain and anxiety.

You can also use imagery as a way to foster positive attitudes and change behaviors. You can accomplish change by preparing—even programming— your mind to help you think more positively. For example, some people feel extremely nervous about having to speak or perform before an audience. First elicit the relaxation response. Then create a mental image of how you would like to speak or perform. If you mentally rehearse the event, visualizing yourself carrying it out with calm self-assurance, the positive mental images can actually enhance your performance. In fact, this method is used by many world-class athletes to practice for competition; they visualize the perfect dive, the highest jump, the fastest race. This use of imagery is fully discussed in the book *Your Maximum Mind,* by Herbert Benson.

As with the other skills you have been learning, you will want to experiment to learn which imagery works best for you. Some people actually use imagery as their repetitive focus for eliciting the relaxation response. Others use imagery immediately after completing the relaxation-response practice as a way of strengthening a positive attitude. Still others recall imagery—perhaps of a safe place—at stressful times during the day.

THE CHALLENGE

> Meditation is not an evasion. It is a serene encounter with reality.
> Thich Nhat Hanh, *The Miracle of Mindfulness*

As we have seen, the relaxation response does not usually occur involuntarily. Whatever method you choose, remember *there is no substitute for regular practice.* The very "busyness" that invades your lifestyle can become the major obstacle to eliciting the relaxation response, but the benefits of this practice depend upon its being done regularly, daily. If you cannot spend the full ten to twenty minutes, at least try a shorter time to give yourself some of the benefits.

The principles of meditation may seem simple, but for many they are a new and challenging undertaking. Some people turn to meditation primarily to elicit the relaxation response; others discover that this inner journey launches them into a lifelong process.

Remember that an attitude of acceptance is both what you seek and what you must learn. Because most people struggle with judgments and expectations, with thoughts and anxieties, you should practice to keep these distractions in check. As you learn to be more accepting of yourself and what happens during meditation, the ability to accept and be flexible extends into other areas of life as well.

As you experiment with these new skills, you will begin to notice the positive, healing effects of eliciting the relaxation response. It becomes a self-reinforcing habit that is not only enjoyable in itself but beneficial to your health. If you practice regularly, you will begin to experience recognizable changes in how you feel, including a reduction in stress-related symptoms and a growing sense of well-being.

Experiment—discover how the techniques described in this chapter may serve as yet another way to extend the benefits of the relaxation response.

Two former patients describe below what they learned through Mind/Body Clinic programs:

> I had a tendency to take everything very personally. If there was criticism, it was a personal attack. Therefore, I was extremely defensive and much too quick to respond before fully understanding what was being said, whether it was positive or negative. I think what the program has allowed me is a certain thoughtfulness, maybe a lessening to some extent, of the defensiveness—and just a little more of going with the flow.—Peter, copy editor, 36

> My change in attitude is the striking thing I got out of the clinic. It gets crazy here at my job, but I'm not reacting as much as I used to. Now I can do a lot and do it easily, whereas before I used to get aggravated and not handle situations as well. Now I am much less agitated, and I don't take it all so seriously. I have a different perspective, so that even when times are very difficult, I see that others are here trying to do the best they can. I think more clearly, and I remember this perspective in relationships and home situations too; they are also affected by this different perspective.—Sandra, television station receptionist, 30

Finally, we strongly suggest that you elicit the relaxation response each time you sit down to read and work with this book. You will reinforce the habit of bringing forth the relaxation response and your learning may be enhanced.

Now, please look at the sample on pages 63–64 and fill out your own Health Commitment.

Olivia Ames Hoblitzelle, M.A.
Herbert Benson, M.D.

RELAXATION-RESPONSE TAPES

The following resource tapes are available through the Mind/Body Medical Institute. If you would like to purchase any of the tapes, please write to

> The Mind/Body Medical Institute
> New England Deaconess Hospital
> 185 Pilgrim Road
> Boston, Mass. 02215

Each tape is $10; please make checks payable to the Mind/Body Medical Institute.

Basic Relaxation Tape (female voice)

Side 1 (20 minutes)
This side introduces a basic relaxation sequence to help you elicit the relaxation response, including some of the key elements such as breath awareness, body scan relaxation, and the use of a focus word. Specific instructions throughout the tape aid in the initial development of your experience of the relaxation response.

Side 2 (20 minutes)
This side offers instruction on awareness, or "mindfulness" of sensations, thoughts, and sounds. It also introduces breath and awareness as "primary tools" that enable you to integrate the relaxation response into daily activities. This side has fewer instructions, allowing you to further develop your relaxation response techniques.

Basic Relaxation Tape (male voice)

Side 1 (20 minutes)
This tape is very similar to the other Basic Relaxation tape; however, this one features a male voice. It also introduces breath awareness and body scan relaxation.

Side 2 (29 minutes)
Side 2 offers frequent pauses to allow you to practice techniques that elicit the relaxation response.

Advanced Relaxation-Response Tape (female voice)

Side 1 (30 minutes)
This side guides you through a body scan and relaxation, leading you into a relaxation response through awareness of your heart and repetition of your focus word. This tape has frequent pauses to encourage you to practice and develop ways of bringing forth the relaxation response on your own.

Side 2 (50 minutes)
Side 2 reinforces basic skills and also guides you through a stretching routine and a series on imagery for healing.

Ocean Waves Tape (female voice)

Side 1 (24 minutes)
Side 1 is a guided body scan relaxation. It incorporates guided visualization of a sandy ocean beach, enhanced by the soothing ocean sounds in the background.

Side 2 (30 minutes)
Side 2 leads you through a series of stretching exercises done in a sitting position. These stretches will encourage a peaceful state of relaxation, awareness, and the elicitation of the relaxation response. This side of the tape does not use ocean wave sounds.

Mountain Stream (female voice)

Side 1 (20 minutes)
This side gently guides you through a series of breathing techniques leading into body scan relaxation. Its purpose is to alleviate tension from each body part and allows you to practice breathing awareness. This side of the tape also includes a word focus exercise.

Side 2 (20 minutes)
Side 2 offers you creative imagery acting as a tour guide on a walk through a forest to a mountain stream, allowing you to escape and become aware of and focus on your senses.

Beach Walk (female voice)

Side 1 (40 minutes)
Side 1 focuses on relaxation exercises, including a long body scan relaxation to relieve tension from every body part. It then leads you through visualization of taking a warm, comfortable bath. The guidance in this tape is very specific, making it quite easy to follow. You may find this longer side useful during medical, surgical, or dental procedures.

Side 2 (20 minutes)
Side 2 directs you through a series of breath and other relaxation exercises that elicit the relaxation response followed by a guided imagery exercise of exploring a sandy beach on a magnificent summer day. (This differs from the Ocean Waves tape because there are no wave sounds in the background.)

Gift of Relaxation/Garden of Your Mind (female voice)

Side 1 Gift of Relaxation (20 minutes)
This side focuses on introducing the basic steps of eliciting the relaxation response. You are quietly guided through body scan relaxation exercise and some simple deep breathing techniques, which are intended to heighten your awareness and enable you to deepen your experience of the relaxation response. The tape ends with positive affirmations, encouraging you to feel good about yourself and be proud of your experience.

Side 2 Garden of Your Mind (20 minutes)
This creative mental imagery exercise begins with body scan relaxation and breath awareness components and incorporates imagery of a lovely garden, one that you have visited in your past or one that you create in your own mind. The tape ends with positive self-statements and encouragement.

SAMPLE
RELAXATION RESPONSE
HEALTH COMMITMENT

Long-Term Goal:
Elicit the Relaxation Response Daily

_____
Signature

_____
Witness

Expected Date of Reaching Goal: _____

Readiness to Change	Short-Term Goals	Comments (supports, rewards, etc.)
Never considered change, need information.	1. Get Herbert Benson's *The Relaxation Response*. 2. Read the chapters in *The Wellness Book* on the relaxation response (chapters 4 and 5).	
Considered change, but not yet committed.	1. Find and talk with people who are long-time mediators to understand benefits better. 2. Talk to professionals who teach various techniques for eliciting the relaxation response about fears, concerns, or skepticism.	
Desire change, need motivation.	1. Do exercises in *The Wellness Book*. 2. Purchase relaxation-response tape to help learn skill.	

(continued)

Readiness to Change	Short-Term Goals	Comments (supports, rewards, etc.)
Attempting change; need structure, support, and skills.	1. Establish a time and place to do relaxation response. 2. Negotiate with family for twenty minutes of free time.	
Change made; need reinforcement.	1. Identify technique that is most helpful and enjoyable in eliciting the relaxation response. 2. Identify, through the use of a daily diary, changes in physical symptoms, thinking, or mood that come from doing the relaxation response.	
Change made; slipping back into bad habits, need renewed motivation and support.	1. Review sections in *The Wellness Book* or review with a relaxation-response teacher the physical and emotional benefits of regularly eliciting the relaxation response. Attend a seminar on this topic. 2. Determine obstacles to eliciting the relaxation response daily. Problem-solve. Do you need to change your time, place, technique, or get support from your family?	

RELAXATION RESPONSE
HEALTH COMMITMENT

Long-Term Goal:

_____

_____ Signature

_____

_____ Witness

Expected Date of Reaching Goal: _____

Comments (supports, rewards, etc.)

Short-Term Goals

PART 2

EXERCISE

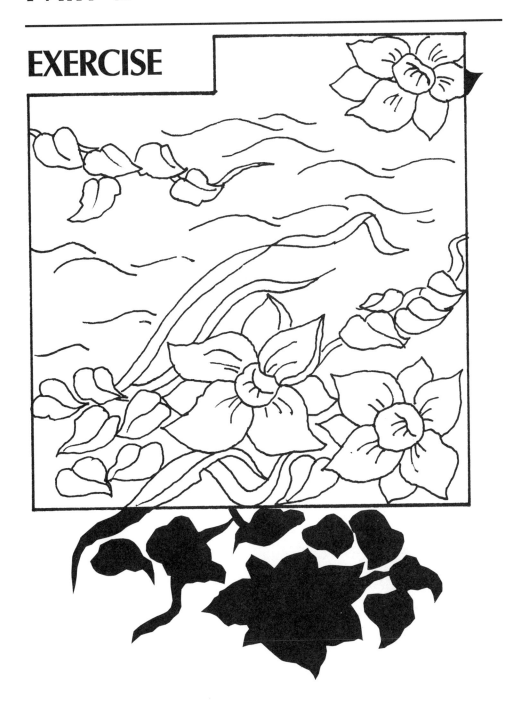

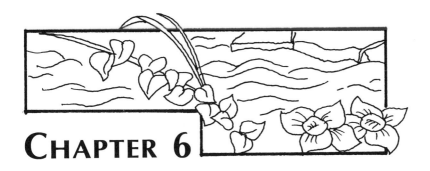

CHAPTER 6

TUNING IN TO YOUR BODY, TUNING UP YOUR MIND

In this chapter you will explore

- your physical cues of stress
- ways to release physical tension
- developing a memory of a relaxed mind/body state
- using awareness of muscle tension and relaxation along with postures to alter your thoughts and feelings
- how to monitor your exercise program, distinguishing stretching from straining or forcing muscles
- using mindful stretching exercises to elicit the relaxation response

You have learned that the mind and body are interconnected. As thoughts affect your body, so too changes in your body have been shown to shape thoughts, feelings, and even body chemistry. In the exercise at the end of chapter 2, "The Mind/Body Model of Health and Illness," the simple act of holding a pencil to simulate a smile or a frown may have changed your mood. This change in mood may have triggered feelings, emotions, and alterations in body chemistry. Thus the posture of your facial muscles, a smile, can initiate a cascade of linked reactions and demonstrate the utility of being aware of your body and the phenomenon of the mind/body connection.

Training in body awareness, as well as in stretching and exercises to elicit the relaxation response are important tools for gaining understanding and influence in your health and well-being. Just as radios, violins, and cars must be tuned to perform well; so too your body and mind require and benefit from attention and refinement.

AWARENESS OF YOUR BODY'S FEEDBACK

High-tech devices called biofeedback monitors measure the various physical effects that stress and relaxation have on your body (e.g., heart rate, skin temperature, or blood pressure). However, you have an innate biofeedback system. The first step in learning to use it is to become aware of your body.

Your body constantly responds to natural biofeedback. Consider messages (biofeedback) regarding hunger and fatigue: when you are hungry you seek out food; when you are tired, you rest. There are also times when you may choose to disregard these physical cues. For example, have you ever chosen not to go to bed, despite exhaustion, in order to finish a project and meet a deadline? You constantly receive messages from your body which you interpret and respond to, choosing your course of action based on internal and external demands.

Unfortunately, many of us have never been trained to pay close attention to our bodies, or have learned to ignore many of its cues. For example, people commonly try to cope with pain by ignoring it. Although ignoring and even denying bodily signals can be a useful coping strategy in the short run, the result of not being aware of your body is limiting and can be harmful. Recall times when you have injured yourself because you did not attend to your body's messages to rest a sore muscle or to get more sleep.

In our clinical program, we often find that people feel disconnected from their bodies. They identify with their mind and its intellectual processes, but have little awareness of their body and the messages it is feeding back to them. One participant in our Behavioral Medicine Clinic said that until now, he thought his body was a pedestal for his head. Little wonder he had physical symptoms of illness!

By developing an awareness of your body, you can become your own "biofeedback monitor." Your choices regarding the day-to-day necessities of eating and sleeping will become clearer, and you will also attain an understanding of the more subtle signals of your body. You can then better interpret and respond to them, choosing the most appropriate course of action.

Awareness contributes to survival. For example, the Eskimos have many different words to describe snow, making fine distinctions between, say, old granulated snow and very old granulated snow. Because they understand subtle characteristics of snow and ice, the Eskimo can survive in an environment hostile to those less aware. Your "hostile" environment is not snow, but it demands a similar alertness from you. You need to understand the subtle characteristics of your internal and external environments. Your internal environment has to do with how your body reacts—where, for example, you feel tension in your body, or what your stressful automatic thoughts are. Your external environment involves your particular triggers for stress—a traffic jam? long lines at the supermarket? seeing the mess in your adolescent's bedroom?

In asking you to pay attention to your body in a new way, we seek to develop distinctions which will increase your understanding of your body and the messages it sends you. Another name for this awareness is *"presence."*

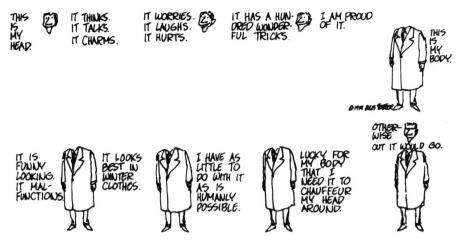

THE PRESENT OF "PRESENCE"

Some young children at play are completely absorbed, enthusiastic, and energetic; they have an astonishing ability to focus awareness on tasks. This power of undistracted observation allows them to learn quickly and easily, and it exemplifies *presence*, or awareness of what is happening in the moment. The practice of mindfulness described in chapter 5, "Eliciting the Relaxation Response," is a way of practicing being present in the moment. In this chapter you will practice being present with your mind/body.

LEARNING BY DOING: YOUR BODY AS A LABORATORY

Physical activity is a good way to increase your awareness. There is wisdom in the Chinese proverb:

> I hear, and I forget.
> I see, and I remember.
> I do, and I understand.

Throughout this chapter we will ask you to perform exercises and carefully observe your experience.

Take a Moment To . . .

Notice where you find tension or anxiety in your body. Can you feel tension in your head? Tightness in your forehead, jaw, or chin? What about the back of your neck, your shoulders, or somewhere else? Are you aware of your face flushing, your heart speeding up, your body temperature feeling either cold or hot? Do you find yourself holding your breath, sighing, scratching yourself a lot, grinding your teeth, clenching your fist? Do you feel a knot in your stomach? Or are your reactions more subtle? Do you find that your mind races or freezes, or you have trouble concen-

THE FAR SIDE   By GARY LARSON

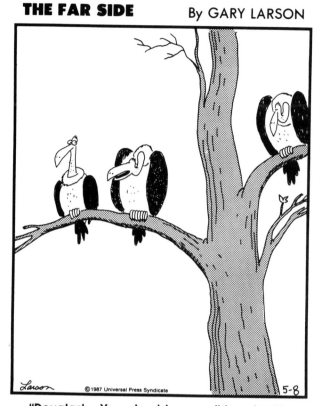

"Douglas! ... Your shoulders aren't hunched!"

THE FAR SIDE © 1987. Universal Press Syndicate.
Reprinted by permission.

trating, sleeping, or sitting still? The muscles throughout your body tend
to hold stress in the form of physical tension, creating "dis-ease." Consider
whether there is a relationship between your characteristic reactions to
stress and any medical condition you may have.

SELF-INQUIRY: PAYING ATTENTION TO YOUR TENSION

When focusing on your body in the previous exercise, you may have become
aware of the discomfort that muscle tension can cause. Less obvious but
nonetheless harmful effects of excessive muscle tension include wasted energy, which may lead to fatigue and other symptoms of dis-ease. In addition,
stimulation of specific muscles has been shown to have specific and potentially
harmful results. In one interesting experiment performed by psychologist
Paul Ekman Ph.D. at the University of California School of Medicine at San
Francisco and his colleagues, subjects were asked to produce facial expressions
that resembled a number of emotions. When the individuals shaped their face
to resemble negative emotions, their heart and breathing rates increased.

Not all muscle tension is undesirable. The muscles tense naturally as a
part of movement. The difficulty occurs when we accumulate excessive muscle
tension and retain it for long periods of time.

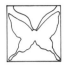

Take a Moment To . . .

Make a fist—very tense and tight—with your right hand (as you did in chapter 2). Notice where you are gripping in your body. What about your jaw? What's happening with your breathing? Now take some natural breaths and release your fist.

While deliberately tensing your hand, you probably also held your breath and clenched your jaw. It is likely you did not recognize this tension until asked about it. The sensations of tension often become "normal" to us, but "normal" is not necessarily healthy. Take time to pay attention to your muscle tension. You may notice yourself building up muscle tension bit by bit throughout the day, finding your shoulders edging up toward your ears and your fists and jaw clenching. Consider the experience of tension buildup and release described by Sheila, a thirty-year-old banker with lower-back pain:

> Last week I had an appointment in Boston at nine a.m. I left my house and got on the subway in plenty of time to get there. However the train was very slow—it moved about three feet every five minutes and I knew I would be late. I realized how tense I was holding my body. I was so frustrated that the train was not moving and it was like I was pushing my body instead of pushing the train. My back pain increased.

Excess muscle tension can also result from using our muscles inappropriately. When injured, we tend to tense the muscles around the site of pain to defend against movement and further injury. Unfortunately, this muscular armoring creates further tension and muscle imbalance.

Al's Experience

For Al, a fifty-year-old insurance salesman, his protective reaction to injury became the primary problem. He came to the clinic to manage pain from an automobile accident. Through body-awareness techniques he realized the initial pain no longer bothered him. However, in adjusting to that initial pain, he had learned to hold other parts of his body tense and now experienced chronic pain from that tension. With practice, he learned to release that tension and his pain subsided.

MOVEMENT AND MEANING

Working with muscle-tension awareness and release is only one part of understanding the connection between your mind and body. There are strong linkages between movement and meaning.

Take a Moment To . . .

Shake your head from side to side five times, repeating, "You are absolutely right." Now, nod your head up and down five times and firmly repeat, "You are wrong!" Can you feel yourself working against a mind/body connection?

A number of studies support the idea that physical postures and tensions are connected to mental attitudes. Expressions can affect the mind and emotions. Dr. James D. Laird, a professor of psychology at Clark University in Massachusetts, reports that when one research subject was asked to clench his jaw, he described automatically feeling angry even though he tried not to. Your body has what Dr. Alan D. Sirota and his colleagues, from Brown University, call a "psychobiological feedback loop": when you change your thoughts and feelings, you change your pattern of muscle use, and this muscle change can in turn reinforce your thoughts and feelings. In this way you perpetuate a particular set of related physical, mental, and emotional reactions.

Take a Moment To . . .

Tighten a group of muscles simultaneously: Furrow your eyebrows as you make your eyes small; clench your jaw and tighten your fists. Hold this for a while. How does it feel? Do you notice how holding muscles tense begins to affect your thoughts and feelings?

READING BODY LANGUAGE: STANCE

The mind/body connection is reflected in language. The word *attitude* means "a position of the body or a manner of carrying oneself" or "a state of mind or feeling with regards to some matter." Thus the word *attitude* describes not merely thoughts and feelings, but also posture appropriate to portraying these feelings.

Similarly, *stance* conveys both postural and emotional meanings. People are described as *upstanding* or *downtrodden* citizens, *stable* or *unstable*. They can be *well-balanced, steady, centered, pillars of the community,* or *off center* and *out of balance.* Sometimes they *dig in their heels.* Body language is revealing when we pay attention to it: we sense another's aggression, insecurity, passivity, dominance, anger, or ease not only from their words, but also from their physical posture and facial expressions.

Take a Moment To . . .

Spend some time seeing what you can infer about others simply by noticing whether their shoulders droop or their chests stick out, whether their jaw is slack or their chin protrudes. Then observe children, noticing the similarities and contrasts to the adults with whom they live.

Children are excellent models because their postures generally reflect their feelings and the moods of those around them. Consider the preschooler who walks with a pounding step and protruding chest; chances are an adult in his family does the same. Children mimic the adults around them, taking on their mental and physical attitudes.

REFLECTIONS ON YOUR REFLECTION

It is usually easier to study others than to study yourself, but in developing a mind/body awareness, the next step is to begin to pay attention to your own body. All thoughts and feelings have corresponding reactions in your body. As you observe your thoughts and feelings and begin to become aware of your body, you will see how thoughts and feelings and your body interact. What body sensations accompany thoughts of unworthiness or fear, and conversely, what messages do you lock into your body if you habitually clench your jaw or stoop over? Sometimes the answer is obvious, but often you must refine your awareness to discern the connection. With increasing discrimination, you gain new control over your body. Look at where you hold chronic tension. What habits of movement have you adopted from families, friends, injuries, and day-to-day tensions? What memories and attitudes does your body maintain?

Take a Moment To . . .

Stand before a full-length mirror and observe your posture:

- Is your pelvis tucked under or tilted forward?
- Do your shoulders droop or does your chest stick out?
- Are you standing on the balls of your feet—ready to run off to do a thousand other things, or are your feet firmly planted?
- Is your chin jutting forward or is it pulled in like a turtle?

Once you have carefully observed your posture, exaggerate the problem areas, such as drooping shoulders and a protruding tummy. How does this feel? What does the mirror tell you about your stance and your attitude?

Now adjust your posture, releasing tension, and notice how this looks and feels.

REEDUCATING YOUR MIND/BODY

Remember that your patterns of tension are not who you are, but rather how you have learned to hold your body. Even if you have held patterns of tension for forty years or more, you are not that tension. Patterns of tension are something you have learned, and therefore they are something you can relearn. Did you know that even your bones reshape and realign themselves based on your patterns of use? If such a "fixed" part of our bodies can and does change, why not your habits of tension?

In the first decade of this century, Dr. Edmund Jacobson, the pioneering expert on relaxation techniques, stressed the value of identifying muscle tension in order to release it and improve both physical and emotional conditions. Famous for developing the techniques of progressive muscle relaxation, Dr. Jacobson did a great deal of research and clinical work showing that thoughts and imagination stimulate affiliated muscles. Special techniques for relaxation can ease this muscular tension. For example, when Dr. Jacobson asked subjects to imagine lifting an arm, corresponding muscle stimulation occurred which subsequently subsided with thoughts of relaxation. In other research, Jacobson found that when muscles relaxed, emotions subsided. In the 1950s, George B. Whatmore, a Washington State physician who researched muscle tension not visible to the naked eye, used electromyographic equipment to measure the motor portion of the nervous system. Dr. Whatmore cites his own research and that of others to show the relationship between muscle tension and mood; for example, depressed patients have increased muscle activity, but when these tense muscles relax, depression decreases. Dr. Whatmore further cites research identifying "on guard" behavior patterns which can be deactivated by relaxation techniques. Many emerging forms of therapy utilizing body massage, breathing, and movement are based on the understanding that decreasing muscle tension changes mental states, thoughts, and even behavior patterns.

Ann's Experience

Ann is a delightful seventy-four-year-old widow who was referred to our clinic for multiple medical problems, including chronic lower-back pain and arthritis. She kept a record of her pain and noticed that it increased with worry, but when she used her breathing to release tension, her pain decreased. She also learned to use her posture to take more control of her situation:

> I notice that if I stand squarely on my two feet, my mind is clearer and I can speak more slowly and directly.

TAKING CARE OF YOURSELF: LEARNING TO BE SOOTHING AND GENTLE

Since your muscle-tension patterns may seem "normal," it can be difficult to let go of that tension with a self-imposed command to "Relax!" One way to find and release your patterns of tension is to practice selectively increasing and letting go of the tension in specific muscles. This method is exemplified in yawning.

Take a Moment To . . .

Score the tension in your face on a scale of zero to ten (ten being as tense as possible and zero being completely relaxed). Now simulate yawning. Close your eyes and yawn three times. Notice what you are doing when you yawn.

Paying close attention, you probably noticed a connection between your breathing and tension. On exhaling, you let go of tension; on inhaling, you may have increased tension slightly as you stretched out your jaw and perhaps tensed the muscles of your forehead. Yawn three times again and notice the differing sensations when you inhale and exhale. When you finish, score the tension in your face again. Did your tension change?

By increasing our awareness of muscle tension, we can be more conscious of the customary tension we find "normal." Then we can return to a "natural" state of physical relaxation by releasing tension each time we exhale.

DEVELOPING CHOICE AND CONTROL

At first, some people in our clinical programs consider the changes they experience after a brief tension/release session to be almost magical because their mind and body and emotions shift so remarkably. But the change is not magic. Rather, the difference is due to the application of important principles and techniques for self-care. Many are age-old and some of them are as simple and natural as yawning when you feel tense. We ask you to try various techniques and choose those that work for you. They only work, however, if you use them.

One common technique is to use tension as a cue.

John's Experience

John, a twenty-year-old car mechanic, came to our clinic after being permanently disabled following a work-related injury to his lower back. Like many of us, he hadn't thought much about life and felt that things just happened. He was always reacting and feeling out of control, often finding himself at a bar drinking without knowing how he got there.

Through his work with body awareness, he began to notice signs of physical tension as cues for emotional stress. Increased pain in his body was a signal that he was holding tension. John would then do relaxing breathing, release the tension, reduce the pain, and, with his mind a little clearer, begin to explore the problem and its solutions. He learned to manage problems before becoming so angry and frustrated that he would return to alcohol for assistance.

> My style is mostly Stop, Breathe, and Relax! This helps to release my tension and I can tune into my feelings and think the problem through.

His increased body awareness thus began a process of expanding personal choice and power. He has returned to school and is applying his self-management skills to starting a career in management at a small technical business.

Another technique is to notice and choose body postures more consciously. The wisdom of this technique is reflected in the common sayings "Put on a happy face" and "Square your shoulders."

Grace's Experience

Grace came to the clinic feeling generally discouraged. A thirty-six-year-old with many talents, she was used to getting what she wanted until a series of disabilities struck her and she found herself overwhelmed. She applied herself to the program diligently, writing extensive journal entries describing the effects of her practices on her mind and body. Initially she observed:

Self-confidence, the ability to get things done, had really gone down the chute almost without my realizing it—so intent was I on how bad I was feeling and which doctor could I go to next for relief.

By carefully monitoring the relationship of her symptoms to her activities and emotions, she began to notice what thoughts and behaviors directly affected her symptoms. She found that stretching exercises early in the morning loosened up her body so that she could go about her activities more comfortably.

Grace also practiced affirmative posture as another way to reestablish control over her life:

I practiced this posture several times, especially during telephone conversations, a few of them very troubling . . . Many previous conversations left me utterly exhausted . . . Interestingly enough, when I stood erect . . . assumed what I would call a confident and assertive pose, the words I was previously at a loss to express came readily to my aid and I was able to disengage myself without rancor or bruised feelings . . .

Through the combination of body awareness and relaxation response, Grace was able to report:

I feel a definite sense of control emerging over the anxiety, and this has done wonders for the level of pain.

HATHA-YOGA

Our clinical programs teach hatha-yoga exercises as one means of developing body awareness and eliciting the relaxation response. Hatha-yoga can easily be modified to an individual's physical restrictions. In addition to some of the more obvious benefits of exercise, yoga can help you realign your bodily posture, release muscle tension, and develop a more subtle control of your body. Yoga is also helpful because it reinforces your experience of maintaining a basic "resting state" in the musculature and the mind while carrying on daily activities.

As you practice these techniques, the memory of muscular relaxation will help you release your physical tension more readily throughout the day. Reflect on your experience of yourself as a relaxed and contented individual, and choose a stance of well-being.

Included in this chapter are three sets of gentle yoga exercises to be done seated, on the floor, and standing. Before you begin, study the general and specific instructions carefully. The first time you practice, allow twenty minutes to a half hour to do one of the sets of exercises. When you become familiar with the poses, you can design your own exercise routine to suit your needs.

Although these exercises have been selected because they are generally simple and safe, please consult with your health-care provider before beginning your proposed exercise practice if you have any medical concerns. Prepare for your exercise by wearing loose comfortable clothing. Remove your shoes and socks. Do not exercise for several hours after eating a large meal. As you start, take a few minutes to notice your breathing, encouraging diaphragmatic breathing.

The suggested exercises combine breathing with slow gentle activity. Never force your breathing, and consciously remind yourself to be aware of your breathing throughout the movement, associating each exhalation with letting go of physical tension. Generally speaking, movements which contract your body or involve bending forward are coordinated with exhaling and those which stretch and open your body are coordinated with inhaling. Although combining movement with your breathing patterns strengthens your focus and sense of calm, some people find this initially too complicated and instead focus on performing the motion correctly while making sure not to hold their breath. In deciding how to proceed, choose those practices which most enhance your sense of calm.

As you exercise, pay attention to your bodily responses. Almost everyone can benefit from this type of gentle exercise, but you should adapt your exercise routine to your specific needs and abilities. For example, any exercise which lowers the head below the heart brings an extra supply of blood to the head. In this kind of exercise, it is important to bring your head up slowly to avoid dizziness. Avoid or adjust exercises which make you feel you are working too hard. See your body as a laboratory in which you can study and learn and gain enhanced control through developing body awareness. *Only do exercises which feel comfortable to you.*

Become absorbed in what you do. Remember, the key elements of eliciting the relaxation response are a focused awareness on a word, prayer, phrase, or motion, and a passive attitude; apply these to the exercises. Take time to take a few deep, easy breaths and return to your starting position after each exercise in order to reestablish a sense of calm awareness. The purpose of these exercises is awareness, not accomplishment.

Remember to move slowly and consciously, letting your body signal what it needs and how it can move most comfortably. A cat needs no lessons in stretching and relaxing; it seems to sense what feels right. When calm, you can use your sense of how to stretch and move.

As you observe yourself, you may notice that you are tensing and working muscles unnecessarily. Isolate and use only muscles that are needed. Avoid any sudden or extreme movement. Forcing and bouncing are counterproductive and can be harmful. Replace these habits with the practice of releasing the tension and allowing the stretch to unfold. As you release your body into the stretch, you can sense a quiet invigoration rather than pain or strain.

More advanced exercises are performed by holding steady in a comfortable position. Whenever possible, keep your eyes closed so that you draw your attention inward to an awareness of where you hold muscular tension and to the physical sensations of muscular relaxation. A sense of inner quiet develops as you hold your poses. In the beginning, poses are held for perhaps a minute or two. As your awareness of your body increases and your body becomes stronger, poses can be held for longer periods of time.

End each of your exercise sessions with five to ten minutes of quiet meditation. We recommend finding a qualified teacher if you would like to learn more than these gentle stretches.

RELAXATION EXERCISES

Seated Poses

These exercises can be practiced sitting either on the edge of a pillow on the floor or sitting forward on a chair with your feet flat on the floor. Sitting forward allows your arms and legs more freedom of motion.

Modify the exercises to suit your own body's needs, and increase the number of repetitions as your body grows stronger and more flexible. The exercises can be done as a complete series or individually at any time during the day when you need to release tension and stiffness and to focus your mind. Between each exercise take a moment to relax, sitting in a resting position with your hands in your lap, your spine straight, and your head upright. Take a few minutes at the end of your exercise to sit comfortably, noticing your breathing and releasing tension with each exhalation. (See fig. 1.)

Feet and leg exercises

Begin each of these exercises with your legs outstretched.

- Alternate curling and stretching the toes (repeat three times and relax).
- Alternate flexing (bending) and extending (stretching) the whole foot at the ankle (repeat three times and relax).
- Rotate the ankles to the right as if drawing circles with your toes (repeat three times and relax).
- Rotate the ankles to the left (repeat three times and relax).
- Alternate flexing (bending) the right knee, drawing the thigh in toward the chest, and then stretching the leg straight (repeat three times and relax). (See fig. 2.)
- Repeat with the left leg, flexing your knee (repeat three times and relax).
- Place your feet flat on the floor and loosen your hips by alternately drawing your arms and trunk back and then reaching out over your legs. Keep your back straight (repeat three times and relax). (See figs. 3 and 4.)

Relax and notice the sensation in your legs and hips.

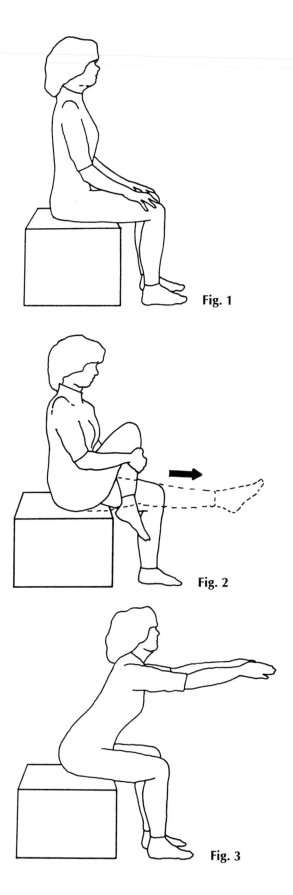

Fig. 1

Fig. 2

Fig. 3

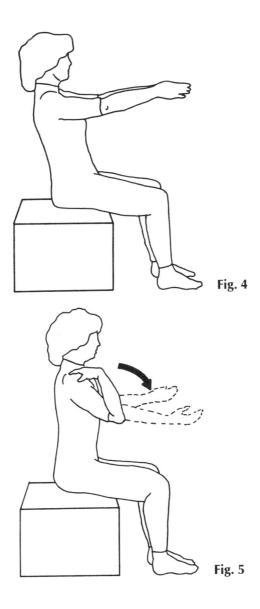

Fig. 4

Fig. 5

Arm and hand exercises

All of these are to be done with your arms extended out in front of you.

- Move your hands up and down, bending from the wrist (repeat three times and relax).
- Alternate stretching your fingers, then making a fist (repeat three times and relax).
- Rotate your wrists first to the right three times, then to the left three times, and relax.
- Alternate bending and stretching your arms at the elbows by bringing your fingertips to your shoulders and then straightening out your arms with your palms facing up (repeat three times and relax). (See fig. 5.)

Relax and notice the sensations in your arms and hands.

Shoulder exercises

- Raise your right shoulder up toward your ear. On an exhale, release your shoulder down (repeat three times and relax).
- Move your right shoulder forward. On the exhale return it to the starting position (repeat three times and relax).
- Move your right shoulder back. On the exhale return it to the starting position (repeat three times and relax).
- Repeat the sequence on the left side.
- Bring both shoulders up toward your ears, tense, and then drop your shoulders down as you exhale (repeat three times and relax).
- Cross your right arm over your chest and under your left arm, reaching back to your left shoulder blade with your right hand. Cross your left arm over your chest, your left hand reaching for your right shoulder blade as if you are hugging yourself. Relax your shoulders down and away from your ears. Take several nice, deep, easy breaths, releasing any tension in your shoulders with each exhalation (fig. 6).
- Repeat but first cross your left arm followed by your right.
- Release your arms and take a moment to study the sensations in your shoulders.
- Place your fingertips on your shoulders. Slowly draw large circles with your elbows, moving with your breathing. Exhale as your elbows come forward, inhale as they go back and your chest expands. Focus your awareness on the expansion of your chest and the release of tension in your shoulders. Draw three circles and relax (fig. 7).
- Reverse the direction of the circles, drawing three more. Again coordinate the expansion of your chest with each inhalation.

Relax and study the sensations in your shoulders.

Head and neck exercises

Hold each of these positions, taking three easy breaths and relaxing tension with each exhalation; then return your head to upright center before doing the next movement.

- Drop your chin to your chest. Feel the weight of your head stretch out the back of your neck (hold and relax for three breaths).
- Look as far as you can over your right shoulder (hold and relax for three breaths).
- Look as far as you can over your left shoulder (hold and relax for three breaths).
- Drop your right ear to your right shoulder (hold and relax for three breaths).

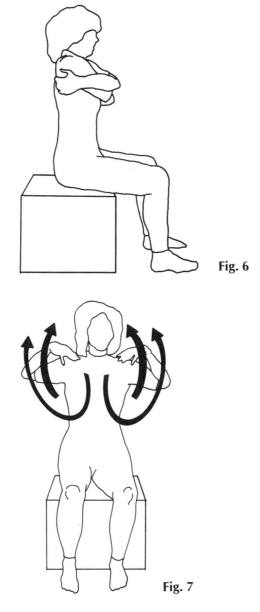

Fig. 6

Fig. 7

- Drop your left ear to your left shoulder (hold and relax for three breaths).
- Clasp your hands behind your neck. Drop your head back. Let your jaw drop open. Relax your whole face. Yawn, stretching your mouth and eyes wide open, then on the exhale release any tension in your jaw and face. Bring your head back to an upright position, and return your hand to your lap. Continue to yawn any time you wish (fig. 8).
- Draw small circles with your chin very slowly, three times clockwise, then three times counterclockwise.

Relax and notice the sensations in your neck.

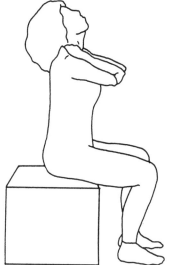

Fig. 8

Eye exercise

Imagine you are looking at a giant clock. Without moving your head, move your gaze upward to look at twelve o'clock. Now look down at six o'clock. Repeat three times, then blink several times, and rest with your eyes closed.

Now look to the right to three o'clock, then move your eyes horizontally left to nine o'clock. Repeat three times, then blink several times, and rest with your eyes closed.

Now slowly move your eyes clockwise around the imaginary clock, starting at twelve o'clock, then preceeding through one, two, three, four, five, six, seven, eight, nine, ten, eleven, and twelve again. Blink several times, then close your eyes and rest them. Now slowly move your eyes counterclockwise. When you finish, blink several times and rest your eyes.

Rub the palms of your hands together until they are warm, then cup the palms over your closed eyes. Imagine the warmth of your hands soothing any tension around your eyes. Take time to feel the sensation of relaxation.

Gentle massage

Notice any residual tension in your face, neck, and shoulders; gently massage the areas of tension.

Cat pose in the chair

Sit forward on your cushion or chair, extending your arms behind you to rest your hands on the floor or the back edge of the seat of the chair. As you exhale, draw in your abdominal muscles as you tuck your head and round your shoulders and torso forward. Your pelvis tilts and your lower back rounds. Then as you inhale, look up to the ceiling, lifting your sternum (breastbone), spreading your chest, pulling your shoulders back, and arching your lower back. (See figs. 9 and 10.) Repeat three times.

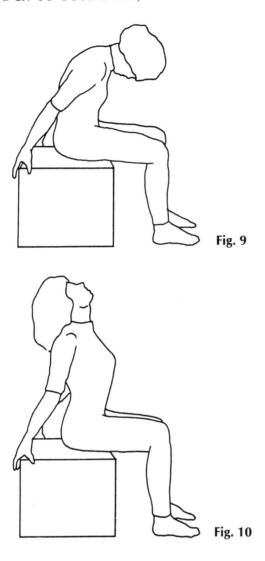

Fig. 9

Fig. 10

Side stretch

On an inhalation, lengthen your torso as you reach up over your head, bending your elbows and clasping them with the opposite hands. On the exhale, bend your torso, head, and arms to the left. Then inhale, stretching up to the center. Exhale as you bend your torso, head, and arms to the right. Maintain an open chest and a lengthened spine as you bend side to side. Repeat three times, alternating sides and moving with the breath rhythm (fig. 11).

Child pose in the chair

Sit forward on your chair or cushion. Imagine your head is so heavy that it slowly draws your neck, shoulders, and torso forward over your legs; your back rounds. Hold this position and breathe softly, releasing tension for about

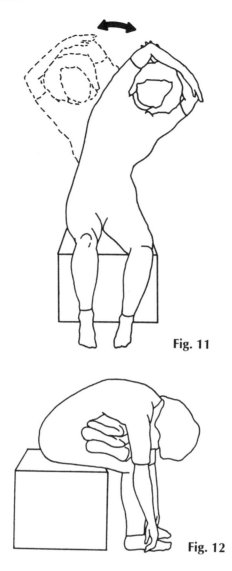

Fig. 11

Fig. 12

thirty seconds. Come out of the pose, rolling gently from the base of the spine, straightening one vertebra at a time. Sit quietly for a couple of minutes, focusing on your breathing and noticing the sensations in your body following this exercise. If you would be more comfortable with upper-chest support for this exercise, try placing a pillow or rolled blanket on your lap, or rest your head on a table, cushioned by a pillow or your forearms.

Attend to your body. What else does it need?

Now sit for a few minutes, observing your breathing and enjoying the sensations of calmness with each exhalation (fig. 12).

Floor Poses

These floor exercises require a belt or strap as well as a mat or blanket to spread on the floor. Repeat the exercises slowly several times. As you strength-

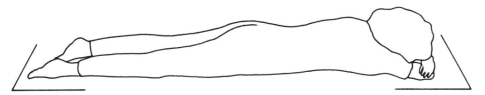

Fig. 13

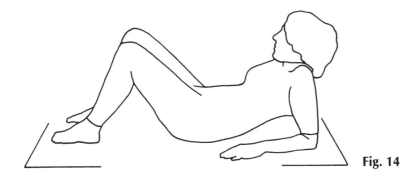

Fig. 14

en your body, you can either increase the number of repetitions, or, in some cases, hold the poses for longer periods of time. Remember to encourage a sense of calm awareness throughout the exercises by focusing on diaphragmatic breathing whenever it is comfortable, and by relaxing between each pose, releasing tension with several deep, easy breaths.

Crocodile

(This is an excellent pose for developing diaphragmatic breathing.) Lie on your stomach with your legs a comfortable distance apart. Fold your arms in front of your body so that your hands rest on the opposite elbows. Rest your forehead on your forearms. Study the sensations of breathing with your diaphragm; notice the rhythm of your breath and how your belly expands when you inhale and contracts when you exhale (fig. 13).

Deep relaxation pose

This is the basic starting position and is used to rest before and after exercises. At the end of a longer series of exercises, rest in this position for about ten minutes, focusing on your breathing rhythm to elicit complete mental and physical relaxation. Assume the position through the following series of movements: Sit on the floor with your legs extended and knees bent. Lean back into your elbows and slowly roll your spine down on the floor beginning with your lower back (fig. 14).

When your shoulders, back, and buttocks support your weight, clasp your hands behind your head and draw your chin toward your chest. Then roll your neck and head to the floor, lengthening the back of your neck. Tuck your shoulders back and down to expand your chest, and bring your hands to rest by your sides with your palms up (fig. 15).

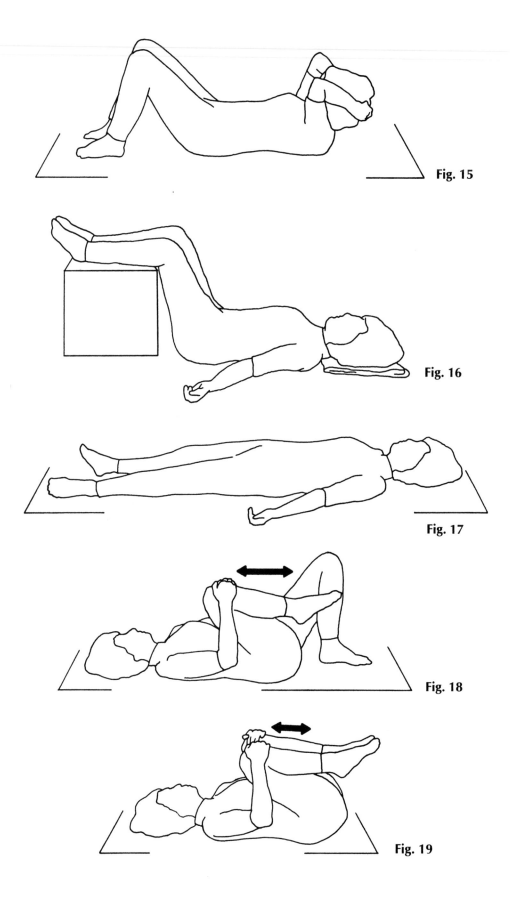

Fig. 15

Fig. 16

Fig. 17

Fig. 18

Fig. 19

If your chin is elevated or you feel a tightness in the throat, place a folded towel under your head until you feel comfortable. If you have a back problem, consider supporting your legs either on a blanket under bent knees or with your calves resting on a chair (fig. 16).

Allow your eyes to close, or fix them on a steady point. Adjust any part of your body that feels uncomfortable. Release your body into the support of the floor; using your exhale to settle into an inner calm. Straighten your legs one at a time, with your feet about ten inches apart and your toes falling outward (fig. 17).

Knee to chest

Begin in the Deep Relaxation Pose (fig. 17). Bend your knees and place your feet flat close to the buttocks, hip width apart. Bring your right knee into your chest, wrapping your hands around your knee or the back of your thigh. Move your knee into your chest as you exhale. Still grasping your leg, move your knee approximately eight inches away from your chest as you inhale. Synchronize the movement with the rhythm of your breathing, repeating six times and then resting (fig. 18).

Repeat six times with the right foot flat next to the buttocks and your left thigh moving toward your chest in rhythm with your breathing.

Bend both knees into the chest, grasping your thighs or knees. Your knees can be close together or separated; find the most comfortable position for you. Exhale and release the tightness at the hip joint as your knees move in toward your chest and your arms bend. Inhale and allow your knees to move out away from your chest about eight inches as your arms extend. Again, the movement of your knees is synchronized with your breathing. Study how these movements gently massage your back and abdomen (fig. 19).

Pelvic tilt

Lie on your back on the mat in the Deep Relaxation Pose with your knees bent and feet flat under the knees. Exhale, and push the small of your back down a few inches into the mat, tightening the buttocks. Inhale, release. Repeat six times, letting your breathing rhythm guide the rocking movement of your pelvis (fig. 20).

Spinal lift

Begin as in the pelvic tilt, with your feet hip width apart firmly pressed into the mat and your arms resting at your sides. Be sure to continue to breathe naturally throughout the exercise. After pressing the small of your back into the mat, tighten and lift the buttocks up. Continue rolling the spine up off of the mat, one vertebra at a time, until your weight rests on your feet, shoulders, and head. Hold briefly. Then, starting at the upper back, roll the spine down one vertebra at a time. Repeat this process three to six times (figs. 21 and 22).

As your body accommodates to the position and your strength increases, gradually increase the length of time you hold your back up. In order to

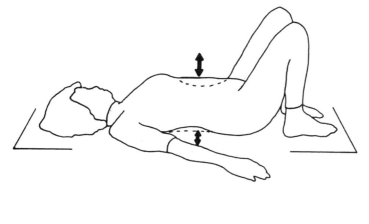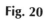

Fig. 20

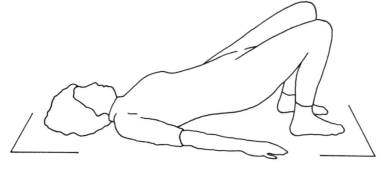

Fig. 21

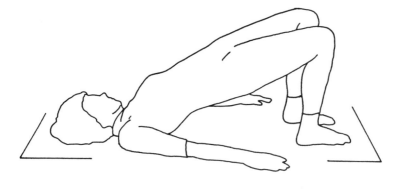

Fig. 22

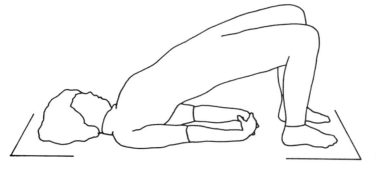

Fig. 23

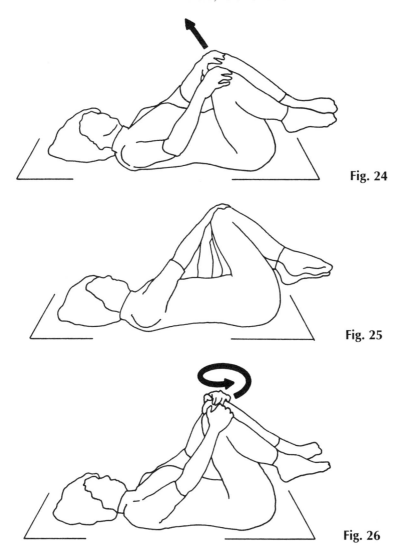

Fig. 24

Fig. 25

Fig. 26

support yourself, draw your shoulder blades together, clasp your fingers together under your buttocks, and stretch your clasped hands toward your feet (fig. 23).

Spine roll

Lie on your back with both knees drawn into the chest, hands clasping the outside of the knees. Roll from side to side gently and slowly so that your spine is softly massaged (figs. 24 and 25).

Next, pick up your head and roll slowly up and down on your spine.

With the knees still drawn into the chest, bring your head back to the mat and move your knees in a circle, first pointing your knees toward your head (twelve o'clock), then to the right (three o'clock), six o'clock, nine o'clock, and back to twelve. This exercise gently rotates the pelvis. Draw three circles to the right, then reverse and draw three to the left (fig. 26).

Hamstring stretch

Start out lying on your back with your knees bent and feet flat, close to the buttocks. Draw your right knee into your chest. Wrap your strap or belt around the ball of your right foot. With your buttocks remaining on the mat, straighten your knee by extending your right foot into the air. Think of releasing the tension in the back of your leg to allow your leg to stretch. Adjust the distance of your leg off the floor so that you feel a gentle stretch in the back of the leg. Take several diaphragmatic breaths, and as you exhale, release any tightness in your body. Notice any unnecessary tension in your face or shoulders. Relax your shoulders to the floor as you hold the position, noticing that effort can be isolated to your leg. You can increase the stretch by drawing your foot closer to your face or by flexing the foot so that the toes point toward your face. Initially, hold this position for half a minute; increase this time with practice (fig. 27).

Repeat, stretching the left leg and keeping the right knee bent.

Inner thigh stretch

From the Deep Relaxation Pose, bend your knees, touching the bottoms of your feet together. Open your knees out to the sides. Release any tightness in your inner thighs as you exhale. As you release the tension, your knees will move toward the floor. If you wish, you can use pillows or blankets to support your thighs (fig. 28).

Sit-up

From the Deep Relaxation Pose, with knees bent and feet flat, lift your arms off the floor reaching toward your feet. Using your abdominal muscles, lift your head and shoulders off the mat as you continue to focus on your breathing. Hold this position approximately thirty seconds. (Increase the time as your stomach muscles become stronger.) Now let your body release down to the mat, and enjoy the support of the mat on your spine (fig. 29).

Twist

A folded towel under your head for support may be helpful in this position.

Lie on your left side with knees slightly bent and feet together. Straighten your arms out to the left. Now lift your right hand off the left, drawing it in an arc over your torso until your arms form a **T**. (See fig. 30.) Follow the movement of your right arm with your eyes and head so that your head turns and rests to the right while your knees are to the left. Relax your shoulders to the floor. Adjust your knees so your spine gets a gentle, comfortable stretch. Initially, hold the position for just thirty seconds while you focus on taking nice, easy breaths and releasing any tension as you exhale. Then arc your right arm back to the starting position. Increase the holding time with practice.

Repeat, starting on the right side. Your knees will be to the right while you head turns to the left.

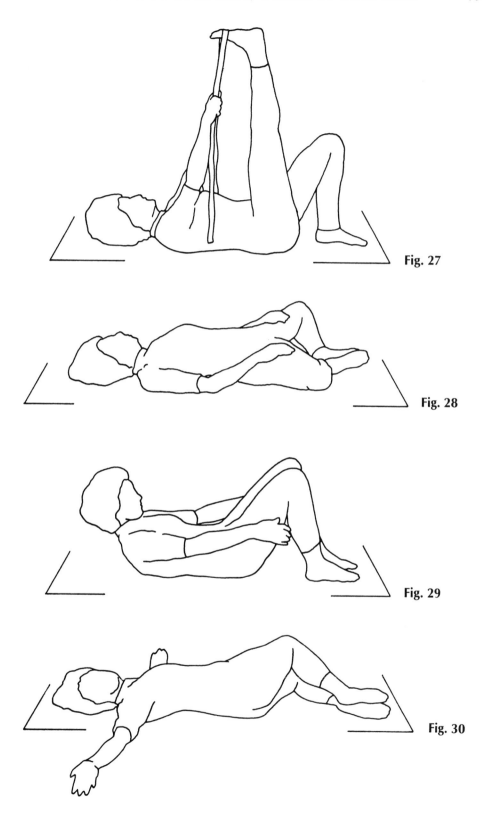

Fig. 27

Fig. 28

Fig. 29

Fig. 30

Three-part breathing

Beginning in the Deep Relaxation Pose (fig. 31), simply pay attention to your breathing rhythm, gradually allowing it to deepen. Now take a slow, complete breath.

Inhale: Expand 1) abdomen, 2) middle chest, 3) upper chest.

Exhale: Contract 1) abdomen, 2) middle chest, 3) upper chest.

Alternate taking a deep, full breath with simple diaphragmatic breathing.

Repeat three times, using the exhale to release your body completely into the support of the mat.

Cat pose on the floor

Begin on your hands and knees, arms straight and hands spread palms down and placed firmly under your shoulders. Hold your knees apart, directly under your hips. Relax your shoulders away from your ears. As you inhale, lift up your head, opening the chest as your belly drops while tilting your pelvis to draw your buttocks up (fig. 32). Then as you exhale, draw your belly in as the back rounds up, the head drops down, and the buttocks tighten; the pelvis tucks under (fig. 33). Repeat several times with your breathing rhythm, imitating the natural fluidity of the cat as it stretches its spine.

Child pose on the floor

Sit back on your heels with toes together, heels separated. If this position is uncomfortable, place a folded towel or blanket under your feet and/or over your calves. (If resting on your heels is still not comfortable without further simple adjustments, review the instructions for the Child Pose in the Chair ([page 87]). One objective of the Child Pose is to develop a sense of safety and security, which you cannot do if you are uncomfortable.)

With your hands reaching to the floor in front of you, lean forward, lengthening your spine as you release your torso onto your thighs. Rest your forehead comfortably on the floor or on a towel or blanket. Now draw your hands back toward your feet to release your shoulders further. Initially, hold this position for just thirty seconds, using the exhalation to release the tension from your shoulders. You may find breathing easier if you allow your back to expand on the inhale (fig. 34).

Draw yourself out of this position very slowly, rounding up from the base of your spine, letting your head hang heavy as your neck is the last to straighten. Close your eyes and notice the effects of this position.

Standing Poses

Mountain

This is a basic resting standing position. Place your feet approximately four or five inches apart (closer if you are comfortable), with the outside of your feet parallel. Distribute the weight on your feet so that only the arch is lifted.

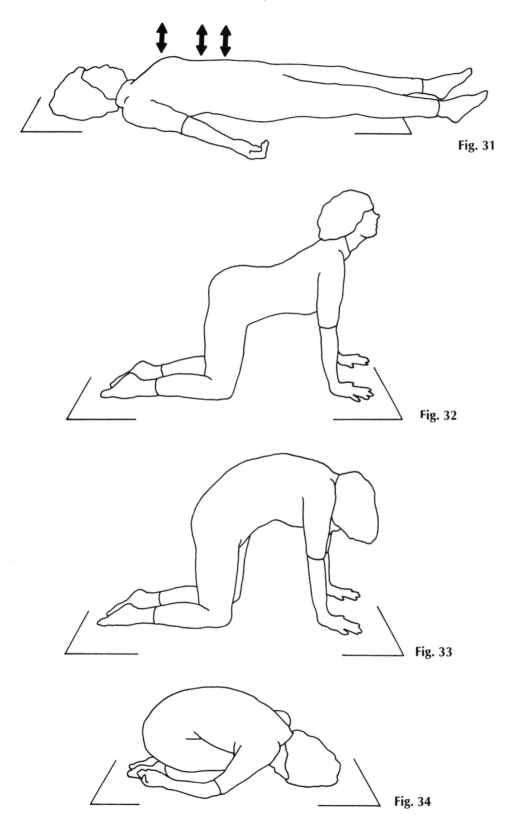

Fig. 31

Fig. 32

Fig. 33

Fig. 34

knee caps lift but do not lock. The weight is neither forward nor back. You might imagine standing with the solidity of a mountain, calling forth that image and your own personal stability to enhance your posture. Adjust your pelvis so it tips neither forward nor back; this angle governs the rest of your posture (fig. 35).

Now think of how the mountain arises out of the earth, and let your own dignity and majesty infuse your posture. Make yourself as tall as possible—perhaps imagining a string drawing you up through the top center of your head. Feel yourself creating spaces between your vertebrae in your back and neck as your spine lengthens. Your shoulder blades draw in and your sternum (breastbone) lifts. Your arms hang loosely by your sides. Relax your throat, jaw, and eyes. Feel simultaneously the stability of your grounded stance and the dignity of your uplifted spine and opened chest as you hold this position, focusing on releasing tension through diaphragmatic breathing.

Corkscrew

This variation of the Mountain Pose is designed to enhance your experience of your body's stability and dignity.

From the Mountain Pose inhale and raise your arms up over your head. Exhale and draw your arms slowly back and down to shoulder level. Hold and breathe, feeling the expansion in your chest. Your hands, feet, and shoulders are pressing down. Imagine your arms as the wings of a bottle opener and your torso as the cork. Inhale, then exhale slowly, pressing your arms down to your sides while your spine gradually lengthens, like a cork popping up (fig. 36).

Close your eyes and allow yourself to experience your body/mind.

Balanced stretching

Beginning in the Mountain Pose, inhale while you raise your arms overhead and rise to balance on the balls of your feet. Exhale slowly as you bring your arms down to your sides and your feet to rest flat on the floor. Repeat three times, letting your breathing rhythm guide your movement (fig. 37).

Balance

This exercise can be done freestanding or with the left side of your body a foot away from the back of a chair or a wall. Your left hand can rest on the chair or wall. Find a focal point for your eyes and assume the Mountain Pose. While your feet remain firmly planted, be aware of lengthening your body up, as if it were rebounding out of the pressure of your feet on the floor. Shift your weight to your left foot. Pick up your right foot and place your right toes on the toes of your left foot. If you feel steady bring your palms together in front of your chest in prayer position or draw them over your head. Breathe comfortably as you balance securely on the left foot, focusing your thoughts and sight on your focal point.

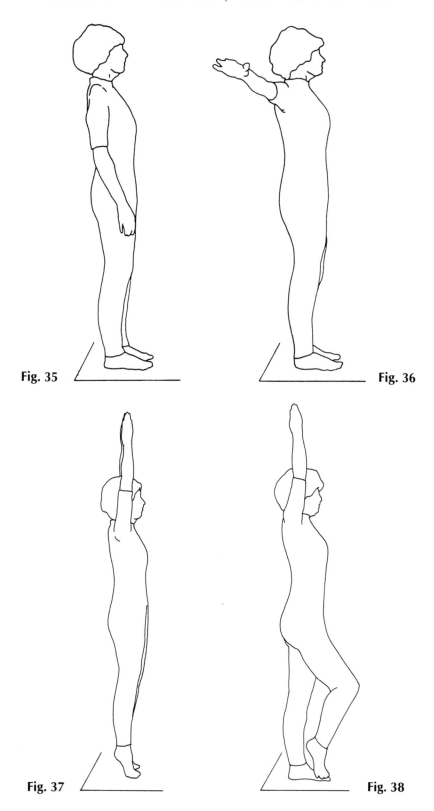

Fig. 35

Fig. 36

Fig. 37

Fig. 38

After holding the pose steadily and comfortably initially for about thirty seconds, return to the Mountain Pose (fig. 38).

Repeat on the other side after turning so that the wall or chair is on your right side.

Deep Relaxation

Remember to assume the Deep Relaxation Pose (fig. 17) at the end of your stretching/relaxation-exercise session. Let your body relax completely into the support of the floor. This can be done in a chair if it is more comfortable. Simply focus on your breath or a sense of inner quiet.

If you prefer, you can mentally guide your relaxation. You might begin the session of deep relaxation with several yawns, then consciously release the tension around your eyes, imagining space around your eyes and cheekbones, resting your eyes in their sockets and relaxing your mouth into a gentle smile, an inner smile.

Continue the deep relaxation by systematically becoming conscious of different parts of your body, either by tensing and then releasing them or by gently shifting your awareness from point to point in your body. Be present to your experience of your body, moment by moment.

Let your body become your teacher. Develop a muscle memory of relaxation so that in time, even the thought of relaxing a body part can induce the sense of relaxation. Finally, notice your experience of your self when your body is relaxed and your mind is calm.

When it is time to shift your awareness gradually back to the room, bring along that inner sense of calm awareness and the understanding that you can return to that state throughout the day with a deep, relaxing breath.

Margaret Flood Ennis, M.A.

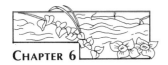
YOGA/BODY AWARENESS

The following resource tapes are available through the Mind/Body Medical Institute. If you would like to purchase one of the tapes, please send a written request to The Mind/Body Medical Institute, New England Deaconess Hospital, 185 Pilgrim Road, Boston, Mass. 02215. Each tape is $10; please make checks payable to the Mind/Body Medical Institute.

Tuning In to Your Body, Tuning Up Your Mind (female voice)

This tape guides you through the yoga stretching exercises that appear in the text. It is designed to be used in conjunction with the illustrations and incorporates detailed instructions for each exercise.

Side 1 (30 minutes)
Side 1 guides you through the chair and standing exercises. The exercises emphasize releasing physical tension, loosening the joints, and realigning posture. The practice session encourages elicitation of the relaxation response through mindfulness.

Side 2 (30 minutes)
Side 2 offers instruction in the workbook exercises that are done on the floor. It includes special instruction in diaphragmatic breathing and three-part breathing and gives guidance for using your breath to enhance your exercise practice. This side ends with an experience of deep relaxation.

Basic Yoga Stretching Exercise Tape (female voice)

Side 1 (20 minutes)
Side 1 encourages you to focus on energizing your body. You are guided through a series of gentle stretches and relaxation exercises to reinforce diaphragmatic breathing. The moderate pace allows you ample time to participate in the activities to enhance your relaxation response experience. Side 1 ends in an exercise to elicit the relaxation response.

Side 2 (20 minutes)
Side 2 encourages you to follow along in a gentle, slow-paced routine of stretching and movement awareness. Its purpose is to decrease muscular tension and elicit the relaxation response.

HATHA YOGA
HEALTH COMMITMENT

Long-Term Goal: _____

_____ Signature

_____

Expected Date of Reaching Goal: _____ _____ Witness

Short-Term Goals	Comments (supports, rewards, etc.)

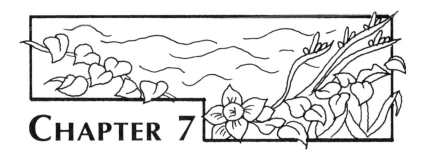

CHAPTER 7

MOVE INTO HEALTH

Those who think they have not time for bodily exercise
will sooner or later have to find time for illness.

Edward Stanley, 15th Earl of Derby

In this chapter you will explore

- the benefits of exercise and an active lifestyle
- motivating yourself to incorporate physical activity into your daily life
- guidelines for a successful exercise program
- how to exercise safely
- using aerobic exercise to elicit the relaxation response

THE SIMPLE TRUTH

This chapter provides guidelines for healthy people to promote health and prevent disease by incorporating physical activity into their lifestyle. The importance of exercise has been recognized for centuries. Numerous studies over the past twenty years confirm that physical activity has a positive effect on longevity and mortality, and lack of physical activity is associated with an increased risk of disease and disability. Much of this information has been gathered from studying the activity levels of various populations, such as London transport workers and British civil servants, San Francisco longshoremen and Harvard alumni. The Framingham Heart Study, which included a broad spectrum of people, was instrumental in linking a sedentary lifestyle to an increased risk of cardiovascular diseases such as heart attacks, strokes, and high blood pressure.

The long list of disorders linked to a sedentary lifestyle includes other cardiovascular diseases, obesity, osteoporosis (brittle bones), and back problems. A sedentary lifestyle is also associated with the inability to cope effectively with stress, increased risk of depression, decreased work productivity, and increased absenteeism from work. Generally speaking, people who exercise regularly, or who naturally include physical activity in their daily routine, feel better mentally and physically, and positively influence the quality and length of their lives.

The problem is that modern, mechanized lifestyles have become too sedentary for our physiology, which evolved to prepare us for physical exertion. Until recently, our daily survival depended on a fair degree of physical fitness. Today, however, you need not be physically fit to drive a car, ride an elevator, hire someone to cut the grass or rake the leaves, or go to the supermarket to forage for dinner. And most people who don't exercise have many excuses that overpower their intent and motivation. You may be familiar with these:

- don't have time
- don't like discomfort
- don't like to sweat
- look ugly in shorts
- I'll do it tomorrow
- the weather's bad
- it's too much like work
- it's boring

Take a Moment To . . .

List any excuses you regularly use not to exercise. Choose from the above examples, or include any "special excuses" of your own!

_____

_____

_____

_____

_____

People also shy away from exercise because of certain basic misconceptions:

- makes you tired
- takes too much time to make a difference
- no pain, no gain
- have to be athletic
- the older you are, the less exercise you need
- all types of exercise result in the same benefit

Take a Moment To . . .

Do you believe any of these misconceptions? If so, list them and the reasons why you think they are valid.

_____

_____

_____

_____

_____

We will address all of these issues throughout this chapter and expect to diffuse, if not eliminate, your excuses and misconceptions.

The bottom line is that you need to exercise everyday to stay healthy. A simple way to begin is to increase the number of healthy activities in your daily routine. For example you could

- play active games with your children
- walk or bicycle to work
- park your car at the back of the parking lot and walk to your building
- climb stairs instead of riding the elevator
- tend your vegetable or flower garden
- cut your grass (and not on a riding mower!)
- houseclean
- walk to do errands

By changing your daily routine in these ways, you not only get some valuable physical conditioning, but you could gain quality time with your family, eat fresh vegetables, save money by not hiring help, and make work seem more like play. With this little extra effort the rewards can be tremendous.

Sam's experience:

Sam used to hate to mow the lawn. It was boring and took too much time away from other activities. As he began to realize that even regular daily activities provided health benefits, his attitude toward mowing the lawn changed.

He did not come to enjoy it, but instead, he began to appreciate the physical exertion of pushing the lawn mower and seeing the finished product of a freshly cut lawn. Further, he knew that he was combining healthy exercise with completing a necessary task.

When visiting his parents during the summer, he even offered to mow *their* lawn. However, his dad likes to keep active, and knows that he can enhance his health and independence with regular exercise. So he continues to mow his own lawn, and when Sam comes to visit, they work on other projects around the house that they can do together.

Take a Moment To . . .

List the healthy activities you could add to your daily life. Choose two, and over the next week make a committed effort to do them.

_____

_____

_____

_____

_____

Exercising regularly can help you embrace a more active lifestyle as you begin to feel better, physically and emotionally. The good news is that your regular, scheduled exercise need only be of "moderate intensity." For example, a brisk walk of thirty-to-sixty minutes three-to-five times a week is a level of exercise attainable by most adults and sufficient to produce the fitness standard that promotes health and decreases risk of disease. "No pain, no gain" is not really the best approach, because "pain" carries with it the potential for actual injury; if you experience pain or extreme discomfort, you are exercising too hard. Health-promoting gains come with moderation, enjoyment, and consistency.

Thus, inactivity puts you at risk for disease, while physical activity can serve as an essential protective mechanism for health. An active lifestyle, however, involves more than simply pedaling a stationary bicycle for thirty minutes, three times a week. An active lifestyle means incorporating a variety of activities into your daily schedule that ultimately extend your capacity for handling the rigors of daily life.

A complete approach to physical fitness includes activities and exercises that improve endurance, strength, and flexibility, as well as body awareness. Using this approach, you can increase your ability to work for longer periods of time without undue fatigue, and with less muscular stress and strain, and also develop an awareness of activity-tolerance that helps prevent potential injury.

By developing an active lifestyle that includes a variety of activities, you can

- strengthen your cardiovascular system
- improve your cholesterol profile
- lower blood pressure
- control blood sugar
- lose weight or maintain your desired weight
- curb insomnia
- facilitate digestion
- delay the disabling effects of arthritis
- increase bone density to help prevent osteoporosis
- improve strength and flexibility

At the same time, medical research indicates that regular exercise leads to many significant psychological changes, such as lessening anxiety, tension, and fatigue; relieving depression; and increasing vigor and self-esteem. Exercise can also help relieve some negative effects of everyday stress, acting as a buffer against stress-related illness, and reaffirming that an active lifestyle is a healthy one. In short, increasing your physical activity is almost guaranteed to make you feel better, look better, and do better.

Looking better

Improved appearance is probably one of the greatest rewards and pleasant side effects of an exercise program. Your body is gradually reshaped as you tone muscle and burn fat. As you increase the percentage of lean body mass (muscle and bone) and decrease the percentage of body fat, your muscles elongate and strengthen while fatty bulges diminish. As you begin to notice and feel good about the changes, your friends' compliments will further enhance your self-esteem.

When trying to lose weight, you should be losing *fat* weight. Approximately 50 percent of American adults are overweight, or, more accurately, "over-fat." Most have failed to lose weight and keep it off. Most have not committed themselves to exercise in their weight-loss program. With exercise, you not only burn calories (and fat), but you also raise your metabolism for extended periods of time after exercising. This means you burn more calories (store less fat) than ever before with regular daily activities.

The best way to lose fat weight and keep it off is to combine nutritious eating with an exercise program that emphasizes prolonged duration, increased frequency, and moderate intensity. Add to this calisthenics and moderate weight training that tone major muscle groups and you will have an excellent formula for increasing your potential to burn calories and lose fat. The key to normalizing body fatness is long-term adherence and permanent lifestyle changes; it cannot be achieved by crash dieting or short-term, high-intensity exercise trials.

Susan's Experience

What finally brought Susan into the Hypertension Clinic was a cholesterol level over 300. She had high blood pressure (140/92) despite two medications, was one hundred pounds overweight, and was sedentary. Working as a librarian kept her inactive most of the day. At age forty, she knew she had to make some changes, but she needed a push. Prior to starting the program, Susan took an exercise-tolerance test, consisting of walking on a treadmill at increasing speeds and inclines. The results showed that although she had a low exercise capacity, her blood-pressure and heart-rate response to exercise were normal, and she could safely increase her exercise practice. In short, she was healthy but her fitness level was poor.

Through the clinic program she learned about nutrition, stress management, and how to elicit the relaxation response, but change was not easy, especially with exercise. She hated walking and used all her old excuses to support her noncompliance. But after learning that exercise combined with nutritious eating would help her lose weight, and after establishing her goals for the program with the clinic team, she decided to give it a try.

She started at a low level: walking twice a week at a slow pace for twenty minutes before breakfast or at lunch. Over time she came to enjoy walking (she missed it if she didn't do it), and she increased her program to forty-to-sixty minutes a day, at the same time increasing her walking pace until she was able to reach her exercise-heart-rate range of 130 to 140 beats per minute.

Through hard work—exercise, diet management, and behavioral change—Susan significantly improved her health profile: she lost over forty pounds, decreased her cholesterol sixty points, and decreased her blood pressure to 121/84 while reducing her blood pressure medication by half. She starts each day now with elicitation of the relaxation response, a healthy breakfast, and a brisk walk. Her goals are continued weight loss and eventual elimination of medication.

Use it or lose it

Aging is a self-fulfilling prophecy, and only you can decide the kind of person you'll become.

Walter Bortz, M.D., *Runners World*

While the aging process is something we all go through, we have unfortunately come to equate aging with physical and mental deterioration; however, this need not be the case. Interestingly enough, the biological changes attributed to aging closely resemble the effects of physical inactivity. Both lists include

- decreased cardiovascular fitness
- decreased muscle mass
- increased body fat
- decreased strength and flexibility
- decreased bone mass
- decreased metabolic rate
- poor sleep habits
- decreased sexual performance
- decreased mental performance

The human body depends on utilizing oxygen for the production of energy. The body's ability to transport oxygen efficiently improves with physical training, whether you are young or old, and normally decreases with age. However, studies have shown that a fit seventy-year-old has the same capacity to transport and utilize oxygen as an unfit thirty-year-old, which suggests that the decrease in oxygen may be less a function of age than of inactivity.

Other studies have demonstrated the benefits of keeping active throughout your lifetime. Senior citizens who remain physically active are less likely to develop osteoporosis and suffer fractures of the spine or hip. In addition, the natural decline of strength and flexibility is slowed with regular physical activity. Fire fighters participating in a fitness program that included time to exercise at work demonstrated a much slower decline in strength and flexibility, as well as a reversal in the decline of exercise capacity normally seen with aging. The lesson? Start exercising now and keep going; don't wait until retirement to develop good exercise habits and you will enjoy a healthier and happier life. A timeless adage advises that old age is the price you pay for the way you live your life.

AEROBIC AND ANAEROBIC EXERCISE

Now that you are familiar with some of the benefits of regular physical activity, the next step is to plan a realistic and attainable exercise program. There are two basic types of exercise: aerobic (requires oxygen) and anaerobic (does not require oxygen). Aerobic exercise (e.g., jogging) elevates the heart rate through sustained activity of moderate intensity. Anaerobic exercise (e.g., push-ups) is quick or of very high intensity. Both offer significant health benefits, but compare the differences in the chart on page 110.

The key differences between these two types of exercise are (1) fuel source and (2) intensity and duration. Any exercise that lasts only a short period of time or is of very high intensity is anaerobic and burns mostly glucose (sugar) stored in your muscles and liver. The initial burst of activity that begins all exercise is anaerobic. As exercise increases in duration and becomes moderate in intensity, aerobic metabolism dominates and a greater percentage of the fuel used comes from fat (fat being what you most want to lose for weight loss).

Two Types of Exercise	
Aerobic	*Anaerobic*
• Large groups of muscles work in rhythmic motion for an extended period of time • Uses oxygen as muscles burn a greater percent of fat for fuel • Many benefits for the cardio-respiratory system • Improves muscle efficiency and tone • Helps lose fat weight • Slow and steady increase in blood pressure and heart rate	• Short burst of activity • Burns mostly muscle glycogen and glucose (sugar) for fuel • Minimal conditioning benefits for the cardiorespiratory system • Improves muscle strength and speed of activity • Ineffective for fat loss, but builds muscle tissue • Disproportionate rise in blood pressure and heart rate

Most forms of exercise are some combination of aerobic and anaerobic. Circuit training—circulating among different exercise machines and stations (i.e., Nautilus) doing high-frequency repetitions against low-resistance weights—is a good example of exercise with both aerobic and anaerobic components. Sports such as tennis, basketball, and racquetball are also examples of activities with both aerobic and anaerobic components. Marathon running is a good example of exercise that is close to 100 percent aerobic, and running the hundred-yard dash is close to 100 percent anaerobic. The following are some good choices for each kind of exercise:

Common Exercise Choices	
Aerobic	*Anaerobic*
walking, jogging, rowing, swimming, biking, aerobics, cross-country skiing	weight lifting, sprinting (running or swimming), calisthenics (push-ups, sit-ups, and pull-ups)

A well-balanced exercise program—cross training—involves doing various types of exercise throughout the week. For example, during one week you could bicycle twice, swim once, and do calisthenics followed by a brisk walk. You may want to add in a game of tennis or go for a hike with friends. A cross-training program increases total body fitness, decreases risk of injury from exercise, and improves long-term compliance by alleviating boredom and maintaining challenge. (Cross-training is different from circuit training. Circuit training is a particular type of exercise that allows you to exercise different muscle groups in the same way, thus increasing overall muscle strength and endurance. You can use circuit training as part of your cross-training experience.)

The key to aerobic exercise is raising your heart rate to a calculated target level and keeping it there with moderate exertion. It does not mean exercising as hard as possible for as long as possible, nor does it mean hours of time. Twenty minutes a day, three days a week, at a comfortable pace is the minimum you need to do, and it is a good place to start.

Aerobic exercise brings cardiovascular benefits that decrease your risk of heart disease, such as lowering cholesterol and high blood pressure, losing fat, and increasing circulation to your heart and exercising muscles. Anaerobic exercise improves and maintains strength, flexibility, and speed, but by itself it cannot produce the desired cardiovascular benefits. Exercise specialists recommend that for a complete approach to fitness, 70-to-80 percent of your total exercise time be devoted to aerobic fitness, with the remaining 20-to-30 percent spent on anaerobic exercise.

Take a Moment To . . .

List the types of exercise that interest you. Work up a weekly schedule that balances aerobic and anaerobic activities.

_____

_____

_____

_____

_____

YOUR EXERCISE HEART RATE AND PERCEIVED EXERTION

Your intensity of exercise is monitored by two key parameters: heart rate and perceived exertion. If you are healthy, with no history of cardiovascular disease or other medical illness, and have no physical disability such as a bad back or knee problems, you can use these parameters to gauge your own exercise. However, if you have known cardiovascular disease or musculoskeletal problems, consult your physician or exercise specialist before developing an exercise program. Heart rate is an objective measure: perceived exertion is subjective. A comfortable, moderate intensity level balances the two.

Your maximal exercise capacity is the most exercise you can do before fatigue makes you stop. The heart rate you obtain with a maximal exercise effort is your maximal heart rate. A generic formula allows us to calculate this rate without an exercise test. The formula is:

$$220 - \text{your age} = \text{maximal heart rate}$$

Remember, however, your exercise should not be at maximal effort. As mentioned earlier, exercise intensity need only be moderate to achieve the health-related benefits of cardiovascular conditioning and weight loss. The general recommendation is that aerobic exercise should be between 60-to-85 percent of your maximum exercise capacity. A good place to start for most healthy people is 50-to-75 percent; the best for fat loss is 50-to-70 percent. The higher end of the range (75-to-85 percent) should be reserved for a training goal; for example, to improve your racing time. An intensity level beyond 85 percent tends to be counterproductive and is more anaerobic than aerobic.

Assuming you are healthy, you would use the following formula to determine your desired exercise heart rate:

$$[(220 - \text{age}) - \text{resting heart rate}] \times \% +$$
$$\text{resting heart rate} = \text{exercise heart rate}$$

Heart rate is also called *pulse.* To determine your resting heart rate (or resting pulse), count the pulse beats at your wrist or neck while sitting quietly for fifteen seconds and multiply the number you get by 4. This will give you beats per minute. Example: Your fifteen-second count is 20. [20 × 4 = 80.] Your resting heart rate is therefore 80 beats per minute.

Example: You are 40 years old, and your resting heart rate is 60 beats per minute; you want to exercise between 60 and 75 percent of your maximal capacity.

The computations are:

a) Subtract age (40) from 220.

$$220 - \text{age} = \text{maximal heart rate}$$
$$220 - 40 = 180$$

b) Subtract resting heart rate from maximal heart rate.

$$180 - 60 = 120$$

c) Multiply 120 times both 60% (.60) and 75% (.75).

$$120 \times .60 = 72$$
$$120 \times .75 = 90$$

d) Now add your resting heart rate to each of the numbers computed in Step c.

$$72 + 60 = 132$$
$$90 + 60 = 150$$

Based on these calculations, your exercise heart rate would range between 132 to 150 beats per minute. When exercising, stop and count your pulse for 15 seconds; multiply that number by 4. If the number you calculate falls between 132 and 150, then you are in your exercise-heart-rate range. For example, your pulse, counted for 15 seconds while exercising, is 35 beats; $35 \times 4 = 140$ beats per minute. You are in your target and exercising at a good intensity.

Take a Moment To . . .

Using the formula above, calculate *your* exercise heart rate range.

a) Subtract your age from 220. This is your age-predicted maximal heart rate (or MHR).

$$220 - \underline{\hspace{2cm}}_{\text{age}} = \underline{\hspace{2cm}}_{\text{MHR}}$$

b) Subtract your resting heart rate (RHR) from your maximal heart rate (or MHR), calculated in Step a.

$$\underline{\hspace{2cm}}_{\text{MHR}} - \underline{\hspace{2cm}}_{\text{RHR}} = \underline{\hspace{2cm}}$$

c) Multiply the number you got in Step b by 60% (.60) and again by 75% (.75).

$$\underline{\hspace{2cm}}_{\text{Step b}} \times .60 = \underline{\hspace{2cm}} \text{ and } \underline{\hspace{2cm}}_{\text{Step b}} \times .75 = \underline{\hspace{2cm}}$$

d) Add your resting heart rate to each of the numbers computed in Step c, to obtain your exercise heart rate (EHR).

$$\underline{\hspace{2cm}}_{\text{Step c (.60)}} + \underline{\hspace{2cm}}_{\text{RHR}} = \underline{\hspace{2cm}}_{\text{EHR}}$$

$$\underline{\hspace{2cm}}_{\text{Step c (.75)}} + \underline{\hspace{2cm}}_{\text{RHR}} = \underline{\hspace{2cm}}_{\text{EHR}}$$

Your exercise heart rate range therefore is _____ to _____ .

This objective measure of your heart rate should be balanced with your subjective feelings of perceived exertion (how hard you feel you are working). Observe your body cues of breathing, arm or leg fatigue, and general fatigue. You should feel as though you are working at a moderate intensity.

What does a moderate intensity feel like?

- You should feel comfortable, with no sensation of pain or strain, and you should feel able to continue for a period of time without an immediate need to stop.
- You should notice some change in your breathing pattern. You should be able to carry on a conversation without breathlessness, but if you can sing, you are not working hard enough.

• You may experience arm or leg fatigue, but not at a painful level; you should feel no immediate need to stop.

The Borg Scale for rating perceived exertion (RPE) is useful for helping you judge your level of exertion while exercising. Developed by Dr. Gunnar Borg, a Swedish physiologist who studied the relationship between heart rate and patient reports of exertion, the scale correlates well with exercise heart rate and is therefore another valid method for establishing exercise intensity.

Borg Scale (RPE)	
6	
7	very, very light
8	
9	very light
10	
11	fairly light
12	
13	somewhat hard (moderate)
14	
15	hard
16	
17	very hard
18	
19	very, very hard
20	

Adapted from G. A. V. Borg, "Psychophysical Bases of Perceived Exertion," *Medicine and Science in Sports and Medicine* 14, no. 5 (1982): 377–81.

A rating of 12-13 (moderate) correlates very well with an exercise heart rate calculated at the 60-to-75 percent level we mentioned earlier. This is the intensity level you want. A perceived exertion rating of 12-13 during exercise indicates a sufficient intensity for both comfort and benefit.

Experience is the only way to become efficient at determining your comfort zone. Not reaching your exercise heart rate despite what you consider moderate activity is nothing to worry about. What is most important is your comfort and willingness to continue. Keeping your heart rate a little lower is better if it means you are able to keep going. Body awareness is an important component of judging your exertion level. Pay attention to how and what you feel, and adjust your exercise accordingly. Remember, the best gains come with moderation, enjoyment, consistency, and long-term compliance. If you allow yourself the luxury of a comfortable challenge, your chances of succeeding will be greater.

Take a Moment To . . .

List those body cues you should be aware of to exercise within a moderate, comfortable exercise intensity.

_____

_____

_____

HOW TO BEGIN

> Whenever I feel like exercise, I lie down until the feeling passes.
> Ascribed to Robert M. Hutchins by J. P. McEvoy
> in "Young Men Looking Backward,"
> *American Mercury*, December 1938

Despite all the health benefits associated with regular physical exercise, many people find it a difficult habit to establish and maintain. Recent estimates indicate that 50 percent of American adults get no regular physical exercise, and of those who begin an exercise program, 50 percent will discontinue it within the first six months.

How many times has someone you know started an exercise program, joined a health club, or started jogging? How often did this new activity last only a week or two? On the other hand, how many people do you know who exercise regularly and have been doing so for years? What's the difference? The answer is simply *motivation.*

To make the change to an active lifestyle, first determine your primary motivation. What need causes you to be willing to exert the effort necessary to make this change? The motivating desire can be negative or positive. It can change as your needs change. And it can be different from that of anyone else you know.

A negative motivation may help you get started, but its influence is usually short-lived. Change to a positive motivation as soon as possible; it is more likely to lead to long-term compliance.

Negative Motivation	Positive Motivation
My father died of a heart attack; I will exercise so that does not happen to me.	I like the way exercise makes me feel, and it improves my health.

Your motivation may change as your needs change. Recognizing this change may help you remain compliant.

Initial Motivation	Ongoing Motivation
I want to lose weight and change my body shape.	I feel so much better with less weight, and I have more energy.

The most successful motivation comes from an inner desire. It is unique to you; it is something you do for yourself and not for anyone else. What works for you may not work for others.

Your Motivation	A Friend's Motivation
With my schedule, exercising at the club is the only time I have to socialize.	With my family demands, exercise provides the only time I have to myself.

Building in positive influences helps to bring about change and keep you motivated. Some suggestions are:

Replace old beliefs with new, positive ones: Instead of saying "I don't have time to exercise," say "Exercise boosts my energy level, so I get more done and have more free time."

Keep the momentum going: When you don't feel like your usual workout, try something at a lower level instead of skipping it altogether. One popular trade-off is instead of running before work, leaving home a little earlier and walking a longer route to work while listening to a favorite cassette.

Keep yourself interested: Alternate exercising alone with exercising with friends. Use after-workout rewards—go out with friends for a low-fat frozen yogurt, enjoy a fruit smoothie, treat yourself to a massage or fifteen minutes in the whirlpool. Use variety—cross training is fun, challenging, and boredom-resistant. Instead of doing a "workout," do a "playout"—don't just sit on that stationary bike, join a friend for a fun ride through the park.

Affirm your right to be happy and healthy: Eliciting the relaxation response and then using visualization helps with motivation. "Seeing" yourself exercise helps to get the momentum going. Affirmations—positive statements that express a feeling of self-worth—work wonderfully, especially when practiced immediately after eliciting the relaxation response and spoken in front of a mirror *with your eyes open.* Examples of affirmations are "Exercise helps me feel good"; "I love to walk"; "I can lose this weight"; "My health is worth this extra effort."

Don't be too hard on yourself: Nobody's perfect. If you slack off your regular program—and we all do!—don't punish yourself. Instead, reexamine your basic motivations and goals, put on your neon spandex or old, favorite, ragged sweat clothes, and just get back on the exercise trail.

Take a Moment To . . .

Think about why you want to begin, or continue, an exercise program. What is your major motivation for wanting to live a healthy, active lifestyle? Stand in front of a mirror with your eyes open and repeat your motivation out loud to yourself several times.

Some other helpful hints that may help you reach your goal of an active lifestyle are:

Pick an activity you like: Aerobic exercise tends to be repetitious, which is why it works, but also why it can be boring. What works for some people is torture for others. Many people bored by running have fun on a rowing machine. Some people enjoy changing their exercise with the seasons. For example, they bicycle in the summer and cross-country ski in the winter. Variety really is the spice of life. Having several options to choose from during the week relieves boredom, provides different exercise benefits, and can satisfy both a "workout challenge" and a "playful mind-set."

Warm-up, stre-e-e-etch, and cool-down: For everyone—but especially for those with muscular tightness or heart disease risks (see Chapter 22, "Heart Disease and Diabetes: Exercise Is for You, Too"), warm-up and cool-down are essential components of your exercise program, not merely options. Both your cardiovascular and musculoskeletal systems will benefit. Your warm-up is a good time to listen carefully to your body to determine how you feel. Be aware of areas of muscle tightness and general energy level to help you prepare for exercise and to modify the goals for that particular session. If specific body areas feel tight, spend extra time stretching them out. Tight hamstrings get injured easily and take a long time to heal. Tight back muscles allow greater freedom of movement when they have been slowly stretched to a more functional length. Always start your exercise slowly, and gradually increase the pace or intensity. Pedal your bike slowly for the first five or ten minutes, or walk several blocks briskly before starting your jog. This will also help loosen up tight muscles (some people prefer to stretch after a few minutes of slow-paced exercise) and help them stretch more easily. Heart muscle also enjoys the challenge of exercise, but it should not be subjected to sudden, extreme demands. The slow progression from easy to more extreme exercise will allow the heart and circulatory system to adjust to the new demands and do their jobs efficiently.

THE FAR SIDE   By GARY LARSON

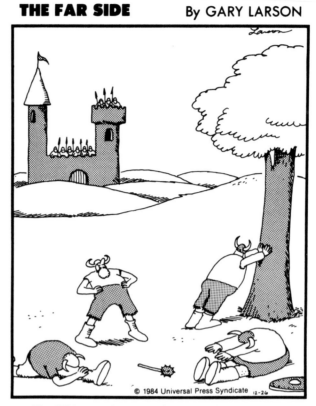

© 1984 Universal Press Syndicate 12-26

**The Vikings, of course, knew the importance
of stretching before an attack.**

THE FAR SIDE © 1984. Universal Press Syndicate.
Reprinted with permission.

Cooling down is just as important as warming up. Your body needs to slow down gradually to its resting level following the challenge of exercise. Stretch out exercise-induced muscle tightness and keep moving to allow your cardiovascular system to readjust. Five minutes of warm-up and five minutes of cool-down are a minimum.

Yoga is an excellent form of exercise to use during warm-up and cool-down. (See chapter 6, "Tuning In to Your Body, Tuning Up Your Mind," for yoga exercises.) Movement into and out of yoga postures provides the necessary stimulation of weight-bearing to help keep bones strong and the movement to stretch and tone muscles. Yoga involves not only movement, but also a mindfulness and awareness of how it feels to move. The yoga philosophy encourages an appreciation of body sensations, slow stretch, and maintenance of proper postures, all of which help to prevent injury and promote health.

Start easily and avoid strain: If exercise is new to you, ease into your program gradually. Start at a low intensity and short duration, and monitor how you feel. As you become more confident and accommodate to the activity, gradually increase the intensity and duration until you reach a level that is

THE FAR SIDE   By GARY LARSON

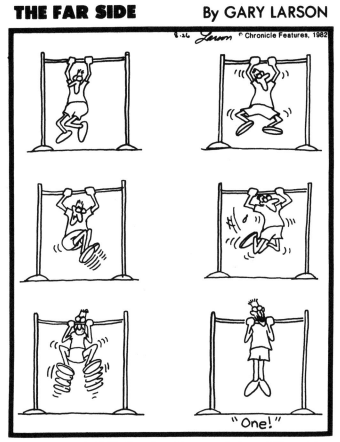

"One!"

beneficial and comfortable for you. Planning to take four to six weeks to achieve your target is quite acceptable. Everyone must start somewhere. So, even if you think you cannot do enough to make a difference, at least get started. You will be surprised by how much you will improve over time. And just as you would not push into your program too fast, sprinting the last hundred meters of a jog is also unnecessary. The key to aerobic fitness is moderation, not strain. Go slowly and set reasonable goals. The goal is to improve your health, not become a track star.

Monitor your inner and outer environment: If you are not feeling well, decrease your exercise effort or skip the session altogether. When you have an infection, a cold, or the flu, your body is being stressed; overexertion will only increase that stress and possibly slow the healing time. Adjust your exercise to accommodate how you feel. Slowly progress to your normal workout level as you begin to recover. Of course, if you are very ill, see your primary health-care provider, and do not resume exercise until you are better.

It is also important to be aware of the environment in which you exercise. Extremes of heat and cold affect performance as your body adjusts to the different temperatures. Air temperature and humidity affect muscle flexibility and the ability to perspire and regulate body temperature. As you warm up, pay close attention to how you feel, wear proper clothing (see below), and adjust the intensity and duration of your exercise session accordingly. Changing the time of day you exercise, adjusting fluid intake, and varying the length of your warm-up and cool-down will help you adjust to changes in the environment and make your exercise more successful.

What to wear: Appropriate clothing can enhance your comfort and help to reduce the risk of injury.

a. *Wear proper foot gear.* Although an all-around shoe with proper support can be adequate, different activities require your foot be supported in different ways. Therefore, when possible, we suggest you wear: jogging shoes for jogging, walking shoes for walking, court shoes for tennis and racquetball. If jogging is your choice, get expert advice on the shoe best suited to your foot structure; e.g., rigid foot (high arch) vs. floppy foot (flat arch). If foot problems have required medical attention in the past, discuss your exercise plans with the appropriate health-care provider.

b. *Wear white socks* to reduce the chance of infections if openings in the skin, such as blisters, abrasions, and pressure points, occur. (The dye from colored socks may leach out with perspiration and seep into openings in the skin.) This is especially important if you are prone to infection due to poor circulation or compromised immune function.

c. *Dress for the weather.* When it is cold, wear several layers of light clothing that can be removed as your body warms. Cotton tends to soak up sweat, which during winter weather can leave you damp and cold, so wear a synthetic material close to the skin. A windbreaker is a good protective outer shell. Wear a hat to reduce loss of body heat through your head. Protect your hands with mittens, old socks, or gloves. Wool socks work well to keep your toes warm. In warmer weather wear a minimum of light, loose-fitting cotton or nylon to enhance air circulation and help the cooling process.

Work out with a friend: As we all know, motivation to exercise can be a problem. One approach to keep you at it is to work out with a friend or group. When one of you wants to roll over and go back to sleep, the other is outside in walking gear throwing pebbles at your window. Exercising with a group provides friendly competition and encouragement to keep yourself moving. So pick a friend who is at a comparable exercise level, or join a group at your local health club and begin to move into health.

EXERCISE AND THE RELAXATION RESPONSE

The relaxation response can be incorporated into your daily exercise pattern. Activities such as jogging, swimming, walking, and bicycling involve rhythmic, repetitive motion and lend themselves well to achieving a focused, passive frame of mind. Once you are comfortable with all aspects of your exercise program, become aware of your breathing and allow it to complement the rhythm of your exercise. Keep your eyes open. Repeat your focus word, phrase, or prayer as you move in time with your breath. Maintain a passive attitude; when you become aware of disruptive thoughts, gently disregard them and slip back into the rhythm of movement, breath, and focus.

Take the example of walking, an activity that lends itself well to eliciting the relaxation response because it involves rhythmic, repetitive motion at a self-paced comfort level. And walking can be done mindfully, with conscious awareness of your safety. You will find yourself more aware of the smell of freshly cut grass, the warmth of the sun, the sight of birds and butterflies, and the gentle flow of thoughts. Of course, not everyone experiences this quieting when walking, and not every walking experience will be the same; but the potential for the experience is there.

An Army chaplain related to us that while jogging, he would repeat a prayer in cadence with his breathing. He felt marvelous, because in true American fashion he was able to complete his prayers, exercise, and elicit the relaxation response all at the same time! Not that we recommend this polyphasic activity for everyone, but it worked for him.

BEFORE EMBARKING ON A PROGRAM

Before beginning a new exercise program, make sure you are healthy enough to handle the challenge. If you are under forty-five years of age, with no known health problems, you can probably begin an exercise program without prior exercise testing, although in all cases *discuss your exercise plans with your primary health-care provider.* As mentioned earlier, begin slowly and progress gradually, staying alert for any signs or symptoms of intolerance. For those over forty-five or who have specific health problems, a maximal-exercise test is recommended. If you have any musculoskeletal problems, such as back, leg, or foot problems, obtain a thorough workup of the problem before beginning your exercise program.

In addition, if you have any of the cardiovascular risk factors or any known metabolic, cardiovascular, or pulmonary disease, it is recommended you have a complete workup, including an exercise test prior to beginning a new exercise program. The exercise test is done for diagnostic purposes as well as to measure exercise capacity. This information is used to develop an individualized exercise prescription. The initial stages of the exercise program should be monitored by the appropriate health-care professionals. (Chapter 22 specifically discusses exercise in relation to heart disease and diabetes.)

NOW, PUT YOUR BEST FOOT FORWARD

The next step is to begin your regular exercise program. Your parameters should include:

F (Frequency):   Three to five times a week of aerobic exercise
                     Two times a week of muscle toning
I (Intensity):   Moderate, by heart rate and perceived exertion
                     Able to complete each toning exercise eight to twelve
                        repetitions
T (Time):   Twenty to sixty minutes, plus warm-up and cool-down
                     Fifteen to twenty minutes to complete a series of eight
                        to ten muscle toning exercises
T (Type):   *Aerobic* (i.e., walking, bicycling, swimming)
                     Muscle toning (i.e., weight machines, free weights,
                        calisthenics)

It all adds up to *FITT* with two *t*'s, which is what you need to be to live the best you can for as long as you can. With these guidelines in mind, you can establish an exercise prescription specific to your needs. However, not only does the prescription need to be suitable, but also your commitment must be firm. It is important to increase activity on a long-term basis; exercise in the short-term is of little overall benefit. To facilitate long-term compliance, you need to be motivated enough to start, enjoy the activity enough to continue, and appreciate the value of exercise enough to start again if you stop.

For those who have never been physically active, deciding to begin an exercise program and committing to it can be particularly difficult. But time and time again, we have witnessed people making such changes: people who hated the idea of exercise, but who slowly came to appreciate the benefits of an active lifestyle. It is gratifying to watch people begin to incorporate exercise into their lives and a pleasure to witness their pledge for a healthier, happier life.

This summary of guidelines will help you maintain a successful exercise program:

1. Choose an activity that is enjoyable; consider cross-training.
2. Adopt a program that is realistic.
3. Consider convenience and affordability.
4. Consider an exercise buddy or group for motivation.
5. Establish a reward system; acknowledge your accomplishment when you achieve one of your goals.
6. If you feel pain, you are working too hard.
7. If you get hurt, stop until you have healed.

8. Fit exercise into your daily schedule; make an appointment with yourself in your schedule book.
9. Find ways to increase physical activity throughout everyday life.
10. Just do it: *You're worth it!*

James S. Huddleston, M.S., P.T.

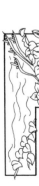

SAMPLE
EXERCISE
HEALTH COMMITMENT

Long-Term Goal:

To participate in an aerobic exercise program 3–5 times per week

_____
Signature

_____
_____
Witness

Expected Date of Reaching Goal: 4 months from now

Readiness to Change	Short-Term Goals	Comments (supports, rewards, etc.)
Never considered change; need information.	1. Attend a lecture on exercise. 2. Explore literature for the layperson on exercise.	
Considered change; but not yet committed.	1. List reasons why exercise is important to you. 2. List reasons why you have not started an exercise program in the past.	
Desire change; need motivation and information.	1. Choose a form of exercise that is fun and enjoyable. 2. Before going to bed, affirm that you will exercise the next day.	

(continued)

Readiness to Change	Short-Term Goals	Comments (supports, rewards, etc.)
Attempting change; need structure, support, and skills.	1. Determine a convenient place and time to exercise three to five times per week. Put it in your appointment book or on your calendar. 2. Exercise initially with someone who is familiar with the principles of exercise so they can provide feedback as you learn about your body's response.	
Change made; need reinforcement.	1. Engage in regular exercise with a friend or group. 2. Participate in a fun run or a walk for a cause, feeling good that you can do it.	
Change made; slipping back into bad habits, need renewed motivation and support.	1. Discuss exercise program with an exercise specialist or your physician. 2. List reasons why you have stopped exercising.	

125

EXERCISE

HEALTH COMMITMENT

Long-Term Goal:

_____

_____
Signature

_____

_____
Witness

Expected Date of Reaching Goal: _____

Short-Term Goals	Comments (supports, rewards, etc.)

Part 3

NUTRITION

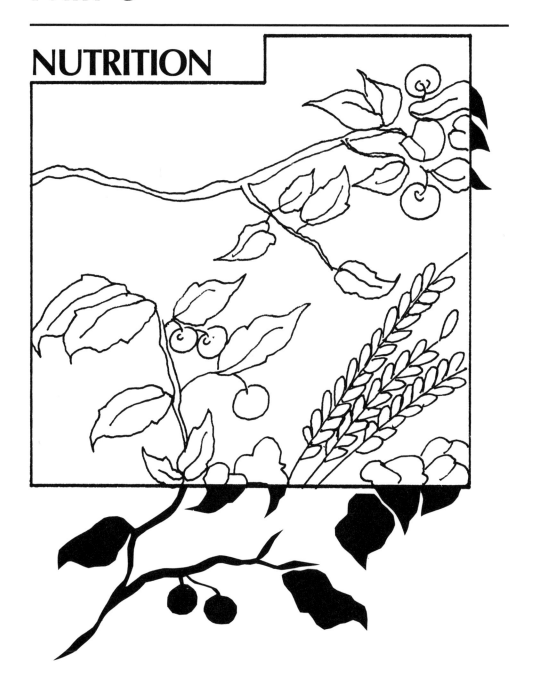

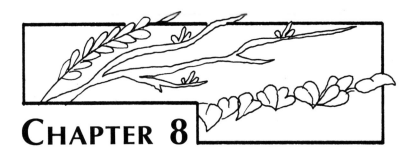

CHAPTER 8

NUTRITION FOR GOOD HEALTH

> There is no love sincerer than the love of food.
> George Bernard Shaw, *Man and Superman*

In this chapter you will explore

- how dietary excesses contribute to major health problems in our society
- specific measures to make your diet more healthful
- sources of caffeine, and a sensible daily limit
- how to evaluate a food label
- behavioral strategies to improve your diet

People today probably have more information about what is "good" for them than ever before. In the past decade, Americans have been deluged with newspaper stories, magazine articles, and books on the subject of nutrition. Every month there seems to be a new best-seller touting a new revolutionary diet plan, and many health organizations publish nutritional guidelines. Yet one of the major health problems in the United States is obesity, and the primary cause of death—heart disease—could be greatly reduced if Americans followed simple nutritional guidelines. In our clinical programs, we emphasize that eating right and exercising are fundamental to keeping healthy people healthy, as well as helping to improve and prevent the progression of some chronic medical problems.

Eating right may necessitate some very specific changes in your diet and may involve limiting certain types of food. Diet can be a difficult aspect of life to change. Food habits are deeply ingrained, and eating patterns are complex. In this chapter, we will look at some basic guidelines and explore some of the pitfalls of trying to choose a healthful diet.

NOURISHMENT

While some people live to eat and a very few eat to live, most of us view food in complex ways that involve much more than simple nutrient intake. Food choices and amounts consumed are strongly influenced by such varied factors as social setting and occasion, by emotions as different as elation and grief, by pleasurable sensations and tastes, individual likes and dislikes, and by cultural heritage and the customs we have grown up with.

Eating is also often a way to cope with stress. Not surprisingly, when food is used in this way, the results carry over into nonfood aspects of our lives. For example, the person who routinely finds his day grueling and difficult, and comes home to a couch, a television, and a large bag of potato chips, is not merely overeating. He may also be skipping the exercise he once did regularly after work. Furthermore, the negative feelings generated by overeating and the sedentary lifestyle serve only to lower his self-esteem and increase his unhappiness. By examining such factors and changing other behaviors as you work through *The Wellness Book*, you can begin to make changes toward healthful eating.

Eating healthfully does not mean feeling deprived. Healthful and delicious foods are abundant; combining them in creative recipes and pleasing meals is also rewarding. See the list of recommended cookbooks at the end of the chapter.

Take a Moment To . . .

Think back over the past day. What meals and snacks did you eat? How did you eat them? Were you hungry? If not, why did you eat?

Richard's Experience

Richard, a thirty-five-year-old physician participating in the Behavioral Medicine Hypertension Program, examined his eating habits for the first time and concluded:

> When I gave any thought at all to what I ate, it was usually just to congratulate myself on how little I thought about food. It seemed that everyone around me was obsessed with food, reading labels, talking about recipes, looking for this ingredient or that . . . I rea-

soned that if I didn't waste time thinking about it, my diet must be fine. When I kept a food record for the Hypertension Program and actually examined what I was eating—lots of fast food, skipping meals; vegetables: what are *they*?—it struck me for the first time that it's essential to put some planning and thought into something so vital as what I eat. It's no longer an area of health that I ignore. I find I now enjoy thinking about what I'll eat, and I notice that when I eat well I feel more energetic.

Most of the time, people eat while doing, or at least thinking about, something else. Did you ever open the mail or talk on the telephone while eating? This habit of distraction contributes to poor nutritional choices and a lack of appreciation for food. As you develop an awareness of what you eat and why, and as you acquire new strategies for coping, you will be able to replace unconscious, poor eating habits with more effective and healthy coping techniques.

The components of food

Foods are composed of many individual nutrients, generally categorized as proteins, carbohydrates, fats, vitamins, and minerals.

Proteins are made up of chains of smaller units called amino acids. Some are broken down and metabolized, while others are rearranged by the body into new and different proteins. Proteins are used for the synthesis of enzymes, hormones, and muscle tissue.

Carbohydrates are broadly classified as simple and complex. Simple carbohydrates are sugars, while complex carbohydrates are made up of chains of sugars. Sucrose, or table sugar, is a simple carbohydrate, while the starch in a potato, rice, pasta, or bread is made up of chains of sugars and is therefore a complex carbohydrate.

Fats, which include both liquid oils and solid fats, are made up of glycerol molecules and fatty acids. Depending on the structure of their fatty acids, fats are classified as either saturated or unsaturated. As will be discussed later, it is the saturated fatty acids that tend to raise the serum (blood) cholesterol level.

Vitamins are food factors necessary in very small amounts for the normal functioning of many biochemical processes. They are essential in the diet because the body is either unable to make them or makes them only in insufficient amounts. Certain *minerals* are also essential in small amounts. Very large doses of vitamins and minerals can be dangerous and should be avoided.

Fiber, the indigestible portion of plant cell walls, is essential for normal gastrointestinal functioning.

The basic food groups

Some foods have higher concentrations of various nutrients than others, and foods are grouped by the major nutrients they provide. Individual foods are categorized into four basic groups: dairy, meat and meat substitutes, fruits and vegetables, and grains and grain products. The meat and meat substitute group, for example, is generally high in protein, while the grain group is high in complex carbohydrates.

Food and health

Until the 1940s, diseases caused by dietary deficiencies were common in the United States. A lack of vitamin D, for example, causes rickets, a malformation of long bones; niacin deficiency causes pellagra; iodine deficiency causes goiter formation; and a diet low in vitamin C results in scurvy. The reduced occurrence of these and other diseases of malnutrition is partially due to the practice of enriching and fortifying foods with essential nutrients (such as niacin, iron, vitamins D and A, and iodine). What has recently become clear, however, is that an *overabundance* of certain nutrients, particularly fat, saturated fat, and cholesterol, can result in illness, and therefore a proper balance of foods is extremely important.

The unhealthy American diet

The typical American diet is high in fat and sodium but low in fiber. Studies of large populations indicate that diets high in fat may influence the development of cardiovascular disease and certain cancers. A high-fat diet combined with physical inactivity favors the development of obesity, which is itself a risk factor for hypertension, degenerative joint disease, cardiovascular disease, and some cancers. Diets high in sodium may be involved in the development of high blood pressure. Diets low in fiber have been implicated in the development of colon cancer.

The American diet, and Western diets in general, are related to a fast-paced, high-stress lifestyle. Many of us rarely sit down for an extended, relaxed midday meal, but instead try to satisfy our hunger in a few minutes. The fast-food phenomenon is no accident—it suits our lifestyle. Fast food, unfortunately, is usually "fat food." A typical fast-food meal of a large burger and fries derives 40 percent or more of its calories from fat. These foods also tend to be very high in sodium and low in fiber.

GUIDELINES FOR HEALTHY EATING

Many health organizations publish guidelines on food choices. Among the best known of these recommendations is the *Dietary Guidelines for Americans*, first issued by the U.S. Department of Agriculture and the Department of Health and Human Services in 1980, and revised slightly every five years thereafter.

Dietary Guidelines

1. Eat a variety of foods.
2. Maintain healthy weight.
3. Choose a diet low in fat, saturated fat, and cholesterol.

4. Choose a diet with plenty of vegetables, fruits, and grain products.
5. Use sugars only in moderation.
6. Use salt and sodium only in moderation.
7. If you drink alcoholic beverages, do so in moderation.

These guidelines are intended for healthy people to promote health and prevent disease. Remember that guidelines are always general; you may need a diet higher or lower in specific nutrients. If you have an illness, particularly one affecting your ability to eat well-balanced meals and maintain your weight, consult with your doctor and, if needed, a registered dietitian. Healthy dietary changes need not be extreme. Your nutritional goals can be small, realistic steps that ultimately lead to variety and moderation in your food choices.

Here are some ideas to help you meet these guidelines:

Guideline 1. Eat a variety of foods

What would be wrong with limiting your diet to a very small number of nutritious foods? First of all, eating the same foods day after day would become monotonous. More importantly, your body needs a large number—over forty—of different nutrients to stay healthy. No small group of foods can provide all of them. Variety is the best way to ensure getting every nutrient your body needs. Furthermore, a diversified diet also helps minimize the risk of toxicities from too much of certain foods.

Use the four basic food groups as a tool to evaluate your diet. By regularly choosing several different items from each group, you will probably eat a well-balanced diet.

Milk group

Dairy products include cheese, yogurt, milk, and products made from milk such as puddings or milk-based soup. Dairy foods are a major source of calcium—the mineral especially important for women in preventing osteoporosis—and are also rich in protein, phosphorous, and riboflavin (vitamin B). You can avoid the butterfat prominent in regular dairy products by choosing nonfat and low-fat products.

Fruit and vegetable group

Fruits and vegetables are major sources of Vitamin C, beta-carotene (also called provitamin A because your body converts it to vitamin A), potassium, and fiber. Try to eat a good source of vitamin C as well as a food rich in beta-carotene at least once every day. See table on p. 134.

Grain group

This diverse category encompasses hot and cold cereals, bread, rice, noodles, and grains such as millet, barley, and oats. These foods are a major source of complex carbohydrates (starch), which should constitute a large portion of our calories. Grains also provide many vitamins and irons, and are an important source of fiber.

Good Sources of Vitamin C

Fruits: oranges, grapefruit, strawberries, tangerines, guava, cantaloupe, kiwifruit, papaya, honeydew melon, mangoes
Vegetables: tomatoes, broccoli, potatoes, brussels sprouts, cauliflower, peppers, collards, kale, chicory greens, kohlrabi

Good Sources of Beta-Carotene

Fruits: apricots, nectarines, papayas, mangoes, cantaloupe, mandarin oranges
Vegetables: spinach, parsley, beet greens, broccoli, sweet potatoes, Chinese cabbage, winter squash, pumpkin, collard greens, chicory greens, mustard greens, turnip greens, tomatoes, carrots, red peppers, kale

---

Meat group

Far more than meat is included here: poultry, fish, shellfish, eggs, nuts, peanut butter, legumes (dried beans and peas), and tofu are also included. These foods are important for their protein and many micronutrients such as iron and zinc.

Healthy adults should eat at least three servings of vegetables, two of fruit, and six of grain products every day. At least two choices should be made daily from both the milk and the meat groups. These are minimums—many people need more to derive enough energy to meet their daily activity needs. The recommended number of servings differ for children, adolescents, and pregnant or nursing women.

For most healthy adults, a well-balanced diet will provide adequate amounts of all needed nutrients; millions of Americans, however, commonly take daily vitamin and mineral supplements. While there is generally no harm in taking a multivitamin supplement, single vitamins and minerals in large doses (megadoses) can be harmful. In some cases, one can interfere with the absorption of another, and they can do damage to various organs, such as the liver. Megadose supplements are no substitute for a healthy diet, and should be avoided.

Guideline 2. Maintain healthy weight

What is a healthy body weight for you? Tables have been compiled that list weights for heights associated with the lowest mortality. Although these tables sometimes present unrealistic goals, they can be helpful. You may be well above your ideal body weight as defined by the height-tables; obesity is defined as being above ideal body weight by 20 percent or more. Even if you do not foresee a large weight loss, you can still set a realistic and reasonable weight-loss goal, perhaps aiming for a weight at which you felt comfortable in the past. If you need help in selecting a weight goal, ask your doctor or dietitian for assistance.

When trying to lose weight, remember these important points:

- *A slow, steady weight loss is best.* Losing one-half to one pound per week is ideal.
- *Do not crash-diet or skip meals.* Such practices provide insufficient essential nutrients. Also, this type of dieting may actually foil your attempts to lose weight, since not eating can lower the metabolic rate, causing you to conserve rather than burn energy (calories).
- *Keep your meals and snacks low in fat.* Fat has over twice as many calories per gram as either carbohydrates or protein; if you eat low-fat foods, you can still eat plentifully but keep the calories under control.
- *Alcohol is nearly as high in calories as fat.*
- *Regular aerobic exercise promotes weight loss.* Evidence is accumulating that people who lose weight and continue to exercise after reaching their target weight are more successful in maintaining their new weight than people who do not exercise. Regular aerobic activity not only burns calories, but it also increases your metabolic rate, causing your body to burn more calories even when at rest. (See chapter 7 on exercise.)
- *Examine behaviors that cause you to overeat.* Do you consistently eat the wrong foods out of habit? Do you use foods as your sole means of celebrating? Do you eat large amounts, without realizing it, while reading or watching television?

By considering these points you can start on your way toward reaching your healthy weight goal.

Guideline 3. Choose a diet low in fat, saturated fat, and cholesterol

Fat is abundant in

- fried foods (like fried chicken and doughnuts)
- rich foods (like super premium ice cream and pastries)
- greasy foods (like spare ribs and bacon)
- added fats and oils (butter, margarine, mayonnaise, oils)

Fat can be hidden, that is, buried where you neither see it nor expect to find so much of it—for example, muffins, hot dogs, and many crackers and sauces are very high in fat. To reduce the fat in your diet, choose simply prepared foods, without rich sauces and gravies. When adding fat or oil, use only a small amount (try thinking *teaspoon* instead of *tablespoon*). Instead of fried food, eat foods that are baked, broiled, steamed, poached, or grilled. Remember: one order of fast-food french fries has about twelve grams of fat; one baked potato (unadorned) has under one gram.

Reducing *saturated* fats is important because they in particular raise serum cholesterol. In fact, saturated fats are more of a culprit than dietary cholesterol.

The major sources of saturated fat in food are animal fats, butterfat (found in dairy products), tropical oils, and heavily hydrogenated oils. To reduce saturated fat, eat chicken and turkey without the skin and fish and shellfish more often than beef, lamb, and pork. Dairy products such as yogurt and cottage cheese are an excellent source of calcium; choose those made with skim milk and 1 percent milk fat instead of those made with cream or whole milk. Replace some of the butter in your diet with less saturated fats and oils such as margarine, mayonnaise, and olive and canola oils.

Avoid products containing large amounts of tropical oils, (coconut, palm and palm kernel oils, and cocoa butter). These oils are frequently used in prepared foods such as nondairy coffee lighteners, whipped toppings, cookies, and crackers.

In the hydrogenation process, liquid oils are made semisolid through the addition of hydrogen atoms. To avoid heavily hydrogenated oils, choose margarines in which the first ingredient is a liquid oil (the second ingredient can be a partially hydrogenated oil), and avoid using solid vegetable shortening.

Cholesterol is found only in animal products—never in a plant product. Foods notably high in cholesterol are egg yolks and organ meats, such as liver. Eat these in moderation.

Guideline 4. Choose a diet with plenty of vegetables, fruits, and grain products

Replace fatty foods with nutritious sources of starch and fiber, mainly grain products, legumes, fruits, and vegetables. To get fiber from grain products, choose whole grains, such as whole wheat or oatmeal breads; try brown rice instead of white. In these grains, the bran is left intact, so you get the vitamins, minerals, and fiber it contains. Breakfast cereal with bran is also an excellent source of daily fiber. Increase your fiber intake gradually, and be sure to include plenty of fluids. This will help avoid gastrointestinal discomfort, which can occur when fiber is suddenly increased.

The many types of fiber can all be classified as either water-soluble or insoluble. Insoluble fiber relieves and prevents certain gastrointestinal disorders, such as constipation and diverticular disease. This type of fiber may also play a role in preventing colon cancer. Wheat bran, whole-wheat flour, and products made from them are very good sources of insoluble fiber. Soluble fiber may help lower Low Density Lipoprotein (LDL) cholesterol—the "bad" cholesterol—which contributes to the formation of plaque in the coronary arteries. Soluble fiber can also slow down sugar absorption from the gastrointestinal tract into the bloodstream, a benefit for people with diabetes. Oats, oat bran, legumes, and many fruits and vegetables are excellent sources of water-soluble fiber. Both types are important and should be included in generous amounts in a healthy diet.

Guideline 5. Use sugars only in moderation

In addition to sucrose (table sugar), other common sugar sources include brown sugar, syrups, honey, jams, and jellies. Ice cream, cakes, cookies, and most other desserts are high in sugar. Many breakfast cereals, particularly those designed for children, are extremely sugary. Soft drinks are loaded with sugar—a twelve-ounce can of a regular cola has forty grams—this is ten teaspoons!

Sugar is by no means a poison, although it is often thought of as such. There are, however, a number of problems associated with an overly sweet tooth:

- Eating too many sugary foods can contribute to dental caries (cavities).
- Sugar often accompanies fat—a pastry or a dish of ice cream has a hefty dose of both.
- Sugary foods too often replace more nutritious fare. This is especially true of soft drinks. Children who drink soda with lunch, dinner, or snacks are missing out on the nutrients they should be getting from milk and juice.

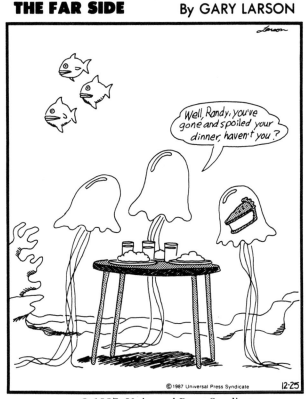

THE FAR SIDE © 1987. Universal Press Syndicate.
Reprinted with permission.

To reduce the sugar in your diet, try eating fresh fruit for dessert. When you buy canned fruit, select the type packed in its own juice rather than in heavy syrup. Replace soft drinks with seltzer or plain water—water is what your body really needs. Add sugar, syrup, and honey in moderation; contrary to popular thought, honey does not have fewer calories, less sugar, or greater nutritional benefit than the sugar in your sugar bowl. Choose a breakfast cereal with six or fewer grams of sugar per serving. Look at the package: information on sugar content is listed under "Carbohydrate Information."

Guideline 6. Use salt and sodium only in moderation

While the exact role of the mineral sodium in the development of hypertension is unknown, certain individuals sensitive to sodium are at risk for developing high blood pressure if they consume large amounts. Dietary sodium comes from three general categories:

- Almost all foods in their natural state contain small amounts of sodium.
- Highly processed foods are usually very high in sodium because of added salt (sodium chloride) and other sodium compounds.
- Added table salt: one teaspoon of salt contains about 2,300 milligrams of sodium.

The Estimated Minimum Requirement for sodium established by the Food and Nutrition Board, National Research, Council/National Academy of Sciences, is 500 milligrams per day; healthy adults should try to consume no more than 2,400 milligrams per day. To reduce the sodium in your diet, use less salt. Instead, flavor your food with herbs, spices, lemon, garlic, onion, and pepper. Avoid excessive use of highly processed foods, such as frozen entrees, canned foods with added salt, luncheon meats, and fast food. Take the time to cook with fresh ingredients.

Guideline 7. If you drink alcoholic beverages, do so in moderation

An alcoholic beverage once or twice a week is considered moderate, although this varies from person to person. While we are not advising daily alcohol consumption, having one drink per day has not been shown to cause nutritional harm to healthy adults. If you are taking any medications, check with your doctor regarding any possible drug-alcohol interactions. Alcohol should be eliminated from your diet if you are pregnant, since it crosses the placenta and can cause damage to the developing fetus.

Alcohol is high in calories. A twelve-ounce can of beer has about 145 calories. One and one-half ounce of gin, rum, vodka, or whiskey has about 116 calories. To reduce calories and alcohol, drink light beer instead of regular (save 40 to 50 calories), or make a wine spritzer—half wine, half seltzer.

CAFFEINE

Caffeine is a drug that affects many systems in the body. Large amounts can cause adverse health effects, including anxiety, restlessness, irritability, sleep disruptions, palpitations, gastrointestinal disturbances, and diuresis (production of large volumes of urine). On the other hand; research on the consumption of moderate amounts of caffeine has yielded many conflicting results. While studies have suggested that moderate amounts may increase the risk of developing cardiovascular disease, fibrocystic breast disease, and several other disorders, other studies have been unable to confirm these negative effects.

Americans consume huge amounts of caffeine, particularly in coffee, tea, and colas. Chocolate also has a small quantity of caffeine. Caffeine is even present in some medications.

Some Common Sources of Caffeine		
	serving size	mg* caffeine
Coffee		
brewed	6 fl oz	103
instant	1 rnd tsp	57
decaffeinated	1 rnd tsp	2
Tea, brewed 3 minutes	6 fl oz	36
Coca-Cola	12 fl oz	46
Coca-Cola, Diet	12 fl oz	46
Chocolate	1 oz	12
*mg = milligram.		

If you drink caffeine-containing beverages, do so in moderation. A reasonable daily limit for adults is 200 milligrams—the amount found in about two cups of brewed coffee. Since caffeine crosses the placenta and enters the fetal circulation, pregnant women might want to avoid or at least limit it because of potential adverse effects on the fetus.

For anyone suffering from anxiety, jitteriness, or sleep disturbances, eliminating caffeine from your diet altogether can be very helpful. Or, if you are using caffeine as a "crutch" to get you through the day (coffee to stay awake in the A.M., to perk you back up in the P.M.), examine and address the problems causing your dependency on caffeine: are you not getting enough sleep? is your day far too hectic? If you decide to eliminate or reduce your caffeine intake, cut back gradually over the course of two to three weeks. One way to do this would be to mix your coffee with decaffeinated coffee and gradually increase the amount of decaffeinated. This can help avoid or lessen symptoms of caffeine withdrawal, which can include headache, fatigue, irritability, and mood swings.

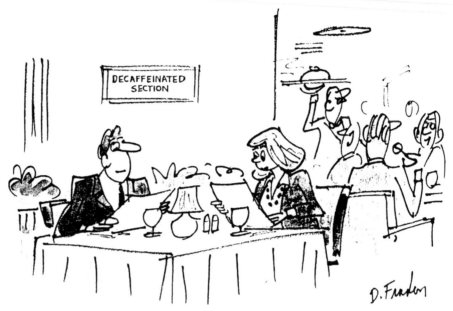

DECAFFEINATED
SECTION

Drawing by D. Fradon. © 1988 The New Yorker Magazine, Inc.

BE AN INFORMED CONSUMER

Before placing an item in your shopping cart, read the nutrition information on the label. Certain words, pictures, the name of the product—even the color of the package—are carefully designed to entice you. Manufacturers of food will, quite understandably, promote the good news (*Cholesterol Free!*) and attempt to hide the bad news (the product may be cholesterol-free but high in saturated fat). Nutritional information usually lists the major ingredients as well as information per serving; quantitative information about the calories, protein, fat, and other nutrients in the product; and percentage of U.S. Recommended Daily Allowances (U.S. RDA) for certain vitamins and minerals (established by the Food and Nutrition Board; National Research Council/ National Academy of Sciences). Be sure to check the manufacturer's definition of a serving; you may have to recalculate if the amount is much more or less than you would normally eat.

The U.S. Recommended Dietary Allowance is gauged for the age and sex that needs the most of that nutrient (very often young men, since they tend to have the highest nutrient needs). You can use the U.S. RDA as an indicator— 10 percent or higher indicates that the food is a significant source of the nutrient in question. For example, if a serving of yogurt contains 20 percent of the U.S. RDA for calcium and 2 percent for iron, it would be a good source of calcium and a poor source of iron.

In the ingredients list, all items must be listed in descending order by weight. If you want to reduce your consumption of something, see if it is among the first five or so ingredients. If not, the product is unlikely to contain an excessive amount of that ingredient. Remember, however, that ingredients lists are not always straightforward. For example, sugar can go by many names, including, *sucrose, fructose, maltose, dextrose,* or *lactose,* depending on its biochemical structure. This means that a product composed with several forms of sugar might have more total sugar than your first glance at the ingredients list led you to believe.

Health claims on food labels

Health claims have proliferated on food labels as manufacturers have jumped on the bandwagon of increased public awareness about food and health. The range of claims now runs from accurate to absurd to deliberately deceptive. The usage of some terms is determined by established guidelines, but a few terms should be approached skeptically. For example:

> *Natural.* The word *natural* does not necessarily mean *healthful.* Many foods that are extremely high in fat, cholesterol, or sugar are entirely natural—consider butter, eggs, and honey. Also, do not fall victim to increasingly sophisticated packaging designed to make everything look as if it was freshly prepared on a farm this morning. Let the nutrition label tell the true story; don't rely simply on appearances.
>
> *Light or Lite.* The word *light* (or "*lite*") on a food label has no legal meaning, although this may change. Light often refers to a reduction in fat or calories—generally desirable modifications—but sometimes the word is used to mean light in color or texture. The only way to know is to read the label.
>
> *Cholesterol-Free.* This claim is extremely popular these days because of public awareness of the role of cholesterol in cardiovascular disease. Before you conclude that a cholesterol-free product must be good for your heart, remember that 1) cholesterol is found only in animal products; the claim is true, but irrelevant when applied to plant products such as corn oil and peanut butter, and 2) to reduce a high serum-cholesterol level, limiting dietary saturated fat is of even greater importance than limiting cholesterol. Scrutinize the label beyond the bold assertion of "NO CHOLESTEROL" and find out how much fat is in the product, and what kind.
>
> *Lean.* When applied to meat and poultry, the U.S. Department of Agriculture (USDA) stipulates that *lean* means no more than 10 percent fat by weight; *extra lean* means no more than 5 percent fat. When applied to foods other than meat and poultry, no established definition exists.
>
> *Diet or Dietetic.* These terms often mean *low-sugar* or *low-sodium* or are used as synonyms for *low calorie* or *reduced calorie. Low-calorie* means no more than 40 calories per serving. *Reduced-calorie* means at least one-third fewer calories than the standard product, and for those foods regulated by the USDA, at least 25 percent fewer calories.

Sugar-free or sugarless. This means the product contains no sucrose (table sugar). It can, however, contain other sweeteners that are calorically equivalent or similar to sugar, such as honey or corn syrup. Therefore, from a nutritional standpoint, some products labeled "Sugar-Free" might as well have sugar in them.

No Preservatives. This means no preserving agents have been added. However, the product may contain additives serving other purposes, like flavorings, thickeners, or emulsifiers. In many food products, preservatives are important in preventing or retarding spoilage.

Take a Moment To . . .

Study the label of a food product you eat often, noting in particular the number of calories and amount of fat and sodium per serving. Is the manufacturer's definition of a serving similar to yours? Observe the name of the product and any claims or pictures on the label. What message, if any, do they convey?

BEHAVIORAL STRATEGIES

If you have tried unsuccessfully in the past to improve your diet, review your goals. Were they realistic?

To develop a workable plan, first identify your long-term goal, then set short-term goals or strategies. If your long-term goal is to reduce the amount of fat in your diet, do not promise "By next week, I'll eat half the fat I now eat." This sounds overwhelming and not at all enjoyable. Instead, give yourself more time and set specific attainable short-term goals that are couched in a positive language. For example:

- "This week, I'll change from whole milk to low-fat milk."
- "Next week, I'll have red meat only twice and eat more chicken and fish."
- "The week after, I'll use only a teaspoon of margarine, instead of a heaping tablespoon, every day at breakfast.

If you recognize that your snacks consist mostly of high-fat, empty-calorie foods, rather than saying "Starting tomorrow, I'll eat healthier snacks," set realistic and achievable goals such as:

- "Starting today, I'll bring two pieces of fruit to work for when I get hungry in the afternoon."
- "I will throw or give away the potato chips and candy at home

since they are my downfall every evening. I will replace them with pretzels and popcorn."

Jeanne's Experience

Jeanne, twenty-five, enrolled in the Behavioral Medicine General Program, explained that she was always ravenous when she got home from work, and often ate several ounces of cheese and handfuls of crackers within minutes of walking in the door. This high-fat snack left her little appetite for dinner. She felt frustrated but had been unable to break out of this pattern. The program taught her how to set realistic goals. First, she would eat a snack every afternoon at three-thirty to prevent losing control later. Second, she would practice eliciting the relaxation response every day when she got home from work.

Jeanne's strategy worked. No longer ravenous when she got home, she was able to give up the cheese and crackers. After eliciting the relaxation response, she was less anxious and calm enough to prepare and enjoy her dinner.

Take a Moment To . . .

Record everything you eat or drink for three consecutive days. Write entries immediately after you eat, and include what you were doing and any companions. Also note your mood (happy, relaxed, lonely, bored, angry?). Use the food record sheets at the end of this chapter.

When you examine your completed record, you are likely to become aware of a pattern that had escaped your attention. If you find your poor eating habits usually occur at a particular time of day, consider the events that lead up to them. Do you let yourself get too hungry? Are you with other people who make the same food choices?

Once you have identified the factors that influence your diet, you can work on changing them. If you find yourself hungry and at the mercy of vending machines every afternoon, packing your favorite healthy snack may be the answer. If you overeat because of loneliness in the evening, you may find that a telephone call to a friend can be far more satisfying than food.

Remember also that eating healthfully need not be a black-or-white affair. If you make healthful choices most of the time, you have room for some indulgences. Food has always been, and should remain, a pleasure. The real challenge is making your day-to-day diet both appealing and healthful.

Healthy dietary changes can affect other issues in your life. Weight loss, for example, can help to enhance your self-esteem and increase your ability to exercise, which, in turn, can help reduce tension and anxiety. In our approach, they all become part of a cycle of positive change.

For nutrition information specific to obesity or eating problems due to cancer, AIDS, or cardiovascular disease, see chapters 9, 19, and 23.

Judith Linsey Palken, M.S., R.D.
Alan E. Shakelford, M.D.

Recommended Cookbooks and Other Resources for a Healthy Diet

American Heart Association. *The American Heart Association Cookbook*. New York: David McKay Company, 1984.

American Heart Association. *The American Heart Association Low-Fat, Low-Cholesterol Cookbook*. New York: Times Books, 1989.

Brody, J. *Jane Brody's Good Food Book*. New York: Bantam Books, Inc., 1985.

Connor, S. L., and W. E. Connor, *New American Diet*. New York: Simon and Schuster, 1986.

Cooking Light Magazine. Six issues published per year. For subscription information write to Cooking Light, P.O. Box 830549, Birmingham, Ala. 35282-9810.

Goor, R., and N. Goor, *Eater's Choice*. Boston: Houghton Mifflin Company, 1987.

Methven, B. *Low-Fat Microwave Meals*. Minnetonka, Minn.: Cy DeCosse Inc., 1989.

Nutrition Action Health Letter. Published by Center for Science in the Public Interest, 1875 Connecticut Avenue, N.W., Suite 300, Washington, D.C. 20009–5728. Ten issues published per year. For subscription information call (202) 667–7483.

Piscatella, J. C. *Choices For a Healthy Heart*. New York: Workman Publishing, 1987.

Piscatella, J. C. *Controlling Your Fat Tooth*. New York: Workman Publishing, 1991.

Stone, M., S. Melvin, and C. Crawford. *Not Just Cheesecake: The Low-Fat, Low-Cholesterol, Low-Calorie Great Dessert Cookbook*. Gainesville, Fla.: Triad Publishing Company, 1988.

Tufts University Diet and Nutrition Letter. Twelve issues published per year. For subscription information write to P.O. Box 57857, Boulder, Colo. 80322–7857, or call (800) 274–7581; in Colorado (303) 447–9330.

Warshaw, H. S. *The Restaurant Companion: A Guide to Healthier Eating Out*. Chicago: Surrey Books, 1990.

SAMPLE
HEALTHY EATING
HEALTH COMMITMENT

Long-Term Goal:
Eat a healthful diet

_____ Signature

_____ Witness

Expected Date of Reaching Goal: _____

Readiness to Change	Short-Term Goals	Comments (supports, rewards, etc.)
Never considered change; need information.	1. Review chapter 8 ("Nutrition for Good Health") and note sections and suggestions that seem pertinent.	
Considered change, but not yet committed.	1. List the benefits of eating well. Think about health, energy level, appearance, and any other factors. 2. Talk to a friend who tends to eat well. Find out what makes him or her want to do it.	
Desire change; need motivation.	1. Determine what foods are problems for me. Remove them from the house. Throw them away if necessary. 2. Affirm daily, in front of a mirror, my right to eat healthfully.	

(continued)

145

Readiness to Change	Short-Term Goals	Comments (supports, rewards, etc.)
Attempting change; need structure, support, and skills.	1. Buy a new cookbook from the list at the end of chapter 8. 2. Select two new recipes to try this week. 3. By the end of this week, be eating at least five servings from the fruit or vegetable group each day.	
Change made; need reinforcement.	1. Browse through any supermarket and select and try two new healthful food items. 2. Reward myself for eating well with a nonfat treat.	
Change made; slipping back into old habits, need renewed motivation and support.	1. Prepare a special dinner for family or friends using some of the healthful recipes that I succeeded with before. 2. Write down everything I eat for three days. Then note specifically how I can improve my food choices. 3. Elicit the relaxation response every day before dinner.	

HEALTHY EATING
HEALTH COMMITMENT

Long-Term Goal: _____

_____

_____
Signature

_____

_____
Witness

Expected Date of Reaching Goal: _____

Short-Term Goals	*Comments (supports, rewards, etc.)*

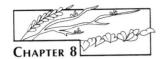

CHAPTER 8

Instructions for Keeping Your Food Record

Record everything that you eat and drink for three consecutive days. You will be less likely to forget anything if you record the food right after you have eaten. Every meal and snack counts, so do not omit even the smallest snack.

Time: The time of day.

Food/Beverage: Everything you eat and drink. Be specific about how it was prepared (i.e., steamed, broiled, etc.)

Quantity: The amount you ate (½ cup, 10 ounces, etc.)

Where: What room you ate in, or if you were at a restaurant, a friend's house, etc.

Activity: Anything else you did while eating, such as reading or watching television.

Alone or with Whom: Alone, or with family members, friends, or coworkers.

Mood: How you were feeling when you ate (worried, tired, bored, angry, happy, sad, etc.).

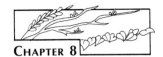

Name _____

Date _____

FOOD RECORD

Time	Food/Beverage	Quantity	Where	Activity	Alone or with Whom	Mood

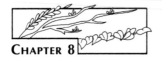

Name _____

Date _____

FOOD RECORD

Time	Food/Beverage	Quantity	Where	Activity	Alone or with Whom	Mood

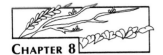

Name _____

Date _____

FOOD RECORD

Time	Food/Beverage	Quantity	Where	Activity	Alone or with Whom	Mood

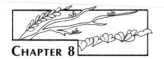

Name _____

Date _____

FOOD RECORD

Time	Food/Beverage	Quantity	Where	Activity	Alone or with Whom	Mood

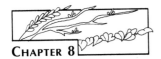

Name _____

Date _____

FOOD RECORD

Time	Food/Beverage	Quantity	Where	Activity	Alone or with Whom	Mood

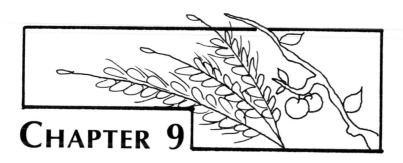

CHAPTER 9

A SENSIBLE APPROACH TO WEIGHT LOSS

Now learn what and how great benefits a temperate diet will bring along with it. In the first place you will enjoy good health.

Horace, *Satires*

In this chapter you will explore

- reducing your dietary-fat intake for successful weight loss
- exercise in a weight-loss program
- behaviors that contribute to overeating
- devising strategies to change behaviors that lead to overeating

Throughout history, the main problem with food has been how to obtain, store, and eat sufficient quantities. Most cultures and religions have evolved rituals that center on ensuring an adequate harvest and giving thanks for what food is available. As problems with food go, obesity is a relatively new one.

Through the millennia during which humans have endured feast-or-famine conditions, the ability to store food energy in the body from one feast to the next was a genetic advantage. As with any other advantage, the ability to accumulate stores of body fat was probably genetically selected for, in that those able to do so survived to pass on their genetic material.

In many parts of the world today, famine conditions render obesity virtually nonexistent. In the United States and other Western societies, we enjoy the unique and relatively new position of having an enormously abundant food supply. Our supermarket shelves are fully stocked with a tremendous assortment of foods. For sweets alone you can choose from a myriad candy bars, cookies, and ice creams of all flavors. In many societies, if you crave a sweet, only one type may be available, and that might be a piece of fruit.

Our marvelous abundance is also a great part of the obesity problem. We have evolved to enjoy the taste of food, yet today, the ability to store excess energy as body-fat stores is no longer an advantage. In fact, an *inability* to store fat efficiently seems to be advantageous.

> Eighty percent fullness is good for the health.
>
> Japanese adage

YOUR MOTIVATION AND GOALS

Obesity is the state of having an excess of adipose (fat) tissues. It is often specifically defined as being 20 percent or more above desirable weight as established by life insurance tables.

If you have decided this is the time to start losing weight, examine your reasons carefully. Having a clear picture of what motivates you now can help if you later need to reaffirm your purpose. Also keep in mind that weight loss is only the first element of proper weight, maintaining the weight loss is the second.

For many, the main reason to start a weight-loss program is the health benefits. Losing excess weight reduces the risk of heart disease, in part by lowering cholesterol and blood pressure. Weight reduction also lowers the risk of non-insulin-dependent diabetes, gallbladder disease, osteoarthritis, and certain types of cancer.

Losing excess weight can also help your emotional well-being. You will feel better carrying less weight, and you will probably be pleased with the result you see in the mirror. Setting and achieving a personal goal generates a great sense of accomplishment. All of these feelings can help reinforce the healthy lifestyle changes you make, and keep you in a positive cycle of healthy behaviors and weight loss.

Take a Moment To . . .

Reflect on your own reasons for wanting to lose weight. You may have many; list three of them:

_____

_____

_____

Before beginning a weight-reducing diet, have a weight goal in mind.

Consult with your doctor or dietitian on the best weight for you. A commonly used formula for determining "ideal body weight" is as follows:

For women: Take 100 pounds for the first five feet, and add five pounds for each additional inch. Once this number is determined, subtract 10 percent and add 10 percent to calculate ideal-body-weight range.

For men: Take 106 pounds for the first five feet, and add six pounds for each additional inch. Once this number is determined, subtract 10 percent and add 10 percent to calculate ideal-body-weight range.

If your ideal body weight seems unachievable to you, set a more realistic goal. It may be the weight at which you were comfortable five years ago, or before you started gaining.

Your weight goal: _____

A healthy short-term goal is to lose one-half to one pound per week. In the first week or two of losing weight, you may lose more than this due to fluid loss. After that, however, losing more than about two pounds per week usually means that lean body mass (muscle) is being lost along with fat. This is not desirable—the goal is to lose excess fat and conserve muscle. With this in mind, look at a calendar and determine when you can realistically expect to reach your weight goal if you lose one to two pounds per week.

Date: _____

Now you have set a realistic weight goal and a reasonable time frame. Do not become angry or frustrated if you have not lost all unwanted weight by next month, or the next holiday. You have a much better chance of maintaining your weight loss if you lose slowly and steadily.

LOSING WEIGHT: THE FACTS

In the short term, losing weight is fairly easy. Diet books abound, many offering quick solutions and each seeming to have its own unique twist. Anyone sufficiently motivated can follow a strict, no-nonsense, low-calorie regime for two weeks. Maybe even a month. Then boredom and the desire for "forbidden" foods set in, motivation declines, and as quickly as it was started, the diet is abandoned. Then come the familiar lamentations: "I can't follow this diet"; "I have no willpower"; "I don't eat *anything*, and still I can't lose weight."

The problem in this classic scenario is that a diet (which may be little more than a simple list of foods to eat and avoid) is expected to cure a weight problem that is probably complex in origin. You gain weight because of your eating habits. To lose weight, you must break some of those habits. Further, if your new diet consists of foods to be eaten every day for breakfast, lunch, or dinner, without deviation, how can you hope to be steadfast for long? The diet may stipulate no dessert except fruit, or no snacks. But you are human; when tempting foods appear, you want them. Having a choice—being allowed an occasional temptation—is much more effective. This approach is called "moderation."

You need not become someone who either eats a pint of ice cream every evening, or who never, ever eats ice cream. You can learn moderation. Moderation means considering issues such as: "Am I hungry for this?" "Is there something else I would rather do than eat this?" "What else did I eat today; do I have room for this in the context of all the other foods I have eaten?"

Losing weight and successfully keeping it off involve making changes in your food choices, activity level, and eating habits.

Stop counting calories . . .

Many dieters rely on counting calories, which are the units used to describe food energy. Calories are found in carbohydrates, protein fat, and alcohol:

> 1 gram of carbohydrate has 4 calories
> 1 gram of protein has 4 calories
> 1 gram of fat has 9 calories
> 1 gram of alcohol has 7 calories

Fat has the most calories per gram; over twice the calories per gram of carbohydrate. A long-popular myth deems starchy foods "fattening." In fact, starch is primarily carbohydrate, calorically among the lowest of the food components. What is fattening is fat—heaped onto foods like the butter on bread or a potato; hidden in foods like chips and dips. To limit calories, limit foods high in fat and also limit alcohol.

. . . Start counting fat

Recent research on weight loss indicates that strictly limiting fat is more effective than simply reducing calories. Calories are not equal once they have entered your body. Fat calories are more easily stored than other calories; this is probably a genetic adaptation to protect against famine. Carbohydrate calories are not stored nearly as efficiently; a larger percentage of carbohydrate is metabolized, or burned as energy.

For these reasons, to lose weight you should limit the amount of fat you eat. No single food need be totally off-limits, but your total fat intake must be low. Start by leaving added fats off most of your foods and experimenting with alternatives:

- instead of butter or margarine, use jam, honey, apple butter, or marmalade

- instead of regular salad dressing, use a low-fat prepared dressing, lemon juice, or a flavored vinegar.
- instead of sour cream, use nonfat or low-fat yogurt

Determine your fat-gram limit. For a healthful diet, no more than 30 percent of calories should come from fat. For example, a woman who needs 1800 calories per day to maintain her weight should calculate her fat-gram limit as follows:

$$1800 \times 0.30 = 540 \text{ (maximum calories from fat)}$$

Then, since every gram of fat has nine calories, the calories from fat are divided by nine:

$$540 \div 9 = 60 \text{ (maximum fat grams per day)}$$

For a man who needs 2200 calories per day, the calculation would be:

$$2200 \times 0.30 = 660 \text{ (maximum calories from fat)}$$
$$660 \div 9 = 73 \text{ (maximum fat grams per day)}$$

Many adults maintain their weight if they eat the amount of fat grams computed by the above equations. To lose weight, fat grams must be further restricted. Women usually lose weight at a maximum of twenty to forty fat grams per day, and men at thirty to fifty per day. Everyone is different, of course; you may be able to eat somewhat more fat grams and still lose weight. To find out, do some careful fat-gram recording and observation of your weight. Add up how many fat grams you ate on several typical days. Analyze the fat grams in any recipes you prepare, then estimate what fraction of the dish you ate. Get a book listing the fat grams in commonly eaten foods; a list appears at the end of this chapter. After you have added up your fat intake for several days, you will be very familiar with grams of fat. You will know, for example, that a slice of bread has one gram of fat, whereas the teaspoon of butter you might spread on it has four.

To start your weight-loss plan, first set your fat-gram limit: Women might begin with a daily limit of thirty fat grams; men with forty. Write down everything you eat, and add up the grams of fat as each day progresses. It is especially important to add up your fat-grams if, for whatever reason, you have a high-fat day. The act of recording what you eat and looking up the fat grams is likely to help you make better choices next time. So if you "lose control" at a party or picnic, don't be hard on yourself. Just keep your record as you normally would, and decide to do better the next day. If your overall diet is healthy and low in fat, occasional indulgences will not destroy your efforts.

You may be surprised to learn how many delicious foods are low in fat. Bread, rice, beans, and pasta are very low in fat; so are most fish, shellfish, skinless chicken, pork tenderloin, and low-fat dairy products. Potatoes are fat-free. Fruits and vegetables are mostly fat-free. You can eat generous amounts of these foods, and still follow a very low-fat diet. This means you should *never* have to feel hungry.

Be sure your diet is well balanced by choosing from all food groups every day. Distribute your meals and snacks over the course of the day. Eating regularly helps to keep your basal metabolic rate up, whereas going for long periods of time without eating will cause you to conserve energy and burn fewer calories because your body "thinks" it is being starved.

When you do add fats to your food, be sure to use a light hand. Every tablespoon of oil, regardless of the type, contains fourteen grams of fat. A tablespoon of regular mayonnaise has eleven grams of fat; a tablespoon of butter or regular margarine has twelve.

Also be aware of hidden fats. A lot of fat can be packed into what seems like a small serving of food! For example, a piece of pie with a double crust has eighteen grams of fat (or more if fat was added to the filling). A hot dog has thirteen. An ounce of cheddar or American cheese has nine. A half cup of ice cream ranges from seven to twenty four depending on the brand and variety. Do not eat an enormous serving of fat without even knowing it! Check your fat-gram counter before deciding on a new food. If necessary, find an alternative that is lower in fat, as in these examples:

- A regular serving of french fries has twelve grams of fat; a baked potato has zero. Decide to have yours baked, even if you have to bring it with you!
- Say good-bye to that muffin in the morning: it has twelve grams of fat. Have a bagel, which has only two.
- Remove the skin from chicken before cooking: three ounces of light meat with skin has over nine grams of fat; without the skin, it has slightly less than four grams.
- A whole egg has six grams of fat. Use two whites instead, and you'll have no fat.
- A cup of whole milk has eight grams of fat; a cup of skim milk has less than one. If you normally drink a cup of whole milk every day and you switch to skim, in just one month you will have given up over 210 grams of fat!
- A cup of fried rice has fifteen grams of fat. An equal amount of white rice has one. Is fried rice worth it?
- A tablespoon of peanut butter has eight grams of fat. Any amount of jam or jelly has zero. Make your next PB & J *light on the PB*!

Even if you opt not to count fat grams now, you can still choose low-fat meals and snacks. The typical American dinner plate tends to be very heavy on protein and fat sources, while accompaniments are given less attention and served in smaller portions. For a healthy, low-fat diet, this must be reversed.

Give lots of space on your plate to starch, whether it be pasta, potatoes, bread, rice, or another grain. Eat lots of vegetables, of many varieties. Put thought and time into the preparation of your grains and vegetables: try them in new recipes; experiment with new seasonings. This will help you to de-emphasize meat, chicken, or fish, which should be limited to three-to-five-ounce servings.

If three to five ounces sounds like a small amount to you, stretch it by preparing casseroles or other mixed dishes. You will be delighted with new and varied flavors if you try low-fat versions of Chinese stir-fries, pasta with clam sauce, chicken, mushroom, and pepper kebabs, burritos, curry with rice, jambalaya, and other recipes. (See the list of creative and healthful cookbooks on page 144.)

Remember, a slow, steady weight loss is best. Your average loss should be one-half to one pound per week. You may lose somewhat more slowly if you are unable to get regular exercise. A more rapid loss indicates that you are probably losing fluid and muscle in addition to the fat stores you want to lose.

The importance of exercise

Part of your weight-loss plan should be an exercise program. Being active will not only help you take off excess weight, but will also help you maintain the loss for the long term. Of course, calories are burned during exercise, but that is only part of the benefit. By regularly performing aerobic exercise, such as walking or biking, you raise your metabolic rate and burn more calories, even when at rest. This effect can last up to twelve hours after exercising. However, if you are over forty-five and do not exercise regularly, or if you have any medical conditions or risk factors for cardiac disease, check with your physician before starting any exercise program.

Exercising regularly while losing weight also helps ensure losing adipose tissue (fat stores) and maintaining muscle mass. Weight loss without an exercise component will involve muscle loss as well as fat.

Since your exercise should be done regularly, it is important to choose an activity that you enjoy and that fits nicely into your routine. For many, brisk walking is the answer—it is easy to do, and inexpensive! Chapter 6 addresses starting and maintaining an exercise program.

Changing your eating habits

First you must understand what causes you to make the wrong food choices. Why is it that one day you feel satisfied eating primarily fruits, vegetables, and grains, but the next day crave junk food and never feel satisfied no matter how much you eat? You may often seek much more than nourishment from food. It may be solace, or a return to a feeling of a better time. It may be a response to boredom: eating can be something different to do simply to occupy your time. If you tend to make poor food choices, try to determine what triggers the problem. Only by understanding the emotions and situations that lead you to overeat can you begin to make changes.

George's Experience

George, a fifty-five-year-old mechanical engineer, looked forward to relaxing at home after a challenging day at the office. Every evening he had an ample dinner, and then ate more even though he wasn't hungry. This was becoming a problem because he was quite sedentary and had been gaining weight steadily. George said, "I eat a big bowl of ice cream every night, sometimes two. I don't know why I do it—I know it isn't good for me to eat so much ice cream—but I seem to have no willpower in the evening."

Close questioning produced more detail. Every evening after dinner, George relaxed in his favorite chair and watched television. After half an hour he would feel bored, and his mind would turn to food. He would wander into the kitchen, get a large bowl of ice cream, and return to the television. Sometimes he went back for seconds. He said, "I just know that ice cream is there. Once I've had one bowl, I might as well have seconds. Of course, by then I feel terrible, but it's too late."

Depicted as a chain of events, George's actions look like this:

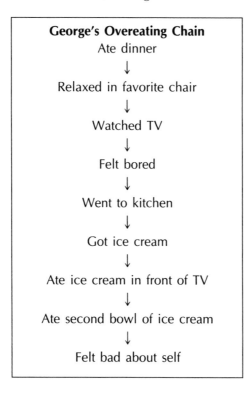

George's Overeating Chain
Ate dinner
↓
Relaxed in favorite chair
↓
Watched TV
↓
Felt bored
↓
Went to kitchen
↓
Got ice cream
↓
Ate ice cream in front of TV
↓
Ate second bowl of ice cream
↓
Felt bad about self

Laying out George's behaviors as a chain makes evident certain points where different choices could change the outcome. At the top of the chain, for example, George could decide that instead of relaxing in front of the television, he would take a walk with his wife and get some much needed exercise.

George could also break his overeating chain further along. He could decide that as soon as watching television becomes boring, he would turn it off and start to read. Selecting a book beforehand would signal his commitment.

The chain could also be broken closer to the bottom. George could decide to continue having his evening snack, but not choose ice cream. First he must get the ice cream out of the house, then shop for healthier snacks.

Ridding the house of ice cream is essential, since George finds it irresistible. Rather than constantly relying on willpower, he could take control and remove the temptation. (George did throw the ice cream down the sink and was surprised to find he no longer thought about it.)

Any one or combination of these options could work for George, since they all lead to the same goal: breaking the chain that leads to overeating.

Your personal overeating chain

When are you most likely to overeat? Every day? Just on weekends? Other specific occasions?

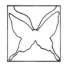 **Take a Moment To . . .**

Write in the chain of behaviors that precede your overeating. Include any emotions that influence your food choices.

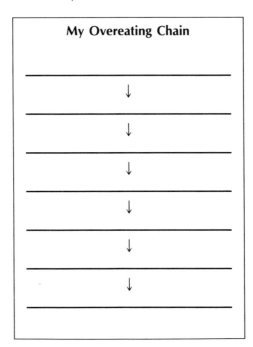

My Overeating Chain
_____
↓
_____
↓
_____
↓
_____
↓
_____
↓
_____

Once you see your overeating chain, determine how you can break it at different points. Try one of your strategies. If it doesn't work, try it again, refining if necessary, or try another strategy. Persistence will pay off.

EMOTIONS AND OVEREATING

Negative emotions often trigger overeating, which in turn leads to further negative emotions.

Kathy's Experience

Kathy, a thirty-seven-year-old dietetic technician, participated in the Behavioral Medicine Hypertension Program. Overweight by fifty pounds, she described her lifelong battle to lose weight, starting during childhood. She was *always* on a diet; she could not imagine either not being on her diet, or being off it and not feeling guilty.

Her diet, a 1200-calorie meal pattern given her in a weight-loss group, was sensible and well-balanced; she felt good when she followed it perfectly. But she felt "bad" when she deviated even a little. She said:

> Yesterday I was good all during the day. I followed my diet. But I went home from work and was craving carbohydrates, as usual. I knew I shouldn't but I had a bagel with cream cheese. I ate it so quickly I didn't even enjoy it. Then, since I had been bad and have no control anyway, I had another one, which I also didn't enjoy. Then I felt really awful.

Kathy had set herself up for failure by resolving to follow a rigid meal pattern indefinitely and by labeling herself as "bad" and "having no control" whenever she deviated. "Good" and "bad" were rigidly demarcated, food was the enemy, and weight control was the lifelong battle. Kathy had long forgotten that food also provides nourishment and pleasure.

Kathy also believed that by going off her diet, even a little, she might as well eat more because she was hopeless, not worth taking care of. This is an example of all-or-nothing thinking, which will be discussed under stress management. Kathy also shared the common misconception that carbohydrates are bad and should be avoided. It is actually fats that are to be avoided because they are efficiently stored as body fat. A bagel would have been a good snack, without the cream cheese. Kathy continued:

> I live alone. I often eat in the evening when I'm lonely. I know I overeat to relieve the stresses of the workday. I always hope food will be a sort of tranquilizer. I always think, before I start, that eating will soothe me. But it doesn't do it. I only feel worse. I feel guilty because I've gone off my food plan.

Time and again, Kathy rediscovered that overeating did not soothe her. It is easy to see why: a lack of food was not the problem. Kathy's problem was loneliness and workday stress.

Though it was easier to turn to food in response to her emotions, Kathy had to develop strategies to alleviate loneliness and the stress at work. She started by prioritizing her projects at work, and becoming more efficient at devoting time to those that were urgent. She later made plans to have dinner two nights a week with friends, and found that this social interaction made her feel better even on the nights that she was home alone.

Once she started to deal with her problems, she stopped using food to fill a gap it could not fill.

EATING MINDFULLY

It is very easy to eat without noticing or appreciating food. We watch television and do other activities while eating, and frequently eat on the run. Think about your last meal or snack: can you recall whether or not you enjoyed it?

Surprisingly, being inattentive to what is eaten does not translate into eating less. Often, the opposite is true. In the above case history, Kathy said she ate her bagel and cream cheese so quickly she didn't even enjoy it. So she ate another.

The healthy alternative is to eat mindfully, which means paying careful attention to what you eat. Look at your food. Appreciate all of its sensory qualities. Enjoy and savor it. If you do so, you will probably not feel deprived if you are trying to eat smaller amounts. Chapter 5, "Eliciting the Relaxation Response," discusses mindfulness in more detail.

Take a Moment To . . .

Try this exercise in eating mindfully.

- Take a piece of bread in your hand. Look at it carefully. What words describe it?
- Hold it up to the light; try to look through it.
- Close your eyes and take a few moments to smell it. See the field from which the grain was harvested and the wheat stalks bending in the wind.
- Run a piece of the bread across your lips; notice the texture.
- Then, very carefully, nibble off a tiny piece. Notice the flavor; think of words that describe it.
- Very slowly, savoring each bite, eat the rest of the piece of bread.

After this exercise you may realize that you have regained a lost skill: how truly to enjoy a piece of bread. Practice eating mindfully at your next meal, and notice in particular how you feel after the meal.

Judith Linsey Palken, M.S., R.D.

Books That Identify and Count Fat Grams

Natow, A. B., and J. Heslin. *The Fat Counter*. New York: Pocket Books, 1989. Lists the fat and calorie content of over 10,000 foods.

Netzer, C. T. *The Complete Book of Food Counts*. New York: Dell Publishing, 1988. Lists the fat, calorie, carbohydrate, protein, cholesterol, sodium, and fiber content of over 8,000 foods.

Pope-Cordle, J., and M. Katahn. *The T-Factor Fat Gram Counter*. New York: W. W. Norton, 1989. Lists the fat, fiber, and calorie content of approximately 1,800 foods.

SAMPLE
WEIGHT LOSS
HEALTH COMMITMENT

Long-Term Goal:
Lose weight—reach and maintain goal of losing 25 pounds

_____
Signature

_____
Witness

Expected Date of Reaching Goal: ___8 months from now___

Readiness to Change	Short-Term Goals	Comments (supports, rewards, etc.)
Never considered change; need information.	1. Review chapter 9, "A Sensible Approach to Weight Loss," and highlight sections that seem relevant and helpful to me. 2. Seek out three friends or co-workers who have successfully lost weight and discuss with them their goals and strategy.	
Considered change, but not yet committed.	1. List five benefits I will derive from losing weight. 2. Take a good, long look in the full-length mirror and ask myself if this is the best weight for me.	Benefits can be related to health, appearance, stamina, and positive feelings of self-esteem.

(continued)

166

Readiness to Change	Short-Term Goals	Comments (supports, rewards, etc.)
Desire change; need motivation.	1. Buy several of the new, low-fat or nonfat foods to replace some of my current staples. 2. Throw away one of my remaining high-fat foods. 3. Every day, eat mindfully at least once. 4. Elicit the relaxation response every day. 5. Before taking second helpings at any meal, wait five minutes and ask, "Am I still really hungry?"	The low-fat or nonfat foods include frozen yogurt, reduced-fat margarine and mayonnaise, and cheese with only two or three grams of fat per ounce. Washing a pint of ice cream down the sink imparts a feeling of true commitment to myself and my goal.
Attempting change; need structure, support, and skills.	1. Set a daily fat-gram limit. 2. Keep food records for two weeks, and add up every gram of fat. 3. Buy a new cookbook that features low-fat, delicious recipes. 4. Write out my own overeating chain.	Rewards— For every day that I am at or below my fat-gram limit, set aside five dollars. This will be a "fun fund" to be used for a nonfood pleasure later.
Change made; need reinforcement.	1. Try two new healthy recipes every week. 2. Give away all my old clothes that are now too large for me. 3. Start a new hobby or activity that will keep me conscious of my new shape (bicycling or joining a hiking group).	Keep a file listing the recipes that I liked, noting if and how they could be improved next time.
Change made; slipping back into old habits, need renewed motivation and support.	1. Resume fat-gram counting, with daily food records. 2. Write out a list of the benefits I noticed when I was eating healthfully. 3. Sign up for a healthy cooking course through a local adult education program. 4. Elicit the relaxation response every day.	I feel more energetic and proud of my accomplishment. I know I am improving my health for the long-term.

WEIGHT LOSS
HEALTH COMMITMENT

Long-Term Goal: _____

_____
Signature

_____
Witness

Expected Date of Reaching Goal: _____

Short-Term Goals	Comments (supports, rewards, etc.)

Instructions for Keeping Your Fat-Gram Record

Write down everything that you eat and drink for four days. Record the number of grams of fat in each item, and total your fat-gram intake for each day.

Purchase a book to count fat-grams as an investment in yourself and your new pattern of healthy eating.

You will find it easier to stay with your fat-gram limit if you record each item and the amount of fat it contains immediately after eating it. Waiting until the end of the day prevents you from budgeting your fat grams appropriately. You may also find that keeping fat-gram records for several weeks or longer can be invaluable to your success in losing weight.

Name: _____   Date: _____

FAT-GRAM SCORE SHEET

Time	Place	Meal	Food: Name and Description	Amount	Fat Grams
					TOTAL:

Place: H - Home
         A - Away

Name: _____ Date: _____

FAT-GRAM SCORE SHEET

Time	Place	Meal	Food: Name and Description	Amount	Fat Grams
				TOTAL:	

Place: H - Home
        A - Away

Name: _____   Date: _____

FAT-GRAM SCORE SHEET

Time	Place	Meal	Food: Name and Description	Amount	Fat Grams
				TOTAL:	

Place: H - Home
         A - Away

Name: _____   Date: _____

FAT-GRAM SCORE SHEET

Time	Place	Meal	Food: Name and Description	Amount	Fat Grams
					TOTAL:

Place: H - Home
        A - Away

Name: _____ Date: _____

FAT-GRAM SCORE SHEET

Time	Place	Meal	Food: Name and Description	Amount	Fat Grams
				TOTAL:	

Place: H - Home
         A - Away

PART 4

STRESS
MANAGEMENT

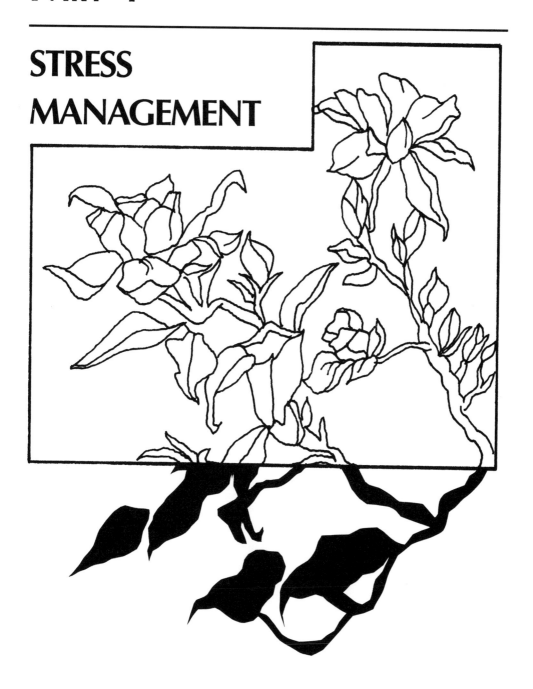

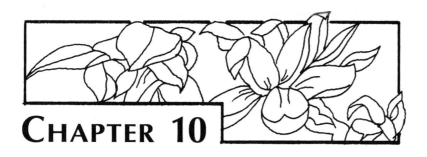

CHAPTER 10

MANAGING STRESS

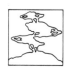

In this chapter you will explore

- what stress is
- more about stress and the mind/body connection
- the strengths you bring to stress management
- a four-step approach to stress management

Stress is part of our lives. Any change is stressful because change requires us to make adaptations. We confront biological and psychological stress, stress in the environment and in our social situations. We have deadlines, people to meet; we face crowded transportation systems; we worry about money. We know all about stress . . . or do we?

In fact, stress can be elusive to define and identify precisely because it is perceived differently by different people. What causes deep anxiety and stress for one person—an approaching deadline at work, for example—can be an exciting challenge and a necessary motivation to do one's best for another. And why is it that some people develop "stress-hardiness"—the ability to experience stress without the accompanying mental or physical stress response.

In deference to common usage, we have chosen to use *stress* to refer to the negative effects of life pressures and events. More precisely, we are writing about *dis*tress. Dr. Hans Selye, the noted Canadian physiologist, demonstrated that to a certain point, stress is challenging and useful. He also observed that when stress becomes chronic or excessive, the body becomes unable to adapt and cope. This is *distress,* and it exacts a toll on your body and mind. Others have also pointed out that stress is both useful and harmful. Drs. Robert M. Yerkes and John D. Dodson, of Harvard University, have demonstrated that as stress or anxiety increases, so do performance and efficiency—but not infinitely. At a certain level, if stress continues to increase, performance and efficiency start to decrease. If stress continues to build, performance and efficiency can diminish significantly, as illustrated in the following diagram.

Yerkes-Dodson Law

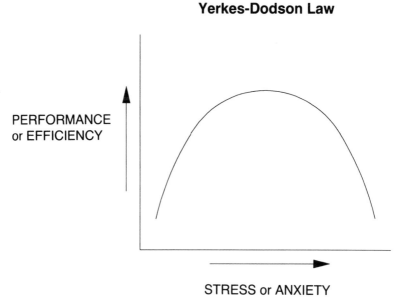

PERFORMANCE
or EFFICIENCY

STRESS or ANXIETY

Adapted from Herbert Benson, M.D., *Your Maximum Mind.*

STRESS-HARDINESS

Chapters 10 through 15 will deal with the harmful effects of stress as well as ways to lessen these effects and cope more effectively. Before becoming immersed in the negative aspects of stress, however, let us examine the benefits of developing a positive approach to stress. Studies by Dr. Suzanne Kobasa, a psychologist at the University of Chicago, and others have shown that some individuals are less vulnerable to stress, and have stress-hardy characteristics which are associated with a decreased incidence of illness as well as decreased absenteeism in the workplace.

In addition to exercise and social support, the characteristics of stress-hardiness are *control, challenge,* and *commitment.* Stress-hardy individuals see stress as a challenge rather than a threat; feel in control of their life situation; and have a sense of commitment rather than alienation from work, home, and family. This makes sense at some intuitive level if you recall the conventional wisdom "If you need something done, ask a busy person." We all know people who approach life with enthusiasm, get involved in what is going on, and welcome learning new things. This zest for living makes them feel vital rather than overcommitted and overwhelmed.

People who enjoy a *challenge* can view stress and the future as a chance for new opportunity and personal growth. If they have a sense of *control,* they know they can make lasting personal choices and influence events around them. And if they have a strong sense of *commitment,* they find it easier to become involved, to be curious and interested in activities and people. Kobasa refers to the personal characteristics of control, challenge, and commitment as the "three Cs." In our clinical experience we have added a "fourth C," *closeness*. People who have relationships and social support feel considerably more stress-hardy than their counterparts who feel isolated from personal contact. If those same individuals also exercise regularly and maintain a healthy diet, the incidence of illness falls even more markedly. Approaching life with the positive attitudes identified as the "four Cs" is healthy and helpful.

Dr. Barrie Greiff, formerly a psychiatrist at the Harvard Business School, also has an interest in the beneficial effects of approaching life positively. He calls the advantageous personal habits which he found correlated with health and happiness the "five Ls of success":

- Learn
- Labor
- Love
- Laugh
- Let Go

These five Ls allow you to embrace life with a sense of involvement, challenge, empowerment, and fun. If you approach each day as an opportunity to *learn* (being open to new experiences), *labor* (at something that satisfies you and brings meaning to your life), *love* (being able to give, recognize, and receive), *laugh* (with yourself and others), and *let go* (of "shoulds" and those things that are out of our control), the stresses you encounter seem more manageable. This is an example of how a positive attitude can affect the way we view a situation as well as our perception of how well we can cope.

Take a Moment To . . .

Reflect on something new and good that happened to you today. It need not be something big. Did you see the sun rise, someone smile, a new spring flower, or the sun set? So many things (large and small) in the course of the day are pleasant.

Was it difficult to conjure up this picture? At the end of the day remembering our litany of stresses is easy, but remembering the good things is often more difficult. Begin now to change this focus on the negative with recalling the positive as well.

THE PHYSIOLOGICAL, EMOTIONAL, COGNITIVE, AND BEHAVIORAL CONSEQUENCES OF STRESS

First, reconsider the simple yet complex question "What is stress?" As we said, the concept is elusive because it is so personal in nature. In addition, what causes stress for you today may not tomorrow. Some define stress in terms of "things" that cause them stress—situations relating to job, family, money, time, boss. Others define stress in terms of how they feel when stressed—pressured, angry, or tense.

More specifically, stress is the *perception* of a threat to one's physical or psychological well-being and the *perception* that one is unable to cope with that threat. And while you may be unable to alter the situation that is causing stress, you can change your perception of that stress and choose a more appropriate response.

As you will learn, you can use various cognitive (mental) techniques to change your perceptions and therefore manage stress more effectively. In fact, you have already started the process of managing stress: eliciting the relaxation response, exercising, and eating a healthy diet all help minimize the effects of stress. The next few chapters will build on this foundation and help you develop specific coping skills to reduce the impact of stress on your life.

As you may recall from reading chapter 4, the fight-or-flight response is a profound set of physiological responses important for survival. Confronted by a stress—either physical or emotional, real or imagined—a part of the brain activates the sympathetic nervous system. Epinephrine, norepinephrine (also called adrenaline and noradrenaline), and related hormones are rapidly released into the body to prepare the body for action.

As illustration, imagine crossing a street and suddenly noticing a car coming toward you. Your brain would instantly receive this message, interpret it as a threat, and send messages to release adrenaline. This adrenaline would increase your heart rate, blood pressure, breathing rate, metabolism, and the blood flow to your muscles, allowing you to run quickly out of harm's way. Once out of danger, the rush of adrenaline would be dissipated by the energy you expended running from the car. You might breathe a sigh of relief. Your heart rate, breathing rate, and blood pressure will usually return to normal, and you would proceed on your way.

Our difficulty in the twentieth century is that many of the stresses we face (relationships, work, family, money, etc.) are not amenable to the physical reaction of fight or flight, yet the physiology elicited by the stress remains the same. In these situations, however, the physical response has no way to dissipate. Imagine driving behind a car which is traveling slowly. You begin to fume because you are "late" and have "important things to do." Your brain receives the urgent message—"going to be late"—and triggers the fight-or-flight response, even though it is not useful in this situation. Without the ability to dissipate the increased adrenaline circulating through your body, you probably remain angry and physically aroused for some time after the incident.

Over time, chronic excessive exposure to stress can lead to physical symptoms and exacerbate many illnesses. Just as stress affects our body, so too it affects the ways we feel, think, and act. Confronted by stress we may feel anxious, helpless, overwhelmed, or angry. Our thinking style can be affected: it may be more difficult to concentrate, think clearly, or make decisions. It is also not uncommon to change our behavior (e.g., smoke more, eat more junk foods, or drink more alcohol) when under stress. See "Stress Warning Signals" (page 182) for examples.

The negative stress cycle

Stress can accumulate as you experience daily hassles. We think of it in terms of a negative stress cycle. An event perceived as stressful or threatening can cause physical and psychological symptoms. These in turn increase our stress. And so the cycle goes: stress makes symptoms worse and the worsened symptoms increase stress.

The Negative Stress Cycle

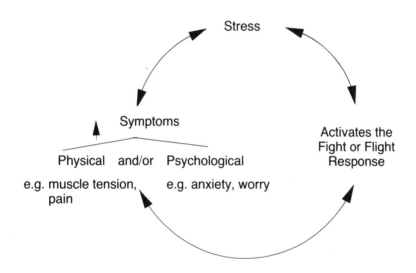

The Negative Stress Cycle can be difficult to interrupt. One good way to avoid the cycle is not to get caught up in the first place. To do this, you must first learn to identify your stress warning signals, which are cues to the development of symptoms. Attending to these cues or signals, you can then recognize when the cycle is about to begin and can choose an effective preventive strategy. Stress warning signals differ from individual to individual, but some common ones are listed here.

Stress Warning Signals

PHYSICAL SYMPTOMS

- ☐ Headaches
- ☐ Indigestion
- ☐ Stomachaches
- ☐ Sweaty palms
- ☐ Sleep difficulties
- ☐ Dizziness
- ☐ Back pain
- ☐ Tight neck, shoulders
- ☐ Racing heart
- ☐ Restlessness
- ☐ Tiredness
- ☐ Ringing in ears

BEHAVIORAL SYMPTOMS

- ☐ Excess smoking
- ☐ Bossiness
- ☐ Compulsive gum chewing
- ☐ Attitude critical of others
- ☐ Grinding of teeth at night
- ☐ Overuse of alcohol
- ☐ Compulsive eating
- ☐ Inability to get things done

EMOTIONAL SYMPTOMS

- ☐ Crying
- ☐ Nervousness, anxiety
- ☐ Boredom—no meaning to things
- ☐ Edginess—ready to explode
- ☐ Feeling powerless to change things
- ☐ Overwhelming sense of pressure
- ☐ Anger
- ☐ Loneliness
- ☐ Unhappiness for no reason
- ☐ Easily upset

COGNITIVE SYMPTOMS

- ☐ Trouble thinking clearly
- ☐ Forgetfulness
- ☐ Lack of creativity
- ☐ Memory loss
- ☐ Inability to make decisions
- ☐ Thoughts of running away
- ☐ Constant worry
- ☐ Loss of sense of humor

Do any seem familiar to you?

Check the ones you experience when under stress. These are your stress warning signs.

Are there any additional stress warning signals that you experience that are not listed? If so, add them here.

_____

_____

_____

_____

_____

Take a Moment To . . .

- Stop.
- Take a breath. Notice your body. Do you feel bodily tension? What

is your posture like? Listen to your thoughts. Are you feeling any of the Stress Warning Signals? Have you experienced them over the past few months?

Learn to heed your early warning signals as cues to prevent you from entering the Negative Stress Cycle.

Challenging myths

Myths or beliefs are explanations we develop, as societies or as individuals, to explain how the world works. They are unscientific, they seem to make sense, and because they are shared by others, we tend to accept them unconditionally. Sometimes, however, our governing myths lead to unwise choices, and at that point should be carefully scrutinized.

MYTH: I must be stressed to succeed.

Some believe, for example, that constant striving, fast-paced lifestyles, competitiveness, and willingness to handle multiple tasks (simultaneously) are the keys to success, even though these characteristics (labeled Type A or coronary prone behaviors) can lead to stress. Studies have shown the opposite. Top-level executives, in one study, did not necessarily have the highest prevalence of these characteristics. Executives who were able to define priorities, delegate tasks, and leave their work behind them at the end of the day were more effective than their counterparts who worked all the time. In accordance with the conclusions of Drs. Yerkes and Dodson, while stress stimulates performance and effectiveness to a certain point, excess stress causes their decline. By using the stress-reducing strategies described in the next few chapters and regularly eliciting the relaxation response, you can enjoy life's challenges without burning out.

MYTH: All stress is bad.

A certain amount of stress is stimulating and makes life interesting: We often do our best work when busy and challenged. However, too much, even of a good thing, is simply too much. The key is balance.

MYTH: If only I could move (change my job) (leave my spouse) (get rid of my boss), then my stress would go away.

If you endorse this myth you will be limited because, in some situations, altering external circumstances solves little. When "stressed" city people move to the country, they can become "stressed" country people. Within reason, our reaction to things (e.g., city life), more than the things themselves, causes us stress. Changing "things" is not always a panacea for stress reduction. As we said earlier, stress is the *perception* of threat to our physical and psychological well-being, and the perception that we are unable to cope. These perceptions can often be changed, and we can choose effective strategies to reduce stress. If we alter our perceptions, we can change the experience of stress and moderate our reaction. So before we go changing jobs, home, or family, we should first look to see if it is possible and realistic to change our perception. If not, then work to change the situation or the environment.

MYTH: There is nothing I can do about stress . . . It's all around me.

Divide and conquer. Looked at globally, stress indeed can become overwhelming. However, when you break global stress into individual stressors, you can learn techniques to manage stress, one step at a time.

And who said stress is an "it"? If you recognize that stress is our perception of a threat, and our reaction to the perception, then logically we can do something to manage our perceptions and reactions. You cannot always control or change a situation, but you can retain control over the way you react to and think about stress.

MYTH: Anyone who makes compromises in order to manage stress is a wimp. I don't want to become a wimp.

This is a good example of all-or-nothing thinking. All-or-nothing thinking in itself can cause stress and make it seem that change is impossible. The challenge is to find a balance that works for you without compromising your standards. A middle ground between being assertive or a wimp, between winning or losing, between black and white does exist.

THE FOUR-STEP APPROACH

The next four chapters build a four-step approach to reducing stress:

- Stop
- Breathe
- Reflect
- Choose

We will introduce this approach now, step by step, so that it will be familiar to you as you read.

Stop

Each time you encounter a stress, Stop, before your thoughts escalate into the worst possible scenarios. We call this "awfulizing" (e.g., your boss buzzes and says he wants to see you, and your thoughts immediately jump to "I'm going to be fired). Simply the act of saying "Stop!" to yourself can help break your pattern of automatic response and interrupt the Negative Stress Cycle at the onset.

Breathe

After you Stop, Breathe deeply and release physical tension. This again is useful in breaking the Negative Stress Cycle. Physically taking a diaphragmatic breath can be important because at times of stress, most people hold their breath. Taking such a breath can elicit the physiology of the relaxation response, and, while you concentrate on it, your attention is momentarily diverted from the stress. Even a momentary interruption is often enough to allow you to focus your attention and proceed to look at the stress in a different way.

Reflect

Once you have stopped the automatic cycle of awfulizing thoughts and taken a deep breath, you can focus your energy on the problem at hand and Reflect on the cause of the stress. Chapters 11 and 12 cover how to appraise situations, identify the stressor and the practical problem, understand where your automatic thoughts and reactions are coming from, and identify the irrational beliefs and cognitive distortions which underlie these thoughts. This process of reflection is an effective tool in understanding the cause of your stress.

Choose

After you have stopped the process of responding automatically, taken a breath to divert your attention from the stress, and reflected on the stress and its cause, it is time to choose how to deal with the stress. Chapter 13 describes strategies for coping and gives many practical suggestions.

 Take a Moment To . . .

Consider once again those things that are important to you, before you become immersed in reflecting on the stresses in your life. A firm grasp of your deeply-held values will help you put your stress in perspective. Many of us run a hundred miles an hour doing what we feel we "must," "should," or "have to," instead of allowing ourselves to do the things we want. Given that we have a limited number of hours per week, it's important that there be a balance between the "shoulds" and "wants." For example, we frequently hear our patients say, "When the kids are grown, I'll go back to school, get a degree, or find a career." When the time comes, often the prospect is too frightening, or we are too old or too tired—and the goals are never met.

What is Important/Meaningful/Valuable to you in life?

For each of the following categories, ask yourself, What do I want for myself, today, next week, a year from now?

Professional/educational/intellectual

Today _____

Next week _____

A year from now _____

Relationships

    Today _____

    Next week _____

    A year from now _____

Creative things

    Today _____

    Next week _____

    A year from now _____

Spiritual

    Today _____

    Next week _____

    A year from now _____

Volunteer/altruistic

    Today _____

    Next week _____

    A year from now _____

Health

    Today _____

    Next week _____

    A year from now _____

Fun/play

    Today _____

    Next week _____

    A year from now _____

Material objects

    Today _____

    Next week _____

    A year from now _____

Which area do you want to work on first? Choose one, and make a commitment to yourself to follow through. Consider T.H. Huxley's advice:

The rung of a ladder was never meant to rest upon, but only to hold a man's foot long enough to enable him to put the other somewhat higher.

At the end of this chapter is an exercise entitled "Challenging Stress and Winning." We will build on it over the next four chapters. Begin now to try out the skills learned here and identify your physical and emotional response to a stressful situation. Think of this process as an enjoyable personal experiment. Recording stressful situations may strike you as simplistic, but it has proven to be an effective technique.

Eileen M. Stuart, R.N., M.S.
Ann Webster, Ph.D.
Carol L. Wells-Federman, M.Ed., R.N.

CHALLENGING STRESS AND WINNING
Stop, Take a Breath, Reflect

CHAPTER 10

Situation Briefly describe a situation that caused you stress this week.	Physical Response Describe how you felt physically in this situation.	Moods and Emotions Describe how you felt emotionally in this situation.

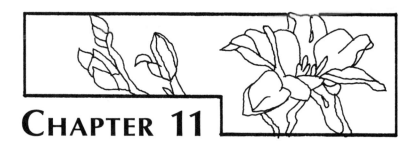

CHAPTER 11

HOW THOUGHTS AFFECT HEALTH

Men are disturbed not by things which happen, but by the opinions about the things. . . . When we are impeded or disturbed or grieved, let us never blame others, but ourselves, that is, our opinion. It is the act of an ill-instructed man to blame others for his bad condition; it is the act of one who has begun to be instructed, to lay the blame on himself; and of one whose instruction is completed, neither to blame another, nor himself.

Epictetus, *The Encheiridion*

In this chapter you will explore

- identifying underlying, negative, automatic thoughts
- thoughts and attitudes which are distorted, exaggerated, or illogical
- challenging negative automatic thoughts

In previous chapters you learned about mind/body connections and were introduced to the concept that stress affects us physically, emotionally, and behaviorally. In this chapter, we introduce an approach called *cognitive therapy* (based largely on the works of psychologists Drs. Aaron Beck and Donald Meichenbaum, and psychiatrist David D. Burns) that can help you work constructively with the thoughts, beliefs, and attitudes that cause you unnecessary stress and problems.

The word *cognitive* relates to what one perceives and knows. Cognitive therapy builds on this definition and is based on two premises:

1. Much of our stress and emotional suffering comes from the way we think (how we perceive the situation).
2. The thoughts that cause us stress are usually negative, unrealistic, and distorted.

Cognitive therapy recognizes that self-defeating thoughts, negative statements, and irrational beliefs adversely affect our mood, behavior, and health.

COGNITIVE RESTRUCTURING

One technique of cognitive therapy, called *cognitive restructuring,* helps us change the automatic way we think. This technique provides a way to learn to recognize negative automatic thoughts and irrational beliefs, notice how these thoughts and beliefs affect our moods, and see how our moods affect our physical condition and behaviors. (The flow can be in either direction. For example, a headache can affect your mood, and this in turn can influence your thoughts. Conversely, focusing on negative thoughts can affect your mood, and this in turn could lead to headache.) By recognizing this cycle of events, you can learn to change some of the automatic thoughts, which will then change how you think, feel, and behave.

The Negative Stress Cycle

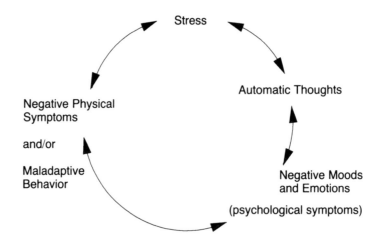

Does the mind have a mind of its own?

Sometimes it seems that way. Most of us have experienced situations that appeared overwhelming or terrible at first, but later turned out to be much less serious. When you look back, you realize your first thoughts were greatly exaggerated or out of proportion to the situation. These immediate, distorted, and negative thoughts are what we call *automatic thoughts.* They are:

- *reflex or knee-jerk responses* to a perceived stressor. They habitually pop into our minds uninvited, rather than as a result of reasoning or deliberation.
- *quick, fleeting,* a kind of shorthand.
- *usually not conscious.* You are often not aware of the difficulty they cause.
- *usually negative, unrealistic and distorted.*

For example, if someone sits in front of you at the movies and starts chatting with a friend, your reaction might be:

"Oh *no!*"
"Why me?"
"Not again!"
". . . should act differently."
". . . should have picked another seat."
". . . always happens to me."
". . . can't stand this!"
". . . won't be able to hear at all."
". . . will talk through the whole movie."
". . . going to be a miserable night."

Your response to the situation is automatic, you don't stop to think or choose, and you end up feeling victimized and miserable. The process resembles a never-ending tape.

Automatic thoughts are similar to personal myths: you believe them unconditionally without really being aware of them or appraising them realistically. You can be very strongly influenced by these thoughts, and they can have a profound effect on how you view daily life.

Mary Ann's Experience

A woman in one of our groups had tremendous fears about speaking to an audience, yet her job required that she talk to various groups. Listen to her automatic thoughts: "Can't do it! I'll forget everything! I'll make a fool of myself. My voice will shake. They'll think I'm pathetic."

You as an observer can see that these thoughts are clearly out of proportion. As a result of her negative thoughts and self-defeating attitudes (also called "self-talk" or "inner dialogue"), she would try to get out of all of her speaking engagements. Through cognitive-therapy techniques, Mary Ann learned to recognize these exaggerated automatic thoughts and learned new ways of thinking and responding.

Cognitive restructuring does not gloss over or deny negative feelings or distress—there are many things in our lives over which it is appropriate to feel anxious, depressed, angry, frustrated, etc. These emotions are often constructive and can motivate you to overcome obstacles and make adjustments that ultimately help you to achieve your goals. What we emphasize is paying attention to how our thoughts influence our feelings in order to avoid *excessive* or automatic anxiety, depression, anger, guilt, etc., so that these emotions are not the only way you feel. When governed by strong emotions *the mind becomes a filter, letting into conscious awareness only those thoughts that reinforce that mood.* Little else is allowed through.

No one wants to be pessimistic, or feel depressed or hopeless. These negative feelings are so powerful we tend to believe they create or cause our thoughts, when in reality the opposite can be true. Negative thoughts actually contribute to painful feelings. According to Dr. David Burns in *The Feeling Good Handbook,* to break out of a negative mood, you must first understand that negative feeling can result from negative thought.

Why are our negative thoughts so powerful?

Consider:

1. Your body doesn't know the differences between things you imagine and things you actually experience. If you recall a scary movie you have seen, you may notice that your heart beats faster or you may get chills. Or if you imagine yourself on a favorite beach, you may feel your body begin to relax and your breath slowing down.
2. We are always talking to ourselves, and the content of that self-dialogue is usually negative. We are engaged in a constant stream of self-chatter, coaching, advising, wishing, criticizing—and after saying something often enough, we begin to believe it.
3. We rarely stop to question our thoughts, and our emotions usually match them. If you tell yourself "I'll never get that job," and you reinforce that thought with feelings of anxiety and doom, your fears seem overwhelming. Thoughts often become self-fulfilling prophecies. If you go to the job interview in this frame of mind, you will probably not present yourself with confidence and self-assurance, and you likely will not get the job.

Because our thoughts feel so right, we develop what Dr. Donald Meichenbaum of the University of Waterloo in Canada calls a *confirmatory bias,* meaning we selectively perceive or attend to things that fit our point of view. This occurrence—a "seek and ye shall find" phenomenon—then confirms our mood.

Susan's Experience

Susan, a patient suffering from chronic headaches, entered our Behavioral Medicine General Program very depressed. Her confirmatory bias was that everything was hopeless, nothing was ever going to change, no one wanted to be with her when she was in pain. She complained of feeling alone and alienated. In her depressed state, her mind became a filter, and she let in only information that confirmed her depression and hopelessness. The more depressed she was, the more headaches she suffered. Further, her depressive attitude was unpleasant for others, so they chose to stay away from her. Susan was creating the very situation she complained of, being estranged and isolated.

At the clinic, Susan began to recognize her negative automatic thoughts and to use techniques described in this and the next chapter to challenge and restructure her thought patterns. These changes, then, had an effect on her depressed mood and feelings of hopelessness, and eventually the frequency and intensity of her headaches decreased.

Working with automatic thoughts

The first steps in beginning to recognize your automatic thoughts are:

- Identify your automatic thoughts in specific situations.
- Do they have a customary inclination, pattern, style? Do they consistently seem to exaggerate or distort the situation?
- Do you usually blame yourself?

The next time you are caught in traffic or on a train stuck between stations, and you feel you are about to explode, try this:

- Stop
- Breathe
  - Release physical tension
- Reflect
  - Ask yourself these questions:
    - What's going on here?
    - Why am I so distressed?
    - Am I late, or am I just racing against time?
    - Is it really a crisis if I'm late?
    - If I am late, what's the worst thing that will happen?
    - Will worrying about it help?

The purpose of this exercise is to begin to change the process of automatic thinking. You can learn to identify automatic thoughts that cause you trouble, see how these thoughts are exaggerated or irrational, eliminate these knee-jerk responses, and then choose how you really want to respond.

Remember, it took years to acquire your scaffolding of worries and anxiety-provoking thoughts—it will take practice to learn to let go of that framework and replace it with a new one. And even if your negative cognitive appraisal of a situation is accurate, still other ways of interpreting a situation may be more effective.

The Opera Singer's Experience

A famous singer relates a telling story. After finishing a performance to a standing ovation, she went backstage. Many people came to offer congratulations and praise, but one person happened to suggest that a particular song could have been done differently. "Instantly," recounts the singer, "I felt my entire performance was off. I *should* have done everything differently. The people who praised me, the people who applauded me were all just being kind. They didn't really think I did well!"

What Happened Here?

What people think and feel and how they behave is based largely on their core of beliefs, attitudes, and assumptions. These beliefs may cause problems, however, when they are viewed as absolutes in all situations, or when they are based on outright misperceptions. Under these circumstances, rigid adherence to these beliefs causes stress that is self-generating. When you stop to think about this story, you realize that we cannot expect people to approve of us all the time, nor can we do everything perfectly at every moment.

The opera singer turned a single negative comment into an absolute statement of truth and rigidly held onto it, allowing it to distort or eliminate the positive aspects of her performance. Furthermore, our beliefs and negative expectations can become self-fulfilling when they distort our understanding of present situations or anticipation of future events.

Review the Negative Stress Cycle on page 195 and see how these beliefs affect mood, symptoms, and behavior.

Attitudes, assumptions, and beliefs that cause us difficulty

Dr. Albert Ellis, a psychologist, developed a model, called Rational-Emotive Therapy, to challenge these exaggerated beliefs and replace them with realistic appraisals. His basic premise was that much, if not all, emotional suffering is due to the irrational ways we construe the world. Ellis referred to all the exaggerated beliefs, mistaken assumptions, and negative attitudes as *irrational beliefs*. He hypothesized that irrational ideas lead to self-defeating automatic

The Negative Stress Cycle

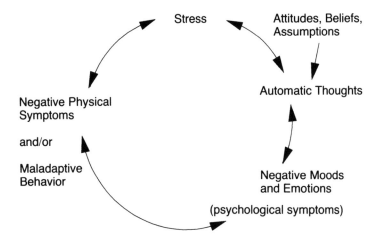

thoughts, which, in turn, distort behavior, limit possibilities, and restrict our ability to cope. Ellis identified ten basic irrational ideas, assumptions, and beliefs. They are listed below.

Irrational Ideas, Assumptions, and Beliefs

- It is an absolute necessity for an adult to have love and approval from peers, family, and friends.
- You must be unfailingly competent and almost perfect in all you undertake.
- Certain people are evil, wicked, and villainous, and should be punished.
- It is horrible when people and things are not the way you would like them to be.
- External events cause most human misery—people simply react as events trigger their emotions.
- You should feel fear or anxiety about anything that is unknown, uncertain, or potentially dangerous.
- It is easier to avoid than to face life's difficulties and responsibilities.
- You need something other or stronger or greater than yourself to rely on.
- The past has a lot to do with determining the present.
- Happiness can be achieved by inaction, passivity, and endless leisure.

You have a right to your beliefs and opinions, and they are not necessarily irrational. The problem is the degree to which these beliefs are held. Seeking love and approval is appropriate; it becomes a problem when we expect it from all people all the time. Now you are probably thinking "That's crazy," I don't expect everyone to love me all the time." In reality it is much more subtle than that. Reflect back on the opera singer. Rationally it is unlikely that she would expect all people to love her all the time. But her reaction to one lukewarm comment caused a cascade of automatic thoughts which indeed reflected this belief.

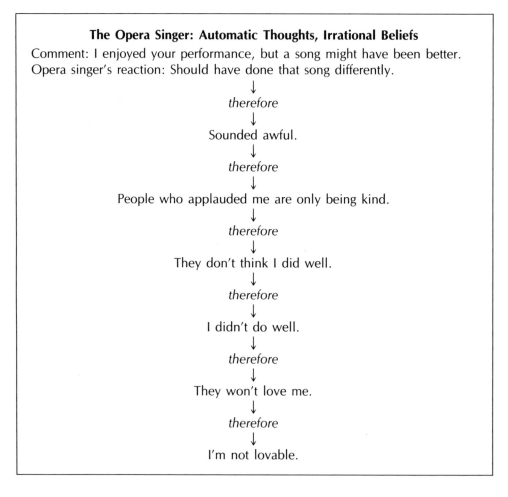

The Opera Singer: Automatic Thoughts, Irrational Beliefs
Comment: I enjoyed your performance, but a song might have been better.
Opera singer's reaction: Should have done that song differently.

↓
therefore
↓
Sounded awful.
↓
therefore
↓
People who applauded me are only being kind.
↓
therefore
↓
They don't think I did well.
↓
therefore
↓
I didn't do well.
↓
therefore
↓
They won't love me.
↓
therefore
↓
I'm not lovable.

Slowly the theme emerges that love and approval are so important to her that she escalates a single criticism into condemnation of herself as "unlovable." This cascade of thoughts was automatic and not always in her conscious awareness. Aspiring to love and approval is not irrational; the degree to which you hold this belief causes the difficulty. Does one slightly negative comment mean she is not a good person? Of course not. And does she consciously believe this? Probably not. But this is a good example of how powerfully underlying beliefs can distort thoughts and behavior.

　　She learned to *Stop, Take a Breath, Reflect* on this cascade of automatic thoughts, and realistically appraise the situation. This allowed the singer to put the comment in perspective and react very differently to this situation in the future.

Take a Moment To . . .

The "Beliefs Inventory" on page 204 is designed to help you identify beliefs that you hold strongly. You may want to stop now and do this self-correcting exercise. The results can be eye-opening.

Once you recognize your pattern of irrational beliefs, the next step is to understand how they precipitate automatic responses. It may be helpful to explore where these beliefs came from. Many are messages you learned from your parents and teachers that you don't need to hang onto any longer. Then you can begin to learn to modify these beliefs to decrease the amount of stress they cause.

An old spiritual teaching story illustrates Epictetus's observation that "Men are disturbed not by things which happen, but by the opinions about the things." Two monks, who had taken a sacred vow of silence and chastity, went for a contemplative walk in the woods. They came upon a young woman who was unable to cross a swollen stream. One, seeing her difficulty, picked her up and carried her to the other side; then both monks continued their walk. That evening, during the brief time when talking was allowed, the second monk rushed over to his friend and said, "How could you have picked up that woman? We have taken a vow of chastity." Whereupon the other monk replied, "That is true, but I put her down on the other side. You are still carrying her." The second monk was so consumed with his opinion (belief) about how the monk *should* have behaved that it became a source of great stress for him all day.

COGNITIVE DISTORTIONS

Another useful model for recognizing and restructuring your automatic thoughts and your exaggerated beliefs is based on the work of David D. Burns. Through years of research and clinical experience, he has found ten general categories of "cognitive distortions," defined as illogical ways of thinking, that lead to negative emotional states. To these, we have added some common self-statements which are also unrealistic. When people can identify their cognitive distortions, they can begin to challenge them.

Common Cognitive Distortions

1. *All-or-nothing thinking.* You tend to evaluate situations in extreme, black-or-white categories. For example, a straight-A student who received a B on an exam concluded, "Now I'm a total failure." The

opera singer who considered her performance a disaster because of one comment was also using all-or-nothing thinking. This type of thinking is often the basis of perfectionism. Any mistake or imperfection is feared as the sign of a complete loser, inadequacy, and worthlessness.

2. *Overgeneralization.* You see a single negative event as part of a continual pattern of defeat. One job interview that does not lead to an offer arouses fears of lifelong unemployment. The pain of rejection is generated almost entirely from overgeneralization.

3. *Mental filter.* You pick out a negative detail in any situation and dwell on it, thus perceiving the whole situation as negative. For example, after a midterm a student becomes depressed because she could not answer twenty out of one hundred questions. When her test was returned, a note said, "Congratulations! You got eighty out of one hundred, by far the highest grade of any student this year."

4. *Discounting the positive.* This is the tendency to transform neutral or even positive experiences into negative ones. For example, upon receiving a compliment, you think to yourself, "They're just saying that to be nice." This is one of the most destructive forms of illogical thinking because the price you pay is the inability to perceive good things in life.

5. *Jumping to conclusions.* You conclude the worst, even though it is not justified by the facts. Two examples:

> *Mind reading.* You assume that someone is reacting negatively to you, but you don't bother to check it out. For example, you leave a message on a friend's answering machine but she doesn't immediately call back; you automatically assume she does not want to talk to you.

> *Fortune-telling.* You anticipate that things will turn out negatively, and you feel convinced that your prediction is an already established fact. For example, a woman waiting to take a routine mammogram assumes she will be told she has cancer. This is often referred to as *anticipatory anxiety.*

6. *Magnification.* You exaggerate the significance of a negative event or a mistake. For example, if your bus is late and you have an important meeting, you say to yourself, "I can't take this." This is an exaggeration—of course you can "take this," you are already taking it. Conversely, you may inappropriately minimize positive personal qualities or events until they appear trivial. For example, when complimented on an outstanding job, you say, "No big deal."

7. *Emotional reasoning.* You consider your emotions evidence of the truth. For example, you say, "I feel inadequate" and you think "therefore I must be a worthless person."

8. *"Should" statements.* You try to motivate yourself by saying, "I should do this" or "I must do that." These statements not only make you feel

pressured and resentful, but also, paradoxically, apathetic and un-motivated. Notice how much better it feels to say, "I want to do that" or "I choose to do this." "Should" statements directed toward others usually annoy them. When the all-too-human performance of other people falls short of your expectations, you feel frustrated, bitter, and self-righteous. You can either change your expectations to approximate reality or always feel let down by human behavior.

9. *Labeling.* This is name calling. When you make a mistake, rather than simply acknowledging this one mistake, you label yourself, saying, "I'm such a jerk" or "I'm so stupid." Or when someone criticizes you, you label them "a loser."

10. *Personalization and blame.* You assume responsibility for a negative event when there is no basis for doing so. For example, a student does not do his homework, but the teacher feels worthless and inadequate because the student is not motivated. This causes unnecessary guilt and self-blame. Conversely, some people blame others for negative events or feelings, even when there is no basis for doing so. For example, a man stalled in his career might say, "If my wife were more supportive, I would be a success."

Maureen's Experience

Maureen's insomnia was worsened by her negative automatic thoughts. Whenever she had difficulty falling asleep, she began to awfulize by thinking, "I'll never fall asleep tonight" or "If I don't get enough sleep, I'll never make it through work tomorrow—I'll be a mess!" After learning that moderate sleep loss rarely affects performance and that anxiety from distorted thoughts can adversely affect sleep, Maureen began to challenge her negative automatic thoughts with more rational coping appraisals. "If I have trouble sleeping, it's not the end of the world," or "Even if I don't get a great night's sleep, I can still perform effectively," or "The less anxious I get, the better I'll sleep." By practicing cognitive restructuring, she did not become as anxious, which enabled her to fall asleep more quickly.

Paul's Experience

Another example of distorted thinking comes from Paul, a person with HIV disease. One day Paul noticed a spot on his arm that looked like a bruise and automatically thought, "Oh no! Now I've got Kaposi's sarcoma [a very serious complication]." He then proceeded to catastrophize and leap to all kinds of conclusions. "It's straight downhill from here. I'll be disfigured. Everyone will think I'm a freak. I'll be fired. Who will take care of me? I'll have to move in with my parents. I'll probably be in the hospital next week."

He continued this type of thinking for two weeks, becoming extremely anxious and depressed. His spot turned out to be a simple bruise.

With training in cognitive-restructuring techniques, Paul learned to cope with the ups and downs of his disease by saying to himself, "I can handle this, it's just a bump in the road." This enabled him to deal with the problem and feel much more in control of his emotions and life.

Challenging cognitive distortions

Now that you have become aware of irrational beliefs and illogical or distorted ways of thinking, you can learn to change some of your own old patterns by "talking back" or challenging your thinking. In other words, "Flip the tape." By choosing how you respond to your thoughts, you can reduce the amount of stress in many situations. These instructions will be covered in the next chapter, but now:

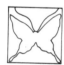

Take a Moment To . . .

Catch yourself in a pattern of negative automatic thinking, and do the following:

- Stop
- Breathe: Release physical tension.
- Reflect: What are your automatic thoughts, irrational beliefs, or distorted thinking styles? Ask yourself these questions:

> Is it really true?
> Am I jumping to conclusions?
> Is it to my advantage to think this way?
> Am I catastrophizing?
> Is there another way to look at the situation?
> Is it really as bad as it seems?
> What's the worst that could happen?
> Can I handle it?

Certain words in your automatic thoughts are "red flags" that can help you catch the exaggerated and distorted thinking that causes you stress. These words include:

Key Words

SHOULD	NEVER
MUST	OUGHT
ALWAYS	

For example, notice the difference in how you feel when you make these two statements: "I *should* be listening to my relaxation-response tape every day" compared to "I *want* to listen to my relaxation-response tape every day."

Through self-monitoring techniques, you have learned to identify stressors in your life and recognize how they affect you physically, emotionally, and behaviorally. You are now collecting more data on yourself by

- first keeping track of your automatic thoughts and irrational beliefs
- then recognizing how these thoughts or statements are distorted, illogical, or exaggerated
- challenging the automatic thoughts and irrational beliefs
- talking back to yourself

Keep in mind that you are trying to change old habits, not an easy task. If these cognitive-restructuring techniques don't work the first time you try, try again. Don't say to yourself, "It didn't work, nothing will ever change." Remember, you are learning a new skill. It's like learning to ride a bike: you did not ride off down the street perfectly balanced on your first few tries. *Practice. Give yourself a chance.*

> Somehow we must develop faith
> And trust in our Self.
> Anything the mind can conceive
> and believe, the mind can "achieve."
>
> The thought manifests as the word.
> The word manifests as the deed.
> The deed develops into habit.
> And the habit hardens into character.
>
> So watch the thought and its ways with care!
> From *A Course in Miracles*

The next step in "Challenging Stress and Winning" is at the end of this chapter. Please take the time to complete the exercise. It is intended to help you identify and challenge the beliefs, attitudes, and distorted thoughts that are causing you problems. On this sheet, keep track of situations that cause you stress, your physical response, your automatic thoughts at that time; notice your emotions in that situation, and how your thoughts were distorted, exaggerated, or illogical. How did this way of thinking affect your behavior? Did you cry, chew your nails, grab a cookie, yell, or light a cigarette? With cognitive restructuring, you will discover that, by changing your automatic thoughts in stressful situations, you can change your moods and feelings as well as your physiology and behavior.

Ann Webster, Ph.D.
Eileen M. Stuart, R.N., M.S.
Carol L. Wells-Federman, M.Ed., R.N.

CHALLENGING STRESS AND WINNING
Stop, Take a Breath, Reflect

CHAPTER 11

Situation	Physical Response	Automatic Thoughts	Moods and Emotions	Exaggerated Beliefs	Behavior
Briefly describe a situation that caused you stress this week.	Describe how you felt physically in this situation.	Write your automatic thoughts in this situation.	Describe how you felt emotionally in this situation.	Write down the exaggerated belief/ cognitive distortion behind your automatic thoughts.	Describe how you behaved during or immediately after the situation.

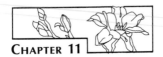   **Beliefs Inventory**

It is not necessary to ponder over any item very long. Check off your answer quickly and go on to the next statement.

Be sure to mark how you actually think about the statement, *not* how you think you *should* think.

Agree Disagree Score

- _____ _____ _____ 1. It is important to me that others approve of me.
- _____ _____ _____ 2. I hate to fail at anything.
- _____ _____ _____ 3. People who do wrong deserve what they get.
- •• _____ _____ _____ 4. I usually accept what happens philosophically.
- •• _____ _____ _____ 5. If a person wants to, he can be happy under almost any circumstances.
- _____ _____ _____ 6. I have a fear of some things that often bothers me.
- _____ _____ _____ 7. I usually put off important decisions.
- _____ _____ _____ 8. Everyone needs someone he can depend on for help and advice.
- _____ _____ _____ 9. "A zebra cannot change his stripes."
- _____ _____ _____ 10. I prefer quiet leisure above all things.
- •• _____ _____ _____ 11. I like the respect of others, but I don't have to have it.
- _____ _____ _____ 12. I avoid things I cannot do well.
- _____ _____ _____ 13. Too many evil persons escape the punishment they deserve.
- •• _____ _____ _____ 14. Frustrations don't upset me.
- •• _____ _____ _____ 15. People are disturbed not by situations but by the view they take of them.
- •• _____ _____ _____ 16. I feel little anxiety over unexpected dangers or future events.
- •• _____ _____ _____ 17. I try to go ahead and get irksome tasks behind me when they come up.
- _____ _____ _____ 18. I try to consult an authority on important decisions.
- _____ _____ _____ 19. It is almost impossible to overcome the influences of the past.
- •• _____ _____ _____ 20. I like to have a lot of irons in the fire.
- _____ _____ _____ 21. I want everyone to like me.
- •• _____ _____ _____ 22. I don't mind competing in activities in which others are better than I.
- _____ _____ _____ 23. Those who do wrong deserve to be blamed.
- _____ _____ _____ 24. Things should be different from the way they are.
- •• _____ _____ _____ 25. I cause my own moods.
- _____ _____ _____ 26. I often can't get my mind off some concern.
- _____ _____ _____ 27. I avoid facing my problems.
- _____ _____ _____ 28. People need a source of strength outside themselves.

•• _____ _____ _____ 29. Just because something once strongly affects your life doesn't mean it need do so in the future.

•• _____ _____ _____ 30. I'm most fulfilled when I have lots to do.

•• _____ _____ _____ 31. I can like myself even when many others don't.

•• _____ _____ _____ 32. I like to succeed at something, but I don't feel I have to.

• _____ _____ _____ 33. Immorality should be strongly punished.

• _____ _____ _____ 34. I often get disturbed over situations I don't like.

•• _____ _____ _____ 35. People who are miserable have usually made themselves that way.

•• _____ _____ _____ 36. If I can't keep something from happening, I don't worry about it.

•• _____ _____ _____ 37. I usually make decisions as promptly as I can.

• _____ _____ _____ 38. There are certain people that I depend on greatly.

•• _____ _____ _____ 39. People overvalue the influence of the past.

•• _____ _____ _____ 40. I most enjoy throwing myself into a creative project.

•• _____ _____ _____ 41. If others dislike me, that's their problem, not mine.

• _____ _____ _____ 42. It is highly important to me to be successful in everything I do.

•• _____ _____ _____ 43. I seldom blame people for their wrongdoings.

•• _____ _____ _____ 44. I usually accept things the way they are, even if I don't like them.

•• _____ _____ _____ 45. A person won't stay angry or blue long unless he keeps himself that way.

• _____ _____ _____ 46. I can't stand to take chances.

• _____ _____ _____ 47. Life is too short to spend it doing unpleasant tasks.

•• _____ _____ _____ 48. I like to stand on my own two feet.

• _____ _____ _____ 49. If I had had different experiences I could be more like I want to be.

• _____ _____ _____ 50. I'd like to retire and quit working entirely.

• _____ _____ _____ 51. I find it hard to go against what others think.

•• _____ _____ _____ 52. I enjoy activities for their own sake, no matter how good I am at them.

• _____ _____ _____ 53. The fear of punishment helps people be good.

•• _____ _____ _____ 54. If things annoy me, I just ignore them.

• _____ _____ _____ 55. The more problems a person has, the less happy he will be.

•• _____ _____ _____ 56. I am seldom anxious over the future.

•• _____ _____ _____ 57. I seldom put things off.

•• _____ _____ _____ 58. I am the only one who can really understand and face my problems.

•• _____ _____ _____ 59. I seldom think of past experiences as affecting me now.

•• _____ _____ _____ 60. Too much leisure time is boring.

•• ____ ____ ____ 61. Although I like approval, it's not a real need for me.

• ____ ____ ____ 62. It bothers me when others are better than I am at something.

• ____ ____ ____ 63. Everyone is basically good.

•• ____ ____ ____ 64. I do what I can to get what I want and then don't worry about it.

•• ____ ____ ____ 65. Nothing is upsetting in itself—only in the way you interpret it.

• ____ ____ ____ 66. I worry a lot about certain things in the future.

• ____ ____ ____ 67. It is difficult for me to do unpleasant chores.

•• ____ ____ ____ 68. I dislike for others to make my decisions for me.

• ____ ____ ____ 69. We are slaves to our personal histories.

• ____ ____ ____ 70. I sometimes wish I could go to a tropical island and just lie on the beach forever.

• ____ ____ ____ 71. I often worry about how much people approve of and accept me.

• ____ ____ ____ 72. It upsets me to make mistakes.

• ____ ____ ____ 73. It's unfair that "the rain falls on both the just and the unjust."

•• ____ ____ ____ 74. I am fairly easygoing about life.

• ____ ____ ____ 75. More people should face up to the unpleasantness of life.

• ____ ____ ____ 76. Sometimes I can't get a fear off my mind.

•• ____ ____ ____ 77. A life of ease is seldom very rewarding.

• ____ ____ ____ 78. I find it easy to seek advice.

• ____ ____ ____ 79. Once something strongly affects your life, it always will.

• ____ ____ ____ 80. I love to lie around.

• ____ ____ ____ 81. I have considerable concern with what people are feeling about me.

• ____ ____ ____ 82. I often become quite annoyed over little things.

•• ____ ____ ____ 83. I usually give someone who has wronged me a second chance.

• ____ ____ ____ 84. People are happiest when they have challenges and problems to overcome.

•• ____ ____ ____ 85. There is never any reason to remain sorrowful for very long.

•• ____ ____ ____ 86. I hardly ever think of such things as death or atomic war.

•• ____ ____ ____ 87. I dislike responsibility.

•• ____ ____ ____ 88. I dislike having to depend on others.

• ____ ____ ____ 89. People never change basically.

• ____ ____ ____ 90. Most people work too hard and don't get enough rest.

•• ____ ____ ____ 91. It is annoying but not upsetting to be criticized.

•• ____ ____ ____ 92. I'm not afraid to do things which I cannot do well.

•• _____ _____ _____ 93. No one is evil, even though his deeds may be.

•• _____ _____ _____ 94. I seldom become upset over the mistakes of others.

•• _____ _____ _____ 95. Man makes his own hell within himself.

• _____ _____ _____ 96. I often find myself planning what I would do in different dangerous situations.

•• _____ _____ _____ 97. If something is necessary, I do it even if it is unpleasant.

•• _____ _____ _____ 98. I've learned not to expect someone else to be very concerned about my welfare.

•• _____ _____ _____ 99. I don't look upon the past with any regrets.

• _____ _____ _____ 100. I can't feel really content unless I'm relaxed and doing nothing.

Scoring the Beliefs Inventory

A. Single dot items

   If the item has one dot (•) and you checked the "Agree" box, give yourself one point in the space provided next to the item.

B. Double dot items

   If the item has two dots (• •) and you checked the "Disagree" box, give yourself a point in the space provided next to the item.

C. Add up your points for items:

   1, 11, 21, 31, 41, 51, 61, 71, 81, 91, and enter the total here: _____ The higher the total, the greater your agreement with the irrational idea that it is an absolute necessity for an adult to have love and approval from peers, family, and friends.

   2, 12, 22, 32, 42, 52, 62, 72, 82, and 92, and enter the total here: _____ The higher the total, the greater your agreement with the irrational idea that you must be unfailingly competent and almost perfect in all you undertake.

   3, 13, 23, 33, 43, 53, 63, 73, 83, and 93, and enter the total here: _____ The higher the total, the greater your agreement with the irrational idea that certain people are evil, wicked, and villainous, and should be punished.

   4, 14, 24, 34, 44, 54, 64, 74, 84, and 94, and enter the total here: _____ The higher the total, the greater your agreement with the irrational idea that it is horrible when things are not the way you would like them to be.

   5, 15, 25, 35, 45, 55, 65, 75, 85, and 95, and enter the total here: _____ The higher the total, the greater your agreement with the irrational idea that external events cause most human misery—people simply react as events trigger their emotions.

   6, 16, 26, 36, 46, 56, 66, 76, 86, and 96, and enter the total here: _____ The higher the total, the greater your agreement with the irrational idea that you should feel fear or anxiety about anything that is unknown, uncertain, or potentially dangerous.

7, 17, 27, 37, 47, 57, 67, 77, 87, and 97, and enter the total here: _____
The higher the total, the greater your agreement with the irrational idea that it is easier to avoid than to face life's difficulties and responsibilities.

8, 18, 28, 38, 48, 58, 68, 78, 88, and 98, and enter the total here: _____
The higher the total, the greater your agreement with the irrational idea that you need something other or stronger or greater than yourself to rely on.

9, 19, 29, 39, 49, 59, 69, 79, 89, and 99, and enter the total here: _____
The higher the total, the greater your agreement with the irrational idea that the past has a lot to do with determining the present.

10, 20, 30, 40, 50, 60, 70, 80, 90, and 100, and enter the total here: _____
The higher the total, the greater your agreement with the irrational idea that happiness can be achieved by inaction, passivity, and endless leisure.

From: Davis, Eshelman, and McKay, *The Relaxation & Stress Reduction Workbook.* 5674 Shattuck Ave., Oakland, Calif.: New Harbinger Publications, 1988. Reprinted with permission of the publisher.

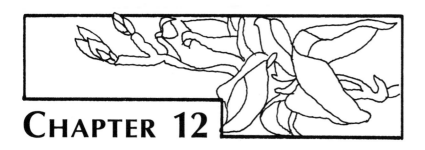

CHAPTER 12

FEELINGS, MOODS, AND ATTITUDES

A pessimist is one who makes difficulties of his opportunities,
An optimist is one who makes opportunities of his difficulties.

Vice-Admiral Mansell, R.N.

In this chapter you will explore

- your patterns of moods, attitudes, and feelings and the important role they play in how you manage stress
- how emotional patterns affect your self-esteem
- how low self-esteem causes stress
- assessing and improving your self-esteem

Chapter 2, "The Mind/Body Model of Health and Illness," introduced the concept that physiology, thoughts, feelings, and behaviors are interrelated and can affect our health. Guilt, anger, hostility, fear, anxiety, and low self-esteem are all feelings which can be influenced by thoughts and behaviors as well as by our physiology; they are important to any discussion of health. We have explained the role of thoughts and behavior in some detail. In this chapter we will focus on how feelings, moods (emotions), and attitudes affect us. We will also present strategies to deal more effectively with these states.

Although cognitive strategies can constructively alter moods and feelings, some individuals suffer from imbalances which are biochemical in origin and require treatment with medication. If you have any questions about this, consult your health-care clinician.

Many people find their emotions troubling, either because they feel out of touch with them, or because they are overwhelmed by them. Depending on your family and cultural influences, you may cope with emotions in different ways. Some families, for example, encourage children to be comfortable with emotions, but many do not.

How we feel about ourselves and the way we express emotions are processes begun early in life. We tend to model ourselves after the significant people in our environment, or we are influenced by their instructions and admonitions. Perhaps your family operated as if no one had any problems and everything was wonderful all the time. Perhaps you had no role models for dealing effectively with problems or for communicating vulnerable feelings openly, consequently you tend to hold things in. In many families, men seem to have the monopoly on expressing anger while women have the monopoly on crying. Some families encourage children to express their feelings, other families believe children should be seen and not heard. What were the emotional patterns and rules in your family? To what extent do you follow them now?

If something is troubling you, you can start from where you are and take the action necessary to change it. Knowing the origins of our emotional conditioning or our negative patterns is not always essential to changing the way we feel or express ourselves.

Feelings of depression, anger, fear, and guilt are all part of the human experience; you cannot expect to prevent those feelings altogether. Many situations cause us to feel sad, afraid, or angry, and these emotions are sometimes appropriate. What you want to prevent is getting stuck in one of these states, so that your mind becomes a "filter," letting into your conscious awareness only material that confirms or reinforces your mood. For example, when depressed, you notice and experience only things that depress you more; nothing fun gets in. You can, however, learn to reduce the frequency, length, and intensity of these feelings. Some of these powerful emotions are discussed in more detail on the following pages.

DEPRESSION

Depression encompasses a number of feelings and behaviors, including feelings of loss, defeat, discouragement, and hopelessness. It can range from "feeling blue" to feeling that life is meaningless. The future is viewed with "doom-and-gloom" pessimism. Depression also involves a loss of self-esteem and concomitant feelings of worthlessness and inadequacy. These feelings may exacerbate both physical and psychological symptoms.

Bob's Experience

Bob, a participant in our Cardiac Rehabilitation Program, was sixty years old and had recently undergone open-heart surgery for a triple bypass. Upon discharge from the hospital following his surgery, Bob became depressed and overwhelmed by his illness. He spent much of the day sitting around having no interest in his visitors and well-wishers. He napped during the day and was unable to sleep at night. His appetite decreased; he skipped the daily walk prescribed for him as well as other activities. He was anxious about his incision, and fearful that his chest pain would recur. His wife inquired about the Cardiac Rehabilitation Program, desperate to help Bob break out of this pattern and begin to take steps toward recovery.

Bob agreed to enter the program. With regular exercise, he developed a sense of confidence that he was strong enough to handle this crisis. He got out of the house, broke the pattern of inertia, and significantly improved his appetite. He began talking to other participants and learned that they, too, suffered from similar feelings of fear, anxiety, and depression. The more he talked and reached out to other members of the group, the less anxious and depressed he felt. Eliciting the relaxation response gave him a tool to decrease his physiological response to stressful situations and become aware of his feelings of loss associated with coronary artery disease. He began to talk with his wife about his illness and all that it meant to him and to them as a couple.

Bob was discharged from the program feeling confident in his ability to cope with the physical symptoms of his illness and looking forward to the future with a new sense of vigor.

People who are depressed have little energy or desire to be active. If you find yourself feeling sad or down, here are some steps you can take:

- Extend yourself and talk to someone.
- Use cognitive-restructuring skills: Ask yourself why you feel sad or down. Can you do anything to change your mood?
- Challenge yourself. Ask if it is realistic to look at the situation differently.
- Begin something "new and/or good" for yourself or someone else.
- Exercise—get some fresh air.
- Start to elicit the relaxation response regularly.
- Go to or rent a funny movie.
- Walk in the sun.

If you have felt depressed for several weeks or months, and all efforts to overcome this mood have been unsuccessful, it would be wise to seek professional help.

GUILT

Guilt implies that you have done something you should not have done or failed to do something you should have. Further, this "bad" behavior shows that you are a "bad" person. The concept of "badness" or self-blame is fundamental to guilt. Without it, we would experience a healthy feeling of remorse or regret, but not guilt.

Remorse or regretfulness stems from an awareness that you have hurt yourself or another, but your feelings do not imply that you are bad, evil, or immoral. Remorse and regret stem from blameworthy behavior, guilt stems from a sense of self-blame, and is often based on distortions of our thoughts.

These distortions that underlie guilt often fall into patterns or themes which you may recognize. One distorted thought is that you have done something wrong. Ask yourself if whatever you are blaming yourself for is really so terrible or wrong, or are you *magnifying* things out of proportion?

Another distortion is *labeling* yourself a "bad person" because of what you did. Labeling is counterproductive because you waste energy on an inaccurate self-perception rather than putting it into problem-solving. *Personalization,* another distortion, is inappropriately assuming responsibility for something you did not cause. A fourth distortion is all of the irrational *"should"* statements that you invoke when you feel guilty.

Once you feel guilty, you get trapped in a vicious cycle.

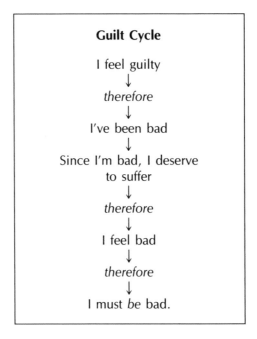

Guilt Cycle

I feel guilty
↓
therefore
↓
I've been bad
↓
Since I'm bad, I deserve
to suffer
↓
therefore
↓
I feel bad
↓
therefore
↓
I must *be* bad.

Self-punishing thinking intensifies the guilt cycle, and guilt-provoking thoughts lead to unproductive actions that reinforce your belief in your "badness."

If you did something inappropriate or hurtful, does it follow that you deserve to suffer? If you answer "Yes," then ask yourself, "How long must I suffer? a day? a week?" Are you willing to set a limit and stop suffering after that? But what is the point of punishing yourself with guilt in the first place? It does not help rectify the original misdeed to think of yourself as a "bad" person.

What is useful and appropriate if you do make a mistake is a process of *awareness, learning,* and *change;* then, if possible, take actions to correct the situation. Does guilt help you to become aware or to learn or change? No. Guilt does not facilitate this process.

Harriet's Experience

Harriet, fifty, enrolled in the Mind/Body Program because of a sleep disorder. By keeping a sleep diary, she discovered that when she awakened in the wee dark hours of morning, she was usually anxious about her relationship with her daughter, who is away at college. She related a specific anecdote about visiting her daughter.

At least once a month, Harriet drives two hours each way to visit her daughter. Each time, her daughter develops a headache and feels so unwell she needs to go to bed. The visits are short and unsatisfactory for both of them.

The particular visit Harriet was describing was worse than usual. Driving home, she felt consumed with guilt because she was giving her daughter these headaches. "What did I do wrong?—If I didn't visit she wouldn't get sick—Why doesn't she like me?—I should have . . ." All the way home she reviewed her mental tape of the visit, her thoughts whirling round and round. Once home, she was unable to sleep all night.

By practicing cognitive-restructuring skills and with the support of the group, Harriet gained insight into her thoughts and realized she was assuming responsibility for her daughter's actions (personalization). No matter how much she loves her daughter, she cannot take charge of her problems. Harriet was able to develop a plan to be loving and supportive of her daughter while at the same time not becoming trapped by her daughter's responses. Harriet decided to be less dependent on her daughter for emotional support. She made specific plans to develop new friendships and other contacts which would satisfy her needs. Over the next few clinic sessions, as she began to follow through on her plan, she reported less anxiety and guilt, as well as an improvement in her sleep pattern.

Most of us feel guilty at least once in a while. But we do have the ability to replace guilt with the capacity to see what we did and to feel genuine regret without labeling ourselves as "bad" or "at fault."

Take a Moment To . . .

When you are experiencing guilt, ask yourself:
1. Did I consciously do something unfair or hurtful that I should not have? Or am I irrationally expecting myself to be perfect?
2. Am I labeling myself "bad" because of this action, or am I magnifying things?
3. Am I feeling realistic regret or remorse which comes from an empathetic awareness of the negative impact of my action?
4. Am I learning from my error and developing a strategy for change? Or am I punishing myself in a destructive manner?

ANGER AND HOSTILITY

Anger is different from hostility. Anger is intense displeasure directed at someone or something specific. Hostility is more global and embraces antagonism, opposition, or resistance in thought and principle.

You experience anger when you feel someone is mistreating you or taking advantage of you. Many people think that holding onto anger demonstrates commitment and a sense of personal pride. Anger can mask feelings of helplessness, insecurity, disappointment, and fear. Anger requires great self-involvement—it requires the feeling of being "right" all of the time.

We are not saying you should always be calm and take everything evenly and quietly. Anger is often appropriate and also serves a purpose: it mobilizes people to change uncomfortable and wasteful situations. However, anger and hostility that are not constructively resolved leave one feeling helpless and out of control. Anger in this case can be thought of as "holding onto a burning ember, waiting to toss it at someone." When you think about it, who really gets burned here?

Certain aspects are key to understanding hostility, according to Dr. Redford Williams, a noted researcher from the Duke University School of Medicine. He identifies these as "cynicism, or a basic mistrust of the nature and intention of others; a more frequent and intense experience of anger; and the tendency to express such angry feelings in overly aggressive behavior." Thus, hostile individuals are more likely to feel angry and upset by the myriad hassles and interpersonal conflicts we encounter every day. Dr. Williams has demonstrated that individuals who are hostile have an exaggerated physiological response to stressful situations and are at increased risk for the development of coronary artery disease.

Every state of mind reflects itself physiologically. Anger or hostility may be reflected in facial expression, posture, social behavior, physiological arousal, and physical symptoms. Angry people may scowl, be impatient, be irritable, and reject the help of others. Most importantly, in the case of hostility, their bodies are in a state of alert, repeatedly triggering the fight-or-flight response with exaggerated physiological reactions. Anger and hostility are detrimental to your health and well-being. Dr. Williams has extensively researched the links between hostility, anger, and coronary artery disease. In fact, he believes that hostility may be the most important component of Type A behavior.

 ### Jerold's Experience

Jerold, forty-five years old, has a ten-year history of hypertension and angina. At the time he entered the Cardiac Rehabilitation Program he was experiencing a significant amount of chest pain on the maximum amount of medication he could tolerate. He had had angioplasty and coronary artery bypass surgery, both of which were unsuccessful in relieving his angina pain. Jerold's symptoms forced him to give up his successful business career. When he started the program he was angry that the world would treat him this way.

Jerold embraced a regular program of exercise and dietary intervention; this gave him some immediate confidence in his ability to accomplish his goals but did not decrease his symptoms. He began to keep a diary of his chest pain and noticed an interesting pattern: his pain occurred much more frequently with stressful situations than it did with exercise or exertion. He then made a commitment to examine his emotions. This was difficult: his entire life he had been discouraged from expressing his emotions, and he was uncomfortable talking about anger.

Jerold began to recognize an emerging pattern of hostility. He found that he was frequently upset and angry about the behavior of others as well as by the hassles of daily life. He began to recognize that he viewed life in general and each day in particular as a battle and a struggle. He was also able to identify the intensity of his anger at being stricken with this disease at so young an age. It had not been in his life plan. These insights in conjunction with the relaxation response reduced his emotional and physical reactivity. People began to notice that he was less hostile and angry in response to stressful situations, and concomitantly the frequency of his chest pain diminished significantly. At the conclusion of the program Jerold still had significant coronary artery disease, but he felt better able to cope with this illness and had a significant reduction in his symptoms.

Most of us feel angry and hostile at times. As with guilt, there are constructive ways to deal with this. First, *acknowledge* the feelings, *reflect* on them, *communicate* them (if appropriate), and *let them go* (if you ultimately want peace of mind). Ask yourself:

Why am I so angry?
Is this really a battle, winner take all?
Is my reaction in proportion to the situation?
Is it helping me?
Is this how I like to spend my time?
Do I want to be right, or do I want to be happy?

One exercise we have found useful is to keep a diary recording your angry thoughts and the events that provoke them. You may be surprised at how often you become angry over what are really trivial events.

> Angels are able to fly because they take themselves so lightly.
>
> Anonymous

FEAR AND ANXIETY

Healthy fear and neurotic anxiety are different. The thoughts that cause healthy fear are realistic: they keep us alert and warn us about dangers. Neurotic anxiety, on the other hand, results from distorted thoughts with little or no basis in reality. This type of fear is inappropriate and unhealthy. When you live your life worrying about and fearing things, you often become unproductive. You focus on "what ifs": "What if I don't get the job?" "What if I make a mistake?" "What if he doesn't like me?" You waste time and energy worrying about future events that may never take place. Or you agonize over things in the past.

Many people whose fears dominate their lives are caught in the "when/then" syndrome: "When my children are grown, then I'll look for a job" "When I finish all these tasks, then I'll be happy" "When I answer all my messages and respond to my mail, then I can concentrate on writing this major proposal." Avoiding fearful things or situations can actually make your problems worse. You give your fears more power. The best way to confront your fears and anxieties is to stop avoiding them. Instead, push through them. Go out and do it!

Helene's Experience

Helene, twenty-eight, made great progress in the Mind/Body Program toward coping very effectively with chronic lower-back pain. Encouraged by this, she began work on her next goal, which was to reenter the work force. Somewhat fearfully, she updated her résumé, networked with colleagues, and applied for a wonderful job in the loan department of a large bank. She was enthusiastic about her prospects until the day they called to congratulate her on being appointed. She fell apart, her pain flared up, she suffered an anxiety attack. She thought: "I won't be good enough—they'll be sorry they hired me—I'll fail—I'll always have pain—I'm going to end up crippled and disabled."

With the help of her clinician, she went through the process of Stop, Take a Breath, and Reflect concerning her automatic thoughts. After examining her thoughts and exaggerated beliefs, Helene decided to reframe the experience. Instead of continuously repeating "I'm so anxious," she would say, "I'm so excited"—and mean it.

Just do it! This may sound strange, but "doing it" precedes feeling better about yourself. In *Feel the Fear and Do It Anyway*, Dr. Susan Jeffers writes that when you do something you have feared, not only does the fear dissipate, but you also feel you have accomplished something. Your big bonus is a boost in self-esteem.

Confronting your fears and pushing through them is called *flooding* or *exposure*. This means exposing yourself to those things that cause you fear, allowing yourself to observe and experience the unpleasant feelings. After a while, your anxiety will decrease and melt away.

Being stuck in any of these emotional patterns affects how we feel about ourselves, that is, our self-esteem. It also influences how we see ourselves in the world and how we cope.

Consider these points:

- What you are today is in many ways due to your past experiences; what you will be, however, is your responsibility.
- Are you limiting yourself with low self-esteem, because of someone else's inaccurate comments years ago?

We all have occasion to feel insecure—a first date, asking for a raise, a job interview, giving a speech. Expecting to meet every challenge with total mastery is perfectionistic thinking and unrealistic. Remember that Ty Cobb, one of the greatest hitters in baseball history, had a lifetime average of only .367. This means he missed two out of every three times at bat. The goal is not to never fall off the horse, but to meet the challenge of picking yourself up and getting back on.

SELF-ESTEEM

> No one can make you feel inferior without your consent.
> Eleanor Roosevelt, *This Is My Story*

Paul's Experience

Paul, a well-dressed sixty-year-old architect, came to the Behavioral Medicine Clinic after a recent heart attack. His history revealed high blood pressure, high cholesterol, and no regular exercise, but when asked to choose a goal, his priority was to lose weight. He was, in fact, only ten pounds over his ideal body weight, but said he saw himself as a "fat man." "I am always struggling with my weight and never feel it's low enough." Upon further questioning, Paul revealed that his mother had frequently told him he was too fat and was often after him to lose weight.

Despite his serious health problem, Paul is most concerned about his "fat" picture of himself. The messages and expectations from his past—that he was fat and should lose weight—remained significant regardless of his reality today.

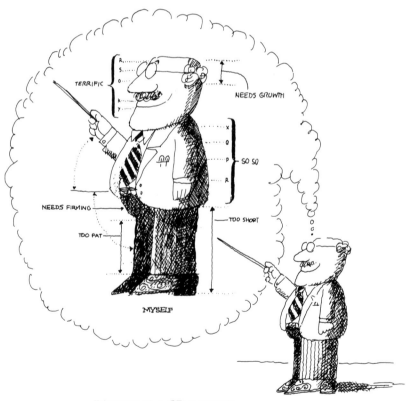

EXAMINING A SELF-IMAGE

Illustration © 1976 by Tom Durfee from *Asserting Yourself*, by Sharon A. Bower and Gordon H. Bower. © 1976 by Addison-Wesley Publishing Company. Second edition published in 1991. Reprinted with permission of the publisher.

Self-esteem is a measure of how good or bad you feel about yourself and how you see yourself in the world. This mental picture is called to mind when you assess your ability to succeed at any endeavor. This image influences your plans, decisions, moods, and behavior.

Messages from the past—from parents, teachers, and friends—often lower our self-esteem in unexpected ways. These personal messages are often reinforced by cultural or societal messages, as in Paul's case, from magazine and television advertisements featuring trim, muscular men leading glamorous lives.

HEALTHY SELF-ESTEEM

Having a healthy self-esteem means accepting one's imperfections. This attitude enables you to have "the serenity to accept the things you cannot change, the strength to change the things you can, and the wisdom to know the difference."

Take a Moment To . . .

Reflect on some of your personal qualities.

List the five characteristics you like most about yourself:

1. _____

2. _____

3. _____

4. _____

5. _____

Do you have any trouble naming five?

LOW SELF-ESTEEM

Because self-esteem is based on your judgment of yourself, not on other people's assessment of your value, it does not rely on your accomplishments. Often enough, even accomplished and famous people hold low opinions of themselves. Even Presidents, heads of banks and large corporations, as well as famous opera and movie stars, all can be beset by insecurities. Inadequate self-esteem results from expectations that exceed your achievements.

Low self-esteem is a fundamental source of stress. This self-imposed stress often manifests itself through perfectionism, lack of self-confidence, anxiety, feelings of jealousy or inadequacy, anger and hostility. It is, however, a source of stress over which you have control.

If you could eavesdrop on thoughts, you would hear people with low self-esteem saying all sorts of negative things about themselves: "I'm going to fail again," "I can't do anything right," "I'll always be like this." The underlying fear is being exposed as inferior to others and, eventually, as unable to cope with new situations. "Face" would be lost in the eyes of friends, colleagues, or family. Underneath your stress, do you find what Dr. David D. Burns calls "silent assumptions"? Some examples from his *Feeling Good Handbook*:

- I must always please people and live up to everyone's expectations.
- If someone criticizes me, it means there's something wrong with me.
- I am basically defective and inferior to other people.
- I must always try to be perfect.

Individuals with "silent assumptions" often become "awfulizers." Haunted by global feelings of fear and anxiety, these people are easily provoked into the negative anxiety cycle, which results in the fight-or-flight response.

Stress caused by low self-esteem can pervade your daily circumstances and bias your interactions with others. This negative view of yourself can be communicated to others even before they have a chance to develop their own impressions.

Fred's Experience

Fred, a forty-five-year-old engineer at a large computer firm, was having difficulties advancing in his career. This created a great deal of stress, adding to a condition of hypertension. When asked to demonstrate his presentation to his bosses, what was striking was how frequently he began his remarks with "You might not agree with me but . . ." or "I don't know if this idea is worthwhile, however . . ."

Low self-esteem limits what you are willing to try and interferes with opportunities for discovery and growth; it reduces stress-hardiness. These attitudes are often chronic and lifelong causes of stress unless the sources of stress—negative thoughts and feelings about yourself—are changed.

Take a Moment To . . .

Assess your self-esteem. Fill out the "Self-Esteem Checklist," developed by counseling psychologists Drs. Nancy and Donald Tubesing, who have published extensively in the field of stress-management education.

SELF-ESTEEM CHECKLIST

AA = ALMOST ALWAYS
O = OCCASIONALLLY
R = RARELY
N= NEVER

1) Do you find yourself bragging or exaggerating the importance of your role?	AA	O	R	N
2) Are you jealous of the possessions, opportunities or positions of others?	AA	O	R	N
3) Do you find yourself judging your behavior by other people's standards or expectations rather than your own?	AA	O	R	N
4) Are you possessive in your relationships with friends and/or family members?	AA	O	R	N
5) Is it difficult for you to acknowledge your own mistakes?	AA	O	R	N
6) Do you resort to bullying and intimidation in your dealings with others?	AA	O	R	N
7) Do you "put people down" so that you can feel "one up"?	AA	O	R	N
8) Are you a perfectionist?	AA	O	R	N
9) Must you be a "winner" in recreational activities in order to have fun?	AA	O	R	N
10) When faced with new opportunities do you feel inadequate or insecure?	AA	O	R	N
11) Do you have difficulty accepting compliments?	AA	O	R	N
12) Do you refrain from expressing your feelings and opinions?	AA	O	R	N
13) Do you shy away from trying new things for fear of failure or looking dumb?	AA	O	R	N
14) Do you neglect your own needs in order to respond to the needs of others?	AA	O	R	N

"ALMOST ALWAYS" or *"OFTEN"* answers to any of these questions may indicate that your level of self-esteem needs attention.

 ©1990 Nancy Loving Tubesing and Donald A Tubesing   Structured Exercises in Stress Management Vol 2 Pg 22

WHOLE PERSON PRESS   1702 East Jefferson Street   Duluth Minnesota 55812 218/728-6807

After reviewing your answers ask yourself the following questions:

1. Is my self-esteem high or low?

_____

_____

2. Is this a problem for me?

_____

_____

3. What can I do to increase my self-esteem?

_____

_____

ORIGINS OF SELF-ESTEEM

Many researchers and therapists believe that insecurity or low self-esteem begins with our family and is a product of our life experiences. Drs. Salvadore Maddi and Suzanne Kobasa, in their book *The Hardy Executive: Health Under Stress*, point to parent-child interactions that foster stress-hardiness. They examined the messages stress-hardy individuals received in their past and found:

- The emphasis was on reward, not punishment. This built commitment rather than alienation.
- The tasks they were given were moderate in difficulty and built feelings of control rather than feelings of powerlessness.
- They were encouraged to look at ongoing changes as full of possibilities, allowing them to feel challenged rather than threatened.

As Maddi and Kobasa have demonstrated, a sense of commitment, control, and challenge leads to a positive perception of stressful events. People with stress-hardy personalities work hard because they enjoy it, not because they are compulsively driven. Even if they don't like their jobs, they find something in them to which they can commit themselves. They make decisions and implement them because they view life as something they can construct. And they are enthusiastic about the future because the changes it will bring seem potentially worthwhile.

Take a Moment To . . .

Ask yourself:

Do you work hard because you enjoy it and are committed?

Do you make decisions and implement them because you view life as something you can construct?

Are you enthusiastic about the future because the changes it will bring seem potentially worthwhile and you see them as challenges, not threats?

If you did not receive stress-hardy messages in your past, you can still develop and add them to your lifestyle. What matters is what you decide to do. You can use the information and suggestions in this book to gain awareness, implement change, and foster growth.

WHAT'S YOUR STYLE?

Your ability to handle stress also depends on how you explain events to yourself (your explanatory style). Drs. Martin E. Seligman, Christopher Peterson, and George Vaillant have been conducting collaborative studies looking at explanatory style. They find that pessimists assign three personal reasons as the cause of a "bad" event: internal (blaming self), global (extending one incident into a general statement), and stable (assuming it can never change). Pessimists tend to think that bad events result from personal failings that are unalterable. Optimists tend to respond to disappointments by formulating a plan or asking others for help.

Dan's Experience

Dan, a corporate manager enrolled in one of our clinics, felt very stressed because an important staff meeting did not go well. He felt he was a "failure," his meeting went poorly because of his personal shortcomings. His reasoning was: "It's my fault; I'm a bad leader" (internal); "I always mess up everything" (global); "I'm always going to be like this" (stable).

We helped him to Stop, Take a Breath, Reflect, and realistically assess the situation. He was then able to see that while he had indeed made a mistake in the way he approached the meeting, he could put it in perspective and recognize the impact of other variables. The staff were on edge trying to meet a rushed deadline; instead of pulling together, they degenerated into petty behavior. Had he not felt personally responsible for these dynamics, he could have dealt with them more effectively.

Drs. Seligman, Vaillant, and Peterson have been tracking the lives and health of ninety-nine male Harvard graduates from 1945 to the present. One of the most interesting findings is that men who were generally optimistic in college are healthier in later life than those who were pessimists. By age forty-five, the pessimists began to have more health problems than their more positive-thinking classmates. Some theories associate a pessimistic attitude with a weakening of the immune system. Others have found that pessimists are more likely to adopt unhealthy behaviors, such as smoking, drinking excessively, and remaining sedentary.

Dr. Seligman argues that your explanatory style can be changed. In a recent study of depressed patients, he found that cognitive therapy changed the patients' style from pessimistic to optimistic. Once you recognize your explanatory style, you can change it, and research is proving it is worth the effort.

IMPROVING YOUR SELF-ESTEEM

The first step to improving your self-esteem is gaining an awareness of the origin of your current level. Insecurity and low self-esteem often begin when people in your life are quick to find fault, criticize easily, are all-knowing, and have difficulty showing love and affection.

You might want to think of your life as a bus with all the significant people from your past riding with you (your mother, father, brother, sister, aunts, uncles, teachers, coaches, friends, priest, minister, or rabbi). When messages from your past—"eat all the food on your plate," "you can't play until your work is finished," "you're going out dressed like that!" "you've got your head in the sand," and so forth—control your life, ask yourself:

- Who is driving the bus?
- Who is in control?
- Whom do I want to drive?

Taking control of the driver's seat means putting the messages in perspective, realizing that you are a child no longer and can make your own decisions, and then moving some of these people to the back of the bus. You may even want to let some or all of them off and never return to pick them up. It is your choice.

 Take a Moment To . . .

Complete the "Messages from My Past" worksheet.

After completing the worksheet, and reviewing what you have written, ask yourself:

1. Do I notice certain characteristics in these messages?

_____

_____

MESSAGES FROM MY PAST

The messages we have received from people who have been important in our lives contribute to our level of self-esteem. These messages can be positive or negative. In the space below, write the messages you recall receiving from people who have been important to you.

Examples

Mother – *"You're so rattle-brained! You'd lose your head if it weren't attached to the rest of you!"*
Father –*"That's my daughter — she can do just about anything she sets her mind to."*
Teacher –*"He's not the brightest kid, but he sure tries hard."*
Others –*"How are you going to get ahead if your head is always in the clouds?"*

My messages from

MOTHER:

FATHER:

SIBLINGS:

CLERGY:

FRIENDS:

TEACHERS:

COACH:

OTHERS:

©1990 Nancy Loving Tubesing and Donald A Tubesing Structured Exercises in Stress Management Vol 2 Pg 23

WHOLE PERSON PRESS   1702 East Jefferson Street   Duluth Minnesota 55812 218/728-6807

Reprinted with permission.

2. Do these messages describe me now?

_____

_____

3. Which ones do I value? Which ones could be eliminated?

_____

_____

4. Are there people on my bus I need to move to the back or drop off?

_____

_____

FURTHER SUGGESTIONS FOR IMPROVING SELF-ESTEEM

> You are not perfect, but parts of you are excellent.
> Ashleigh Brilliant, historian and author

If you are insecure, face the issue. Bringing it out into the open makes it possible for you to examine what needs to be done. For example, a successful corporate lawyer with significant coronary artery disease insisted he could not quit his stressful job because his family needed the income. Upon further examination, however, he discovered his self-esteem depended on his identity as a lawyer. If he quit his job, his sense of self-worth or security would be shattered.

Stop, Breathe, Reflect. "What are my 'silent assumptions' about myself? What steps must I take to challenge them?" Affirm to yourself that you count.

Everyone is entitled to their own opinion. Unless you decide their opinion is worth more than yours, no one can put you down.

Most of us think we are not physically attractive, not pretty enough, thin enough, our bodies are not in perfect shape. Just remember, mistakes and failures are normal. Sometimes you will need to forgive yourself for merely being human. As Dr. Burns points out:

> Even if you behave badly, it won't do much good to write yourself off as a "bad person." You will simply waste time and energy ruminating about how lousy and terrible you are. This will only incapacitate you and make the problem worse. In addition, this is very self-centered because you're entirely caught up in yourself! Genuine self-esteem is based on humility and an acceptance of your shortcomings. This makes it possible to assume responsibility for your actions, to feel remorse, to apologize and make amends, and to get on with productive and joyous living.

Make your own decisions, and trust yourself.

Reach for your highest potential. Changing your behavior, however, takes more than just well-meaning intentions. Old habits and ways of thinking about yourself will take time to change.

Set realistic goals and plug away—the battle is often uphill, but can be won. We have seen many patients in the Behavioral Medicine Clinic significantly transform their old thoughts and behaviors in ways they never would have thought possible.

Act and speak as if you are worthy of respect. You are.

HOW OUR ATTITUDES, MOODS, AND FEELINGS AFFECT OUR ABILITY TO COPE

If you are an anxious awfulizer plagued by global feelings of fear, you are interfering with your ability to "roll with the punches" and may experience increased physical symptoms and behaviors which are not healthy. Remember the Negative Stress Cycle.

Healthy self-esteem gives you the "hardiness" to greet stressful events as challenges to be met rather than as threats to be feared, which in turn begins the Negative Stress Cycle. If your self-esteem and sense of mastery are low, your ways of coping—behaviors that you use for protection against threat—will often be ineffective. When you cope effectively you can view life's challenges as ways to grow and learn. According to psychologists M. Robin DiMatteo and Howard S. Friedman, "Coping mediates the impact that stressors have on a person's health."

Even small changes in your thinking can profoundly improve your self-esteem and ability to cope. This subtle shift in thinking affects your attitude and can mean the difference between viewing yourself as stress-hardy versus helpless and hopeless. We see such changes every day here in the clinic. Chapter 13 discusses coping. Keep in mind how your thinking, and, therefore, your view of yourself in the world, affects your ability to entertain and risk new ways of coping with old problems.

The Negative Stress Cycle

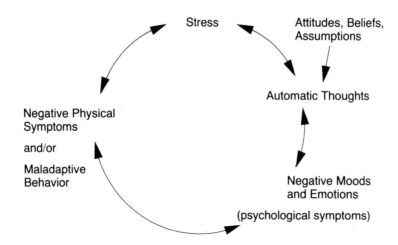

The exercise "Challenging Stress and Winning" appears at the end of this chapter. Please take the time to complete this exercise. Again, identify a situation that causes you stress, your physical response, your automatic thoughts, your irrational beliefs and behaviors. Pay particular attention to how you feel emotionally in the situation and whether your self-esteem is involved.

Carol L. Wells-Federman, M.Ed., R.N.
Ann Webster, Ph.D.
Eileen M. Stuart, R.N., M.S.

CHALLENGING STRESS AND WINNING
Stop, Take a Breath, Reflect

Situation	Physical Response	Automatic Thoughts	Moods and Emotions	Exaggerated Beliefs	Behavior
Briefly describe a situation that caused you stress this week.	Describe how you felt physically in this situation.	Write your automatic thoughts in this situation.	Describe how you felt emotionally in this situation.	Write down the exaggerated belief/cognitive distortion behind your automatic thoughts.	Describe how you behaved during or immediately after the situation.

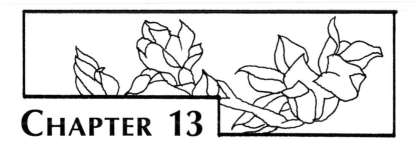

CHAPTER 13

COPING AND PROBLEM SOLVING

God grant me the serenity to accept things I cannot change, courage to change things I can, and wisdom to know the difference.

Reinhold Niebuhr, American theologian

In this chapter you will explore

- skills to deal more effectively with stress
- a variety of approaches to coping
- how to recognize the emotional hook and the practical problem when problem-solving

We introduced the concept of successful coping in chapter 10 when we described those individuals who possessed the characteristics of "stress hardiness." We said that people who (1) exercised, (2) had a good network of social support, and (3) possessed the characteristics of the "three C's" (challenge, commitment, and control) were more likely to be stress hardy and to feel that they were coping well. They were less likely to suffer from stress-related illnesses. Dr. Victor Frankl identified similar characteristics in survivors of the holocaust in his book *Man's Search for Meaning*. He described these "survivors" as individuals who had a sense of life-meaning and purpose. They had the ability to remain flexible and committed and to use a variety of coping techniques. These are important considerations to keep in mind as you begin to consider new, more effective ways to cope and solve problems.

In this chapter, we will provide you with specific exercises to help you to learn a variety of coping skills. These skills will build upon your basic beliefs regarding life-meaning and purpose. They should allow more variety and flexibility in the way you cope with stressful situations.

PRACTICAL PROBLEMS AND EMOTIONAL HOOKS

Stressful situations can be thought of as having two components: the practical problem and the emotional "hook." To illustrate this, let us look at the following scenario, which Mike, a forty-seven-year-old businessman who had had a recent heart attack, described one evening in the clinic.

> I was in the checkout line in the grocery store, worried about being on time to an important engagement, and someone cut in front of me. My response was instantaneous. My body reacted: my heart started racing, my muscles tensed, my chest tightened. My mind reacted: "Not fair, why me, ought not to, nerve of him, bad, late, awful, terrible!" Angrily, I declared, "Hey, don't you know that the line forms in the rear? What's the matter with you?" Even though the man moved to the rear of the line, I left the store feeling angry and upset, and still felt this way several hours later.

Mike's reaction is instantaneous, but exactly *what* is he reacting to? The practical problem is clear: he is running late and someone has just delayed him further. The emotional hook, however, is more subtle. The clinician had him Stop, Breathe, and Reflect on how his automatic thoughts, exaggerated beliefs, and distorted thinking contributed to his response. Mike found that he was really angry that this *inconsiderate* person, who *ought* to know better, cut in front of *him* when he was already pressed for time. To his surprise, he realized that the stress here was not so much time but his expectation about how other people should behave.

Mike's anger was not an effective way to cope, although it resolved the practical problem—the man moved to the back of the line and Mike was no longer inconvenienced or held up. So why was it not effective? Because the solution did not address the emotional hook, which was causing the real stress for him, and because several hours later Mike still felt angry, upset, and had a tightness in his chest. This type of physical response, as you know, can have a deleterious effect on health if it occurs regularly. It is the chronic, excessive exposure to stress which is associated with stress-related symptoms and illnesses. For these reasons, exploring strategies to deal effectively with stress is important to your health.

In the clinic that evening, we took Mike through a series of questions to help him develop a less stressful strategy for coping. As you read Mike's answers, think about how you might respond in a similar situation.

Define the problem to be solved.

- I am late to something which is important to me.
- I need the man who cut in front of me to take his proper place behind me.

Define the emotional hook.

- He's inconsiderate.
- He should know better.
- I'll never be on time.
- Why does this always happen to me?

The emotional hook is all of the automatic thoughts—shoulds, nevers, alwayses, musts, and oughts—that often not only make the practical problem worse, but keep us from seeing solutions.

What are some possible solutions? Consider all possibilities.

- Tell him to go to the end of the line.
- Ask him to go to the end of the line.
- Let him know in no uncertain terms that I am annoyed with his inconsiderate, irresponsible behavior.
- Get the cashier to tell him to move.
- Ignore the situation.
- Call my appointment and tell them I will be late.

List the pros and cons for all the possible solutions.

Which seems to be the most practical and desirable solution? The solution Mike chose as most desirable was "Ask him to go to the end of the line."

Pros: He moves and I am not late.

Cons: I won't have the satisfaction of telling him how rude he is.

Try the most acceptable and feasible solution. Allow yourself to be flexible.

Several weeks later Mike reported that in a similar situation, he had asked a man to move—and he did. Mike Stopped, Took a Breath, Reflected, and Chose how he wanted to respond. He asserted himself without getting caught up in shoulds, oughts, and musts. Because he *chose* how he wanted to act, Mike left the store, and the situation behind. This response was unusual for him, and he was pleasantly surprised that it worked without the accompanying physical and emotional arousal.

In essence, Mike separated the practical problem (having the man move so he would not be late) from the emotional hook (all the feelings he had about the man, his behavior, and its implications of disrespect for Mike), and Mike *chose* how he wanted to respond.

In this case, Mike decided that the real issue was the practical problem of being late and that his feelings about the man needed no action beyond recognition. In other stressful situations, the emotional hook is the primary issue and the practical problem is incidental. Successful coping addresses both components.

Take a Moment To . . .

Imagine yourself in the shopping line. Someone cuts in front of you. How would your react? Would you get caught by the emotional hook?

_____

_____

_____

If so, how would you deal with the emotional hook?

_____

_____

_____

What practical steps could you take?

_____

_____

_____

COPING AND PROBLEM-SOLVING SKILLS

Many techniques can be used to cope with stressful situations. Work to develop a variety of coping strategies, because what works in one situation may not work in another. Above all, remember that coping is the art of finding a balance between acceptance and action, of letting go and taking control.

If you feel that you can cope in a stressful situation, this minimizes or buffers the harmful effects of stress. You no longer feel threatened but simply challenged, and this has a different physiological effect. The experience which you are gaining by regularly eliciting the relaxation response gives you the skills to distance yourself from automatic thoughts, exaggerated beliefs, or distorted thinking, and to *choose* how you want to respond. The following skills provide a variety of coping strategies from which to choose. Careful thought needs to be given to each situation in order to choose the most effective technique.

Distraction.

Put aside a problem or stress until it can be dealt with more effectively. We call this the Scarlett O'Hara of coping techniques—"I'll think of it all tomorrow." For example, the stress created by a delayed flight might be handled with a good magazine. Or, if you are ready to confront an issue with someone, and they are not, it might be more effective to wait until tomorrow.

Used properly, this technique is not procrastination, which puts off confronting an issue because delay is easier than dealing with it.

Direct action.

Just do it! Acting directly on the problem can mean, for example, changing a behavior (such as stopping smoking or starting an exercise program), confronting a problem, changing an environment, connecting with friends, or volunteering, to name just a few. Witness the power of direct action in the book *Feel the Fear and Do It Anyway.*

However, just as fear of action can be self-limiting, acting without discrimination can be just as limiting. Consider the situation of being angry with a friend and wanting to hash out the problem immediately (direct action). Your friend is upset and not ready to resolve the issue right now. In this case, insisting on direct action is ineffective and premature, even if it is your preferred coping style. Pausing to Stop, Breathe, and Reflect often allows you to see possibilities differently from whatever you are most accustomed to.

Pro and con list.

Another way to take a different perspective on a problem is to list the pros and cons of possible solutions. For instance, after fighting over whose family they would share the Easter holidays with, John and Mary were so angry they were not speaking to each other. To deal with this standoff, Mary made a pro and con list of possible solutions. She could persist in her anger and let it escalate, refuse to see her husband's point of view (making him angrier), or refuse to go anywhere that day. However, they could also compromise and have both sets of parents at their own house, visit both families briefly that day, or go to mutual friends. By creating this list, Mary saw that she had some options. She was able to discuss the problem calmly, and they both agreed to have all the parents at their house.

Relaxation.

When you feel stressed, do something you enjoy or find relaxing. At the end of a busy day, for example, you might take a moment to elicit the relaxation response or go for a run before settling into the evening. Studies have shown that individuals who take time to play, laugh, and relax are, in fact, more productive and content.

Reframing.

Sometimes called *situational redefinition,* reframing is the ability to look at an event from a different perspective. The classic example is a glass filled to midway: is it half full or half empty? In describing a failed project, a patient who had originally been very stressed by "failure" reframed the experience with the familiar saying:

I'm not a failure if I don't succeed . . . I'm a success because I tried.

Looking at the situation in this way, he no longer felt bad, and he was free to reexamine the project for possible new solutions.

Affirmations.

> Nothing erases unpleasant thoughts more effectively than concentration on pleasant ones.
>
> Hans Selye, M.D., stress researcher

An affirmation is simply a positive thought, a short phrase or saying that has meaning for you. It can be a common adage such as "One day at a time," or something that specifically addresses your life. You can create your own affirmation, using these guidelines:

Creating Affirmations

- Select an aspect of your life that is causing you stress.
- Decide what you want to have happen or how you would like to feel in a situation.
- Articulate this goal as a first-person statement: "I can have a relaxed body and a focused mind" or "I am confident in my work."
- Always state affirmations in the present.
- Always phrase affirmations in the positive.
- Repeat the affirmation to yourself and notice how it feels.
- Repeat your affirmation often during the day, perhaps before or after eliciting the relaxation response, or as part of a breathing exercise.

An especially effective time to use affirmations is immediately after eliciting the relaxation response; when your mind is quiet, you are more receptive. Some people write their affirmations on a card and keep it in a conspicuous place—on a mirror or on their desk at work. If advertising works on us, why not use the same techniques to improve the inner environment of our minds! Some examples of affirmations are:

- "I can handle it."
- "I accept myself as I am."
- "I am peaceful."
- "I am becoming healthy and strong."
- "I would rather be happy than always right."
- "Let it be."
- "I am finding the best job for me."
- "I am doing the best I can."

Using affirmations is an effective tool for reframing negative self-talk into a positive message, thus reducing the stress born of undermining thoughts. In a short time affirmations become second nature.

> Assume a virtue, if you have it not.
> That monster custom . . . is angel yet in this. . . .
> For use almost can change the stamp of nature,
> And either master the devil, or throw him out
> With wondrous potency.
>
> Shakespeare, *Hamlet*

Social support.

Family, friends, coworkers, and professionals can be a supportive network during times of stress. Talking out your problems is beneficial. Not only do you get to let off steam, but you also hear different perspectives from others. In one study, employees with a network for social support had less incidence of minor illness and absenteeism. Another study, done in Sweden, found that individuals with strong social support had less heart disease.

Spirituality.

Call on your personal belief system. Some people describe this as fundamental to their coping with daily hassles as well as life crises. In chapter 5, we discussed how a personal belief system could be used to elicit the relaxation response and how eliciting the relaxation response enhances spirituality.

Catharsis.

Find a form of emotional release. Sometimes a good cry—or laugh—will release emotional energy and can be a good cure for a stressful situation.

Journal writing.

Keeping a journal or diary of your thoughts and feelings is another way to cope with stress. Write things down and get them off your chest. Dr. James Pennebaker, a psychologist in Texas, has found that writing in order to get in touch with our deepest thoughts and feelings can measurably improve physical and mental health. We suggest getting a special notebook and colorful pens for your journal. Write about those things that cause you stress, and see if this helps you find another perspective. But write about life's pleasures, too.

Acceptance.

We opened this chapter with the words of Reinhold Niebuhr describing the "serenity to accept things I cannot change" (acceptance), "courage to change things I can" (direct action), "and wisdom to know the difference."

Successful coping is a matter of the wisdom to achieve the delicate balance between acceptance and action, of letting go and taking control. It is also the art of choosing the right strategy at the right time. At times it is neither wise nor possible to act immediately in the face of stress. In such cases, distraction, relaxation, humor, or acceptance may be most effective until the situation allows you to act directly. There are also times when distraction is ineffective, when you need to act directly. You would not say "I'll think of it all tomorrow" when your house is burning down. Each coping strategy is effective in some situations and ineffective in others. Successful coping depends on your taking the time to: Stop, Breathe, Reflect on your automatic thoughts, beliefs, attitudes, and assumptions, and Choose the most appropriate coping strategy for that situation. Unfortunately, there is no universal strategy or cure for stress.

As you read about various techniques for coping, did you find a style that seemed familiar to you? Often we tend to use one style consistently, whether or not it works! The next time you encounter a stress, experiment with a different coping strategy and see what happens.

To increase your skills for effective coping and problem-solving, *each time you encounter a stressful situation,* apply the four-step model we have been building upon.

Stop

Breathe
- Release physical tension.
- Use your breath and relaxation-response techniques to stop your automatic reactions.

Reflect
- Appraise the situation.
- What is the concern?
- What are your automatic thoughts and exaggerated beliefs?
- What is the emotional hook?
- What is the practical problem?
- Am I threatened?
- Am I exaggerating this stress through negative thinking?

Choose
- What do I want?
- What can I do, what coping techniques would work here?
- Do I have the time, skills, and personal investment to achieve a practical solution?
- Do I need to temper my emotional response before I can act responsively, practically, and appropriately?
- Am I avoiding the best solution because it will be difficult for me?
- What is possible?
- What is my decision?

Now do it!

Sally's Experience

Sally, a fifty-year-old insurance agent with irritable bowel syndrome, was asked to take on some new responsibilities when a colleague abruptly quit. Sally was flattered and pleased, and she worked hard to accommodate the additional tasks. When it was time for her annual review, she was rated Above Average, but no mention was made of her new responsibilities. Worse, her boss had checked the box saying "Job description appropriate."

Sally reacted immediately. Her stomach churned, her heart raced, she felt hurt, angry, and sick. She left the meeting saying nothing, but she raged over the injustice all day.

Later, she was able to apply the four-step approach to coping that she had learned in our Behavioral Medicine Clinic. She Stopped and Took a Breath. In this way she was able to elicit the relaxation response, release physical tension, and halt the cascade of awfulizing thoughts.

The next step was to Reflect or appraise the situation: What is the concern? what are my automatic thoughts and exaggerated beliefs? Her automatic thoughts poured out: "Not fair, no respect, worked hard; again, why me, always me?" She realized her expectation was that if she worked hard she would *always* be respected, rewarded, and treated fairly by *all* people. Note: the key here is the *always* (degree), not the belief itself.

Now she was ready to Choose: what do I want? what can I do? what is possible? what is my decision? Sally remembered the two components of stress. The emotional hook required that she confront her expectations of her boss and discuss with him what she perceived as his lack of respect for her as a person and her contributions to the company. The practical problem was the need to redefine her responsibilities in order to acquire formal authority and respect as well as financial reward.

She decided to request a meeting with her boss the next day. She prepared her arguments carefully (direct action), redefined the experience as an opportunity and learning experience (reframing), sought support from coworkers and family (social support), took a long run the evening before (distraction/relaxation), and decided to let go of a sense of personal injury (acceptance). As the plan took form, her stomach pain began to subside, and she felt less angry and hurt.

The meeting was a success: Sally was well prepared and calm, and her boss readily agreed with her. In fact, he spent most of the meeting talking about how he was so overwhelmed that he couldn't keep track of everything that was going on. She got the new job description, the raise, and she felt great about herself.

Sally told the group that this was a very different way of coping for her. In the past she would have said nothing and been sick for a week. She was very pleased with her new approach and the positive outcome for her.

In Sally's story you can see that successful coping includes both emotional and practical aspects. It involves the ability to use a variety of coping techniques and also requires the ability to be flexible and willing to try new ways.

Richard's Experience

Richard, thirty, had been diagnosed with brain cancer shortly after moving to Boston to enter a doctoral program. While he was completing a rigorous course of chemotherapy his wife divorced him, and he could attend classes only part-time. He joined our Behavioral Medicine Cancer Program three months after he was diagnosed.

After five clinic sessions, in which he learned to elicit the relaxation response, use visual imagery, perform goal-setting exercises, and use basic cognitive-restructuring techniques, he came to the group and reported that he needed to resume chemotherapy because of a recurrence of his cancer. Depressed and defeated, he said, "This wouldn't have happened if I had done more." The group encouraged him, telling him what an inspiration he had been to them, given the seriousness of his experience and his ability to maintain such a positive attitude throughout.

After leaving the group that evening, he Stopped, Took a Breath, and Reflected on all the positive things he had done for himself already. He had accepted his diagnosis but retained a fighting spirit for those things he could fight. He had thoroughly investigated all of his treatment options and become involved in the decision-making about his treatment plan (direct action). He had returned to his exercise program and enrolled in a gourmet cooking course—he decided that if he was going to be single, at least he would eat well (humor)! He joined a Bible class which gave him a source of support. He also returned to writing and playing music (distraction and relaxation) and gave a concert for children at a Christmas party (social support and altruism).

After reviewing his accomplishments, Richard realized that he had indeed been successful in coping with his initial diagnosis. He *chose* to view the recurrence as one more challenge and felt confident he could succeed again. His daily affirmation was "I got through this successfully before, I can do it again." He reached out for support from his fellow group members by asking them to visit him when he was in the hospital for his next series of treatments. He completed the treatments with minimal side effects and returned to the seventh clinic session feeling encouraged and with a greater feeling of control.

At the final session of the cancer program, he brought his guitar and played a song that he had written and composed. The lyrics inspired us, as we hope they will you.

I'm Living for the Day

Sometimes I can't believe
the way I've led my life,
so preoccupied with things from day to day.

It felt like life was just a problem
from one minute to the next.
Why did they always seem to come my way?

But now I'm living,
living for the moment.
Won't let a minute, an hour, a day
pass me by.
There's no time like now
to do the things we wish we'd done.
That is why
I'm living for the day.

If I had only known
just a short while ago,
the problems that I had were oh so small.
If I had stopped for just a minute,
maybe then I'd have seen
there really was no problem at all.

At least now I've begun
to realize
that things like worry, hate, and guilt
do not belong
'cause every precious moment
is like a gift from God.
You've got to make the most of every single one.
I have to see it as a challenge,
a race where I'm in control.
You gotta take the reins and
hold them tightly in your hands.
I've heard it said you can do
the things you set your mind to do.
How was I to know if it was true?

If there was just one thing I could say to you,
you can't have thoughts
of how and what you didn't try.
So why not grab the moment when you've got so much
to lose,
and no one else but you to answer why.

But now I'm living,
living for the moment.
Won't let a minute, an hour, a day
pass me by.
There's no time like now
to do the things we wish we'd done.
That is why
I'm living for the day.

Richard Fennell

Richard's experience is uplifting and educational. He made use of a variety of coping strategies, and most importantly, he did not hesitate to reach out for support.

Take a Moment To . . .

Stress busters are the resources and tools available to you in stressful situations and that keep you healthy, relaxed, and strong. As a reaffirmation of your own abilities, list your own stress busters below:

Stress Busters

1. The skills and strategies I use to manage my stress:_____

_____

_____

_____

2. Experiences in my past that helped me learn about myself:_____

_____

_____

_____

3. Values & beliefs that nurture me:_____

_____

_____

_____

4. The daily activities that support my healthy lifestyle:_____

_____

_____

_____

5. People who support me:_____

_____

_____

_____

THE HELP AROUND YOU

> Only connect! . . . Only connect the prose and the passion, and both will
> be exalted, and human love will be seen at its height. Live in fragments
> no longer.
>
> E. M. Forster, *Howards End*

Another aspect of coping is to recognize and use the support and help
around you. You may have very strong positive beliefs—spiritual or
intellectual—that form the basis for your personal strength. You may gain
perspective from the arts—literature, music, theater, dance. You may have
strong family support, or significant support from longtime co-workers and
friends. Sometimes it makes sense to seek professional help from counselors,
social workers, or therapists. You will gain strength if you can recognize these
supports and begin to use them.

CREATIVE THINKING

> The problems that exist in the world cannot be solved by the level of
> thinking that created them.
>
> Albert Einstein

Creative thinking can be a great asset in effective coping and problem-
solving. Through cognitive restructuring and eliciting the relaxation response,
you have learned to disengage from a conditioned and distressing chain of
thought. Now the object is to engage your imaginative and intuitive resources
as a way of strengthening and enhancing your mental freedom.

When you elicit the relaxation response, your creative abilities are enhanced. You look at the world differently—with a fresh perspective. You can
strengthen this new perspective by using these tools:

- Belief in your ability to think creatively. Be aware that you can
  consciously call on your creativity to solve problems or develop
  new ideas.
- Absence of judgment. Recognize the negative thoughts and self-
  judgments that interfere with your creative abilities.
- Observation. Become aware of the "observing self," the part that
  takes over when you open the door to creative thinking. Eliciting
  the relaxation response allows you to become more open and
  aware of new possibilities and new paradigms for solving problems.

• Questioning. Creativity begins with questioning, not with defining expectations or narrowing possibilities.

The goal is to allow creative thinking to break through negative, unproductive thought patterns and to open the door to new possibilities. When you practice the relaxation response and the methods of cognitive restructuring, you will begin to see a change in your patterns of thinking. Gradually, new patterns will displace the old as creative, positive thinking becomes more natural to you.

Before moving on to the next chapter, stop and complete the exercise "Challenging Stress and Winning," on pages 244–45. In addition to identifying stressors, physical response, automatic thoughts, and irrational beliefs, you now have the opportunity to envision a more effective response. You may be surprised at how creative and innovative you can be.

Eileen M. Stuart, R.N., M.S.
Ann Webster, Ph.D.
Carol L. Wells-Federman, R.N., M.Ed.

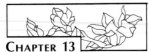
Situation	Physical Response	Automatic Thoughts	Moods and Emotions
Briefly describe a situation that caused you stress this week.	Describe how you felt physically in this situation.	Write your automatic thoughts in this situation.	Describe how you felt emotionally in this situation.

(continuation)

Exaggerated Beliefs Write down the exaggerated beliefs behind your automatic thoughts.	*Behavior* Describe how you behaved during or immediately after the situation.	*More Effective Response* Describe how you might think or act differently that would help you cope more effectively.	*Potential Outcome* Describe how this might make you feel and behave.

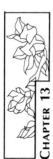

SAMPLE
STRESS MANAGEMENT
HEALTH COMMITMENT

Long-Term Goal:
To manage the stress in my life efficiently and effectively

_____
Signature

_____
Witness

Expected Date of Reaching Goal: _____

Readiness to Change	Short-Term Goals	Comments (supports, rewards, etc.)
Never considered change; need information.	1. Read chapters 11–15 in _The Wellness Workbook_ to identify all the factors that could be contributing to stress and distress. 2. Attend a lecture on "How Stress Can Affect Our Lives and Our Physical/Mental Health."	
Considered change, but not yet committed.	1. Identify my particular stressors. Can I avoid them? Do I create or contribute to them? 2. Make a list of stress warning signs (physical and psychological signs of distress).	

(continued)

Readiness to Change	Short-Term Goals	Comments (supports, rewards, etc.)
Desire change; need motivation.	1. Take fifteen minutes: imagine what life would be like without daily hassles, worries, and constant change. 2. Find a friend who has successfully managed stress and inquire about what worked and what didn't.	
Attempting change; need structure, support, and skills.	1. Elicit the relaxation response daily and use mini-relaxation responses throughout the day whenever I experience stress warning signs. 2. Participate in a stress management course.	
Change made; need reinforcement.	1. List the positive changes, e.g., decreased symptoms, increased energy, since beginning to manage stress in my life. 2. Keep a diary. Document those times I've managed stress effectively. Identify what I was thinking/feeling. What direct action did I take and what was the outcome?	
Change made; slipping back into bad habits, need renewed motivation and support.	1. Elicit the support of friends to remind me to Stop, Take a Breath, and Reflect. Choose a plan of action whenever this happens. 2. Teach a friend how to elicit the relaxation response. Inform him/her of benefits.	

247

STRESS MANAGEMENT
HEALTH COMMITMENT

Long-Term Goal:

_____

_____ Signature

_____

_____ Witness

Expected Date of Reaching Goal: _____

Short-Term Goals

Comments (supports, rewards, etc.)

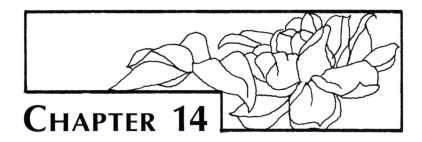

CHAPTER 14

COMMUNICATING

Do not find fault before making thorough inquiry;
first reflect, then give a reprimand. Listen before you
answer, and do not interrupt a speech in the middle.
   Do not wrangle about something that does not concern you, nor interfere in the squabbles of sinners.

Ecclesiasticus 18:13

In this chapter you will explore decreasing stress by

- improving your self-esteem and your relationships
- expressing your likes and dislikes, accepting compliments, saying
  how you feel, and asking for what you need
- expressing yourself in open, honest, and appropriate ways
- acting out of choice
- becoming aware of your nonverbal communication

Communicating, the process by which information is exchanged between
individuals, powerfully influences our lives. Effective communication is important in avoiding stressful situations, as well as in resolving situations once they
arise. An amazing amount of stress can be eliminated from your life if you
examine how you communicate with people around you. The way you communicate and how people respond to you is rooted in and also affects self-
esteem.

Communication is verbal. It is what you say and how you say it. Communication is also how you listen, hear, and understand.

Communication is also nonverbal. Your body language, eye contact, and
your actions are powerful components of communication. Remember, "Actions speak louder than words."

The way you communicate affects the way others respond to you. Effective communication is usually open, honest, and appropriate; it enhances self-esteem, nurtures relationships, and helps in coping with stressful situations. Ineffective communication blames, denies, and attacks, injuring self-esteem, to say nothing of relationships, and can actually increase the stress in your life.

Effective communication is assertive, which simply means you speak and act from choice. It is the ability to separate the issue from the person. If you Stop, Take a Breath, Reflect, and then Choose how you wish to proceed, you can communicate in a directed, assertive manner. You may choose to take direct action, or you may try other ways to cope, but the choice comes from a calm center and is directed toward resolution of the problem. It is not controlled by automatic emotional reactions—the emotional hook. When we get caught in the hook, our verbal and nonverbal communication often turns negative and attacking. We then tend to speak and act either passively or aggressively.

More often than not, an aggressive person is caught by the emotional hook, although sincerely believing that he or she is constructively facing the practical problem. Aggressive responses come from automatic reactions and often read as "I count, you don't count." Passive responses, which are also automatic reactions, often sound like "I don't count, you do."

Assertive responses are arrived at by choice. They take into account the situation, as well as the person to be communicated with. They are open, honest, and appropriate. Assertive communication usually reflects a tone of "I count and you count."

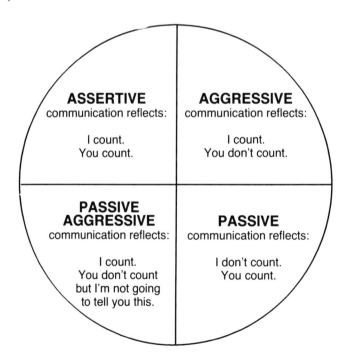

At the Behavioral Medicine Clinic, we have found that helping patients with stress-management problems usually means working with them to improve their communication skills. Dr. David D. Burns ascribes two "properties" to effective communication: "You express your feelings openly and directly and you encourage the other person to express his or her feelings." People hooked on the emotion often feel vulnerable and refuse to share their feelings openly or listen to what the other person has to say. When you feel communication is being hampered by emotion, use the four-step model:

- Stop
- Breathe
- Reflect and look for your emotional hook.
    Am I responding to the real problem or my irrational belief/ distorted thought?
    Do I need to "win" this conversation?
    Am I afraid to show any sign of weakness?
    Do I feel compelled to tell this person how wrong they are and set them straight?
- Choose how you want to respond.

Ultimately, effective communication reflects your ability to act out of choice and helps you deal with difficult situations by letting you express feelings without losing control of them.

One caveat. Being an effective communicator does not mean always being in control or always answering correctly and without emotion. That would be just another trap—the need to be perfect. We all have faults, self-doubts, and moments of sensitivity. These times, however, are often the impetus for growth and understanding.

Any change in the way you have been behaving and communicating is a challenge that must be met with genuine commitment to the task and forgiveness when you stumble. Keep trying and keep practicing. This will enable you to eventually replace old patterns with new, more effective ways of behaving and communicating.

EXPRESSING YOURSELF

Self-expression—when it is open, honest, and appropriate—usually feels good to you and the other person. Effective communication means that you can express your likes and dislikes, accept a compliment, know when to say yes and when to say no. It also means you say how you feel when it is appropriate, you ask for what you need, and usually keep your word.

Take a Moment To . . .

Reflect on the times when self-expression seemed easy and comfortable to you.

In what situations is it easy to express yourself openly, honestly, and appropriately (work, home, play)? Be specific.

_____

_____

_____

_____

With whom do you find it easy to express yourself openly, honestly, and appropriately (spouse, child, boss, colleague, friend, parent, etc.)? Be specific.

_____

_____

_____

_____

Communication Strengths
Check the areas in which you feel confident.
I can

_____ usually express myself in an open, honest, and appropriate way with most people.

_____ express my likes and dislikes easily.

_____ comfortably accept compliments.

_____ comfortably disagree with someone.

_____ say no.

Congratulations on all the ones you checked! What about the ones you did not check? Need some help? Read on.

When is it difficult to express yourself appropriately? When do you become angry or hostile? blame yourself or others? deny your feelings or theirs? Be specific.

_____

_____

_____

_____

In what situations do you have the most difficulty expressing yourself openly, honestly, and appropriately (work, home, play)? Be specific.

_____

_____

_____

_____

With whom do you have the most difficulty expressing yourself openly, honestly, and appropriately (spouse, child, boss, colleague, friend, parent, etc.)? Be specific.

_____

_____

_____

_____

Difficult communications often result from or are caused by disagreements or conflicts, especially with those you feel close to. Conflicts usually arise because of the differences in expectation or from insecurity that generates a need to "win" to boost self-esteem. Your ability to communicate is impeded when you feel threatened, hurt, or vulnerable.

As we have been discussing, the way you perceive a situation will affect the way you respond to the situation. If you feel threatened, hurt, or vulnerable in response to a stress, the fight-or-flight response is activated. You may feel anxious, nervous or tense. Your heart rate may increase, your blood pressure may go up, your breathing may become shallow and more rapid. As depicted in the following diagram, your response to a stressful situation is based on

The Negative Stress Cycle

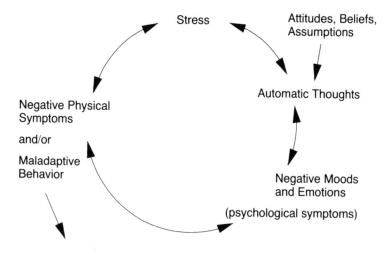

attitudes, beliefs, and assumptions underlying your automatic thoughts which, in turn, can cause negative moods and emotions, negative physical symptoms, and maladaptive behavior. This maladaptive behavior can manifest itself as ineffective communication.

Perceiving a situation as threatening because of your irrational beliefs or distorted thinking can lead to a communication battle. For example, if you think another person is wrong and your thoughts are distorted by all-or-nothing thinking, your communication will be geared toward having to "win" the argument. Becoming hooked by "I'm right, you're wrong" interferes with your ability to hear what is being said and prevents you from dealing with the practical aspects of the issue that need to be resolved. This type of communication pattern is ineffective and actually creates more stress.

EFFECTIVE COMMUNICATION

To help patients with ineffective communication and coping we teach several communication techniques that address the most common problems.

Just say "Thank you."

Someone compliments you on a job well done, which you worked hard on, and without hesitation you say, "Oh, it was nothing." Sound familiar? Do you have problems accepting compliments? You somehow have developed the idea that self-denigration is the polite response. Is it? Stop and reflect.

Discomfort with compliments often reveals low self-esteem or self-worth. Is your automatic, knee-jerk response "I don't deserve a compliment"? Does it feel awkward to have been noticed? Deflecting a compliment can be a double-edged sword because it often draws more attention than if you just said "Thank you." It belittles the other person's taste as well as yours!

The reason we address the inability to accept a compliment first is that the problem is very common and often easy to correct. The week's "homework" we assign to clinic patients with this problem is simply to say "Thank you" to any compliment they receive. The second part of the assignment is to become aware of how that makes them feel. The third part is to observe the reaction of the other person.

At the next clinic session, most patients describe how good just saying "Thank you" feels, even if it is a little awkward to master at first. They also report that the reaction of the compliment-giver is usually a smile.

Could you be better at saying "Thank you" when complimented?

Take a Moment To . . .

Reflect back on receiving a compliment this week:

• How did it make you feel?

- How did you respond?
- How did the person who gave the compliment respond?
- Next time you receive a compliment, Stop, Take a Breath (savor the moment), and say "Thank you."
- Keep practicing; if you say it long enough you will believe it (as with affirmations). As Hamlet says, "Assume a virtue, if you have it not," and soon that virtue becomes "a kind of easiness."

Look for the Win-Win solution.

Do you tend to believe you are right and the other person is wrong, or to blame the other person for the situation? Such thinking reflects the "I count, you don't" attitude and forces both of you to defend yourselves and your own turf. This is counterproductive and creates more stress than it resolves.

John's Experience

John, a forty-seven-year-old editor at a local publishing house, enrolled in our Mind/Body Clinic for lower-back pain, was having problems with his sixteen-year-old son. They regularly got into arguments and disagreements over housekeeping chores that would quickly escalate until one of them (usually the son) would storm out of the house, leaving many bad feelings.

John recounted how, three weeks ago, the son agreed to put out the rubbish every Thursday evening. Since that time, however, the son had "forgotten" each week.

The conversation the next morning at breakfast:

JOHN: You're totally unreliable! You said you'd put out the rubbish one night a week and you've forgotten three weeks in a row! You make me so angry. I can't count on you for anything! You never clean your room either. You're always doing this."

SON: "Dad, you're always after me about something. I can never please you. What's the big deal about the rubbish, anyway?"

And on and on until John's son stormed out of the house.

What went wrong? How could John have resolved this problem so that the son would understand he meant business, but without escalating a transgression into a war?

Dr. Donald Meichenbaum refers to this escalation as "kitchen sinking." This is our tendency to bring in past material that doesn't even relate to the present problem.

For a Win-Win communication, remember:

If you must resolve a problem, do so immediately: The next morning was too late, and certainly three weeks should not have gone by before John called for a discussion. Be specific about what the person did, stick to the problem or behavior, and discuss the issue as soon as possible.

Acknowledge and express your feelings: John could not acknowledge his own anger and frustration and instead blamed his son ("You make me so angry"). Do you express your feelings openly, honestly, and appropriately? Do you own the feelings as your own? Do you say you are angry, hurt, or sad when you are? Do you think it wrong to have those feelings in difficult situations? Somewhere in your past you may have learned that having or expressing feelings is inappropriate.

Reflect on your emotions and behavior during a disagreement. Are you angry or nervous? Are your muscles tight? Is your stomach in knots? Reflect on your automatic thoughts, irrational beliefs, and distorted thinking style. Where is your anger coming from? Do you also suffer by believing that having these feelings makes you imperfect, vulnerable, or weak; do you want to deny them quickly?

As discussed in chapter 12, "Feelings, Moods, and Attitudes," having a wide range of emotions and feelings is healthy. What is important is to express these feelings appropriately and not become trapped by negative moods or emotional hooks. Anger can be appropriate as long as you take responsibility for your feelings and reactions. Recognize that no one can make you angry. You can, however, feel angry when someone is rude or irresponsible.

Use "I" statements rather than "You" statements. This is an effective format for expressing your feelings, opinions, and beliefs. The premise is that you have stopped and reflected on what these feelings, opinions, and beliefs truly are. Instead of starting the reprimand with a confrontational "you," John could have started with a matter-of-fact "I" statement, for instance: "*I feel* angry *when you* forget to take out the rubbish *because* we had an agreement and I expect you to keep your word."

This is an assertive statement that expresses your feelings and opinions, reaffirms your identity and rights, and establishes the reason and immediacy of the subject. It begins with your emotional state up front, identifies the specific behavior in question, and finishes with an expression of your views. Assertive communication is not judgmental; you are merely expressing your views about a specific subject (I count, you count).

The general format is:

>   I feel (emotion)
>   when you (the behavior)
>   because (your explanation)

Reaffirm the person: John needs to let his son know that he disapproves of the behavior, not his son. Be sure to let the other person know you value him. Separate the person from the act and stick to dealing with the problem. You need to communicate forgiveness. We all need to know we have been forgiven for our mistakes and shortcomings. All too often this is not communicated, and people (especially children) go away feeling that they are bad, will "always" be like this, will "never" learn, and are unworthy individuals. These thoughts and feelings promote insecurity and low self-esteem.

If you are open and honest in communicating your feelings and able to acknowledge the person when it is over, you are more likely to have a Win-Win communication, avoiding conflict and the subsequent physical symptoms. You may also be nurturing a greater sense of security and self-esteem.

One final caution: When it's over, it's over! Resist bringing up past transgressions and mistakes. Stick to the current problem or situation and deal with that.

Stop, Breathe, Reflect on your feelings, opinions, and beliefs in a certain situation; Choose how you want to respond. To have a Win-Win communication, sometimes you must ask yourself "Would I rather be right, or would I rather be happy?"

Say what you need and be specific. Know your intent.

Do you play the mind-reader game? Do you use "vague" language, hoping the other person will know what you need or want without having to say it? That way you avoid being rejected or having to hear the word *No*. When people cannot read your mind or anticipate what you need, you become resentful and blaming, usually because of your belief that others "should" know what your needs and wants are.

Barbara's Experience

Barbara, thirty-eight and married, suffers from tension headaches. Now that her three children are teenagers, she has decided to return to nursing school.

At the clinic she shared with the group that her family was not "cooperating" now that she was in school. She had sat down with them before the semester began and explained that she understood this would be a change for the whole family. She would not be at home as much and would need their cooperation and help with household chores. At the time they readily agreed to help, but, as situations came up, they had not followed through.

Anger and frustration were evident when Barbara described how they had not gotten the groceries, done the dishes, made their beds, or taken out the garbage according to their agreement. They ended up arguing a lot, and her tension headaches were interfering with her ability to study.

What went wrong? We asked Barbara for her automatic thoughts. On reflection, Barbara said her thoughts were: "My family should know what needs to be done and not have to be told each time. They don't care about me, don't support my going back to school, don't love me. I've done so much for them—why can't they do for me? I've sacrificed so much—why can't I have my turn? They're selfish. I've failed as a mother. I've failed . . ."

We then asked Barbara to identify the practical problem. She stated simply that she needed help with specific tasks at home.

Making a vague request such as "Will you cooperate, help, or support me?" almost certainly prevents being rejected. It also, however, forces you to rely on others' anticipating what you need and want and makes others responsible for your happiness. When you want cooperation, help, and support, specify what that means to you unless you have mind readers in your family. You must take responsibility for being specific and asking for what you need. By doing so, however, you risk hearing *No*. Then you must remember they are rejecting the task, not you. Negotiate.

Further, don't mix apples and oranges. Because they say no or do not follow through, don't assume they are bad or don't love you. Perhaps they did not understand the ground rules. Perhaps they are busy with their own priorities. Perhaps they forgot. Perhaps . . . By finding out why they acted a certain way, without being hooked by the emotions, you are freer to explore alternatives and resolve the problem.

Barbara's Experience (continued)

Barbara's homework assignment was to reconvene the family conference. She would identify specific tasks she needed help with and present what she felt was a fair and equitable division of labor—prepared beforehand. She would compromise when necessary. We also suggested that a few reminders might be necessary since behaviors are hard to change (as she was well aware). With some gentle coaching, both she and her family developed a Win-Win situation. Barbara was able to get the help she needed, the children felt good about their value in the household, and her headaches were much less frequent and no longer interfered with her studies.

Sometimes you may have trouble asking directly for help because you may not be consciously aware of what it is you need. This usually results in an uncomfortable or unsatisfied feeling at the end of a conversation.

Rose's Experience

Rose had a benign lump removed from her left breast. She still had incisional pain a few weeks after surgery, so she went to her doctor.

ROSE: Doctor, I still have pain in my incision.

DOCTOR: I'll give you another prescription for pain medication.

After the visit, however, Rose felt unsettled and upset. She felt her doctor had not listened to her. Allowed to go unchecked, this anxiety became a Negative Stress Cycle. The incisional pain and uncertainty increased her anxiety, which, in turn, increased muscle tension, which increased her pain. Upon reflection, she realized that what she really wanted from the doctor was reassurance that this continued pain did not mean she had cancer or any change in her general health. Once she was aware that what she needed was reassurance, she could be specific.

Notice the difference in her next conversation with the doctor:

ROSE: Doctor, I still have incisional pain and it's three weeks since my surgery. I need to know if there is something seriously wrong with me. Could this mean I have cancer after all?

DOCTOR: Rose, I'm sorry to hear you still have pain. The pain is to be expected with this type of incision. I want to reassure you that your tumor was benign—you do not have cancer. Healing takes time after surgery. Let me examine the incision to make certain everything is healing properly.

Rose's intent was to get reassurance and her statement reflected her intent. If you feel uneasy, angry, or upset after a conversation, chances are you did not get the information you needed. Stop and reflect. Do you need help, understanding, advice, truth, permission, reassurance, or to be listened to? Then make certain your statement reflects your need. One way of knowing your statement matched the intent is that you got the information you wanted.

However, do not confuse getting the information you want or need with getting the answer you want. If, for instance, Rose was told that, indeed, her pain was due to cancer, she would have felt uneasy, angry, or upset, and appropriately so. But these feelings would not have been due to inappropriate communication. Again, the importance of precise communication reinforces the need to Stop, Take a Breath, Reflect, and be clear about what information you are seeking and how to process the information once you receive it.

Challenge yourself today to state as clearly as you can one simple request. Make certain your statement reflects your intent. Reassess at the end of the day: how well did you do? how did it feel? did anyone say no? how did that feel? Practice tomorrow with two clear, simple requests.

Know when to say yes.

Do you habitually say yes to too many tasks and too many people and often feel overwhelmed? Do you confuse saying no with rejecting someone? "If I say no, they will think I don't (love, respect, value, care for) them."

Saying yes from an exaggerated desire to please rather than from choice often creates feelings within us of resentment and blame. "Why me? Can't they see I'm too busy? They ask me because they know I always say yes." Always saying yes places your well-being in the hands of others. You assume they should be able to see your needs, therefore it is their responsibility to take care of you. You lose your autonomy and, perhaps, ultimately your self-respect. And they get a blaming, resentful husband, wife, father, mother, co-worker, or friend.

Say yes to the person, but no to the task. Be sure that the person understands you are rejecting only the task. You can say "Thanks for asking . . ." or "I would love to help you out, but . . ."

Scenario. Your neighbor and best friend has agreed to pick up the neighborhood kids from the movies tonight. It is her turn. You have had a very busy day at work, your husband is working late, and you are expecting a friend to visit. And, oh yes, you have covered for her before.

[*Telephone rings:*]

FRIEND: Nancy, this is Pat. Listen, something's come up and I can't pick the kids up from the movies tonight. Would you mind helping out and getting them?

Stop.
Breathe.
Reflect on your automatic thoughts.
Choose how you want to respond.

YOU: I'm sorry I can't help out this time. How about asking Stephanie or Molly?

FRIEND: Stephanie is out of town, and Molly filled in for me last time.

YOU: I'm sorry, I can't this time, Pat. I am glad to help you out if I know in advance and can plan to do so.

Take a breath; let it go.

You are declining this specific request and were able to say no to the task but not to her.

If you find yourself getting "caught" in the request and having difficulty breaking the yes habit, try this. Become aware when someone is making a request. Then, Stop, Take a Breath, Reflect. Whenever possible, give yourself some space, put some time (an hour or day or week) between the request and your answer. Say you must check your calendar, or check with your boss, secretary, wife, husband, or family, and you will get back to them. Breaking old habits and ways of responding is often very difficult. Give yourself the challenge of putting some space between the request and your answer.

Actively listen and acknowledge what the other person said.

When I ask you to listen to me and you start
giving advice,
You have not done what I asked.
When I ask you to listen to me and you begin to
tell me why
I shouldn't feel that way,

you are trampling on my feelings.
When I ask you to listen to me and you feel you have
to do something
to solve my problems, you have failed me,
strange as that may seem.
Perhaps that's why prayer works for some people.
Because
God is mute and He doesn't offer advice or try to fix
things.
He just listens
   and trusts you to work it out for yourself.
So please,
just listen and hear me.
And if you want to talk,
wait a few minutes for your turn
and I promise I'll listen to you.

Anonymous

Active listening means devoting your attention to what someone is saying. It requires you to listen with an open mind uncluttered by inner dialogue. Concentrate on understanding what the other person is saying, not on phrasing your response. Repeat what the other person said and infer his or her feelings. Active listening can improve your ability to hear because you are focused on the other person, not on what you are thinking. It can also influence how the other person responds. The other person doesn't feel like he or she is just going through the motions and may appreciate being heard and understood.

Active listening is related to many of the techniques we teach in *The Wellness Book*. It is an important part of uncovering automatic thoughts and exaggerated beliefs and choosing an effective way to respond. Eliciting the relaxation response reveals how much distraction is part of an active mind. Using a mini creates a more relaxed state that allows you to listen to yourself and your body.

Active listening can also be called "mindful listening." In practicing mindfulness, you have been working toward becoming more attentive to detail and nuance, more able to filter our "noise." As you work to become a more active listener, apply this same mindful attentiveness to the people around you. You will begin to listen not merely to the words people say, but also to the meaning and emotional content behind them.

Add a dash of empathy. . .

> You can experience compassion for others only when you are
> compassionate with yourself.
>
> Anonymous

Empathy is the capacity to understand another's thoughts, feelings, and actions, and to communicate this understanding back to the other person.

Since communication by definition is "a process by which information is exchanged between individuals," to communicate effectively you must have empathy, the ability to take into consideration the other person's perspective.

Empathy has been shown to have many beneficial effects. It may counter anxiety and depression as well as improve communication skills, interpersonal effectiveness, social skills, and social perceptiveness. It can also improve stress-hardiness, self-acceptance, and altruism. Conversely, a lack of empathy has been associated with both defensive and aggressive behavior.

Can empathy be learned? The answer is fairly simple. If you want to understand another's experience, then you have the potential to learn empathy. Be sure to recognize that communication—because it takes place between two individuals—is not completely within your control. No matter how empathetic you are, the other person must want to be understood. Take, for example, a friend who is angry with you but cannot admit it. You ask, "Are you angry with me for something I said?" If he responds, "I'm not angry, whatever do you mean?," empathy is blocked from the outset.

If, on the other hand, your friend is willing to address the issue, then he might say, "Yes, I'm really mad at you. You were supposed to pick me up at the bus yesterday. Where were you!? I waited an hour for you." Your response to such an accusation is critical. Instead of getting hooked by your defensive emotional reaction, you can choose to operate from empathy; you can try to understand your friend's anger. Use the four-step model.

Stop
Take a Breath
Reflect

- What are your automatic thoughts/exaggerated beliefs/distorted thinking patterns?
- Whose perspective are we dealing with (yours or theirs)?

Choose

- I choose not to react defensively.
- I will try to understand the other perspective.

Ask yourself the following questions:

1. What *thought* is the person conveying? "I waited an hour for you at the bus stop."
2. What *feelings* is the person conveying? Anger at being treated unfairly and disrespectfully, anger at having wasted time, fear of abandonment, depression from loss of affection or attention, or guilt that he may have misunderstood the arrangements and was "wrong."

The simple practice of asking yourself these two questions provides you with a very different perspective as you begin to formulate your response. Further, the other person's actions may offer some clues that will help you correctly identify the predominant feeling or combination of feelings.

Now what? Once you have considered the other's thoughts and feelings, you must identify his or her response to your action (e.g., anger), and determine if you are correct.

Restate your interpretation of the other person's thoughts and feelings: "You waited an hour for me at the bus stop [the thought]. I can understand that this would make you angry [the feeling]."

Possible responses:

"I was so worried something happened to you."
"Darn right. I'm still angry!"
"I wasn't angry, I was scared. Did you ever wait in a bus station at that hour of the night?"

This variety of responses demonstrates the importance of confirming your assumptions about the other person's thoughts and feelings. You will probably be surprised to see how often we misinterpret others' thoughts and feelings. By recognizing possible reasons for the other's response and acknowledging the truth in their statement, you are likely to be able to continue communicating rather than reacting defensively. You can now proceed to resolve the practical problem.

Pay attention to your body language.

Our facial expressions, voice quality, the movements of our arms and legs, our posture and eye contact, all contribute to the message we are communicating. You read about this in detail in chapter 6. For open, honest, and appropriate communication, unfold your arms and legs, face the other person squarely, and look her frequently in the eye. If you want to invite interpersonal interaction, lean forward slightly. This kind of "open" posture conveys the message "I am friendly and interested in what you have to say, and I welcome an opportunity to have a conversation with you."

Stop—Take a Breath—check your body language.
Look—at the other person
Listen—to what they have to say

THE CHALLENGE OF EFFECTIVE COMMUNICATION

Set yourself a realistic goal to change how you interact with someone in a given situation. Record this goal on your Health Commitment at the end of this chapter. Now review your strategies to achieve this change. Be sure to express your feelings openly and directly, and to encourage the other person to do the same. You may have to do this several times before communications improve. Other people need time to get used to the changes we are trying to make. You may have to be a "broken record" and repeat yourself again and again.

Do not expect to feel calm and assured at all times. This is an unrealistic expectation and perfectionistic thinking. At times you will feel nervous and uncertain, especially during difficult conversations or crises. Watch your feelings and reactions; acknowledge them and do your best.

Sometimes you will feel vulnerable and afraid to be open with your feelings for fear others will think you weak. Sometimes you will feel you have tried everything but remain convinced the relationship cannot be saved. Sometimes you will lose your temper and feel out of control. Sometimes you may feel stuck. But these are the moments of growth and opportunity. Sir Winston Churchill understood the value of practice when he said, at a commencement address: "Never give in, never give in, never, never, never." He then took his seat.

Carol L. Wells-Federman, M.Ed., R.N.
Eileen M. Stuart, R.N., M.S.
Ann Webster, Ph.D.

HEALTH COMMITMENT
COMMUNICATING

Long-Term Goal:

_____

_____

_____
Signature

_____
Witness

Expected Date of Reaching Goal: _____

Short-Term Goals

Comments (supports, rewards, etc.)

265

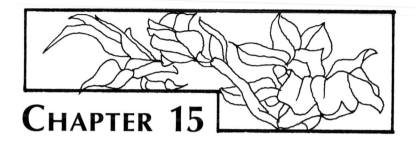

CHAPTER 15

JEST 'N' JOY

There ain't much fun in medicine, but there's a heck
of a lot of medicine in fun.

> Josh Billings, American humorist

In this chapter you will explore

- how thoughts, feelings, and behaviors interrelate
- humor as a coping strategy
- how your physiology is enhanced by using humor
- a variety of techniques to build more humor and optimism into
  your life.

What is humor? A funny story, a practical joke, or a slapstick skit? One
way to view humor is as a coping skill that involves your thoughts, feelings, and
behaviors. The result may still be a funny story, a practical joke, or a slapstick
skit, but when humor is used to help us cope, it also becomes an expression of
joy, optimism, compassion, hope, love, equanimity, and playfulness in the face
of a potential threat. Simply put, it can be an attitude of self-acceptance which
strives to affirm life. We complete the process of stress management with
humor because it allows us to see a silver lining behind each dark cloud, offers
us insight and subsequent freedom from negative self-talk, and can even bring
us closer to others.

As George Vaillant wrote in his book *Adaptation to Life,*

> Humor is one of the truly elegant defenses in the human repertoire. Few
> would deny that the capacity for humor, like hope, is one of mankind's
> most potent antidotes for the woes of Pandora's box.

Take for example the following humorous account of a trip to the super-market:

> Two women who have never met are in the same aisle in the super-market. The first woman observes that the second woman is pretty stressed out. In fact, she is so stressed out that she can't even find the item she wants on the shelf. She begins to talk out loud.
>
> SECOND WOMAN: I can't stand these crowds. You can't find any-thing. Do you believe it, every time I come in here it fills up with people. *(She sighs, clearly annoyed.)*
>
> FIRST WOMAN: *(Enjoying the opportunity for humor.)* I know, isn't it strange, the same thing happens when I come in here, too.
>
> SECOND WOMAN: What do you mean? *(She asks suspiciously.)*
>
> FIRST WOMAN: The managers are clearly busing people in . . . to see us! We're famous. There's only one thing to do. We'll buy the place. You take the bakery, I'll take the fruit section. *(She smiles as she dons a pair of ridiculous Groucho Marx glasses.)*
>
> SECOND WOMAN: *(First looks puzzled, then shocked, then gradually begins to laugh louder and louder. At last she gives a sigh of relief.)* Thanks, I needed that.
>
> Both women proceed on their way, feeling a lot more relaxed and open to life's possibilities.

Humor is the shortest distance between two people.

Victor Borge

What kind of thinking is behind each woman's communication? Do you identify with the first woman . . . with the second woman? The second woman is expressing an irrational belief, that is, everything bad happens to me. The first woman appreciated the feelings of tension and frustration expressed in the thought, "every time I come in here it fills up with people" and provided humorous relief through exaggeration. Her intention was not to ridicule. On the contrary, it was to shift the focus from negative self-talk to levity. In this scenario, the gentle playfulness of humor helped to bring the irrational thought to light in a positive way. It is compassionate and empathetic. Ridicule is another matter. To differentiate laughing with someone from laughing at someone, Dr. Joel Goodman contrasts ten characteristics.

Humor Versus Ridicule	
Laughing with	**Laughing at**
1. Going for the jocular vein	1. Going for the jugular vein
2. Based on caring and empathy	2. Based on contempt and insen-sitivity
3. Builds confidence	3. Destroys confidence through put-downs
4. Involves people in the fun	4. Excludes some people

5. A person makes a choice to be the butt of a joke (as in "laughing at yourself")

5. A person does not have a choice in being made the butt of a joke

6. Amusing—invites people to laugh   .

6. Abusing—offends people

7. Supportive

7. Sarcastic

8. Brings people closer

8. Divides people

9. Leads to positive repartee

9. Leads to one-downmanship cycle

10. Pokes fun at universal human foibles

10. Reinforces sterotypes by singling out a particular group as the "butt"

Reprinted with permission from Volume 1, no. 3 of *Laughing Matters* magazine, edited by Dr. Joel Goodman and published by the Humor Project, Inc., 110 Spring St., Saratoga Springs, N.Y. 12866.

SITCOM OF THE MIND

One way to begin seeing that life is a source for humor is to become an observer to the "Sitcom of Your Mind." Automatic thoughts that express irrational beliefs might resemble comic routines on television. If you are like most of us, the following situations will sound familiar.

The traffic jam

You are running late to an important meeting when suddenly you notice the traffic up ahead has slowed down. You automatically say, "Oh no!" Anxiously, you think "I knew it. This always happens to me whenever I'm in a hurry. I'll never make it now. Why do all these people have to be on the road at this hour. Don't they have anything better to do? This world has too many people in it. I'm stuck now. I'll never get there on time. I'll look like a fool showing up late."

The humorous reframe from oh no! to ah-ha!

Say your monologue out loud, with exaggeration, optimism, equanimity, or absurdity—play with it. Consider these reframes:

"I knew it, this always happens when I'm in a hurry. Hey, this happens heven when I'm not in a hurry. It always happens. It must be me. I attract people. They probably want to see what I'm wearing. I'm never going to make it. I can hear the news reports now. Man (woman) found petrified in car with hands gripping steering wheel and face fixed in angry stare. Another casualty of the dreaded traffic jam known to claim the lives of ten thousand Americans each day."

The relatives

You may have family members who feel compelled to share their superior knowledge and expertise. Their advice is so frequent and consistent that you know what they will say before you even see them. They sound something like this: "Why don't you settle down and get married?" "Have you lost weight yet? Just a few pounds and you'd look gorgeous." "Those children of yours need a little discipline. You'll be sorry if you don't . . ." "You still hate your job? You should . . ."

The humorous reframe from oh no! to ah-ha!

"What harm is there in listening to my relative's advice? As the old saying goes, 'Even a blind pig finds an acorn once in a while.' The next time a relative says something ridiculous, I'll just picture a blind pig rooting around for that acorn." This reframe helps you become less defensive and more open to others' suggestions. Over time you'll learn to take in what's useful and passively disregard the rest.

Another humor technique useful in situations beyond your control is literal interpretation. Mindy Cohen, R.N., relates this technique in her article "Caring for Ourselves Can Be Funny Business." A man at the back of a long and slowly moving supermarket line kept yelling to the cashier, "Hurry up! Get this line moving." Finally, the cashier, responding "literally," called out, "All right, everyone in line, start dancing!"

> There are three things which are real: God, human folly, and laughter. The first two are beyond our comprehension. So we must do what we can with the third.
>
> Ramayana as paraphrased by John F. Kennedy

THE POWER OF PLEASURE

Humor and pleasure can be tremendous stress buffers. Just as the experience of or even the anticipation of stress can trigger the stress response, an experience or anticipation of pleasure can trigger a stress buffer. For instance, optimism has been associated with longer life and less illness in studies by Dr. Christopher Peterson and his colleagues. How a positive attitude affects our health is unclear, but an understanding of the process is emerging. We now know that merely watching a humorous video alters your physiology beneficially. In a study led by Dr. Lee S. Berk, a professor of preventive medicine at Loma Linda University School of Medicine, two groups of subjects were compared: one watched an hour-long humorous video, the other engaged in a neutral activity. After these sessions, several hormones known to increase during the classical stress response were measured; the levels of the humorous-video group were found to be significantly lower than those in the neutral activity group.

Furthermore, all the subjects knew their group assignment beforehand. A comparison of stress hormones made prior to the selected activity revealed that those anticipating the humorous video had lower levels than those anticipating the neutral activity. Thus, these findings not only support the stress-reducing benefit of engaging in humor, but also the benefit of its anticipation.

Humor as a powerful coping strategy

Research suggests that people who use humor suffer less fatigue, tension, anger, depression, and confusion in response to stress. In other words, you are less affected by stress when you are able to recognize and use humor in daily life. Fortunately, because it is cognitive, this magnificent coping aid is under your control. Just remember it is a learned skill perfected only through repeated use.

Three mechanisms have been suggested to explain how positive emotions, such as humor, result in successful coping. First, humor gives you a break from ongoing stress and buys time for creatively altering your otherwise automatic stress response. Second, humor restores or replenishes depleted emotional resources. Third, humor acts to sustain you so you are better able to persist in coping.

> It is my belief, you cannot deal with the most serious things in the
> world unless you understand the most amusing.
>
> Winston Churchill

The stress-buffering effect of humor has also been shown to enhance immune function. Among people reporting high daily stress, those who use humor to cope have higher levels of an infection-fighting substance known as immunoglobulin A, compared to those who do not use humor. Another study found immunoglobulin A increased after subjects watched a humorous video, but did not increase in subjects who watched an instructive video. Stress is known to be detrimental to the immune system, but these findings show that humor may help shield us against some of its ill effects.

> A person without a sense of humor is like a wagon without springs—
> jolted by every pebble in the road.
>
> Henry Ward Beecher, nineteenth-century American clergyman

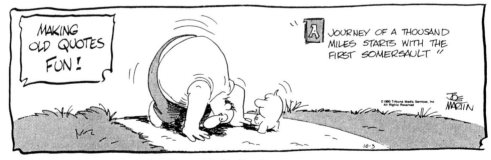

Reprinted by permission of Tribune Media Services.

THE DOMINO EFFECT OF THOUGHTS, FEELINGS, AND BEHAVIORS

In previous chapters, the relationship among thoughts, feelings, and behaviors has been described in detail. We will now explore how humor and optimism influence these relationships.

- Thoughts influence feelings and behaviors.
- Behaviors influence feelings and thoughts.
- Feelings influence thoughts and behaviors.

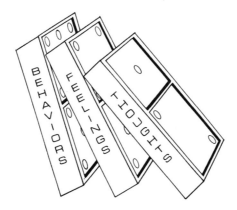

Thoughts influence feelings and behaviors

We usually express our thoughts in words. However, the words we speak and hear often profoundly influence our thoughts, which, in turn, create corresponding feelings and behaviors.

Take a Moment To . . .

Carry out this exercise, which illustrates how thoughts transform our feelings and behaviors. Read the following words slowly to yourself.

GLOOM	DESPAIR	MELANCHOLY	DARKNESS	TEARS
HARDSHIP	LOSS	SORROW	SADNESS	ANGUISH
DREAD	DEPRESSION	TORMENT	PAIN	TROUBLE
FEAR	FRUSTRATION	REJECTION	REGRET	MISERY

How do you feel?

Now read this next list slowly:

JOY	CHEERFUL	MERRIMENT	JOKING	GIGGLES
SILLY	LAUGHTER	CHERISH	FUN	GLADNESS
JOLLY	HILARIOUS	PLAYFUL	EXUBERANT	PLEASURE
BRIGHTEN	ENERGIZED	AMUSEMENT	GENTLE	WARMTH

How do you feel?

Many of us begin to feel the emotions these words denote. The first list invokes feelings of loss and sadness. Your body may become tense; you may find your shoulders becoming rounded, your gaze shifting downward, legs crossing, or your muscles tightening. The second list can be an antidote; your negative feelings and body postures can change into positive ones. In fact, in general you feel and look better when you have pleasant thoughts. So choose your words with care and heed the warning—frequent use of some words is "hazardous to your health."

Many statements you speak or hear, like the words in the exercise, promote feeling anxious, fearful, or sad. They may even create feelings of self-defeat, victimization, or loneliness. The following are some common negative thoughts we play over and over in our minds like a cassette tape on automatic.

You never know . . .	It's always me . . .	I'm just a worrier . . .
It's not fair . . .	I'm not lucky . . .	Why me . . .
I should have . . .	I'm so tired . . .	What a loser . . .
Nobody cares . . .	If only . . .	My life is a mess . . .

Take a Moment To . . .

Write down five of your negative tapes. Now reframe your tapes into funny talk. Follow the examples listed below.

You never know. ANSWER: What it is I need to know I don't know, so if I know, how will I know that I know?

I should have. ANSWER: I should stop shoulding on myself!

It's always me. ANSWER: Always. And I only volunteer 90 percent of the time. Who's responsible for this? I've got a volunteer monkey on my back.

Why me? ANSWER: Why not one of the other superheroes like Wonderwoman, Superman, Zoro, or Batgirl?

_____

_____

_____

Spend a few hours one day this week monitoring the language you use in everyday conversation. Listen very carefully to your words. Are they negative and self-defeating? "I can't, this is terrible, it's awful, this is the worst, how could they, I should have, I must." Cognitive therapist Dr. Albert Ellis humorously refers to the frequent use of the word *must* as "musturbation." Remember, musturbation is an activity with no relief.

Harnessing humor to change thoughts

Humor is not a gift you either have or not, it is a skill. Like any skill, it improves with practice.

One simple way to develop your use of humor is to create suitable affirmations. Repeating a funny phrase to yourself several times a day is likely to result in four benefits. It will 1) make you laugh; 2) inspire your use of humor; 3) increase your recognition of humorous situations; and 4) increase your appreciation for the humor of others. Another way to use affirmations to develop your sense of humor is to choose a phrase that affirms your need for humor. For example, if you do not perceive yourself as humorous, create an affirmation that provides this perspective, such as the examples below. And, of course, you can always create your own humor-enhancing affirmations.

- I possess humor
- Life is full of comedy
- My life is fun
- I'm playful
- Joy and pleasure are my birthright
- I'm amused forty times a day
- I'm an inspiration to myself
- Life is too short to take too seriously

Affirming these beliefs will likely increase your awareness and use of humor. Eliciting the relaxation response immediately before reciting these beliefs will enhance their benefit. In fact, coupling these techniques acts like a magnet. Within a short time you are likely to recognize situations, people, and belongings that spark humor and joy.

> When you smile, things seem to smile back.
> Allen Klein, *The Healing Power of Humor*

Opening your eyes to humor can change your lifestyle

Mindfulness is necessary for humor. In fact, your humor potential soars with full awareness of the present, especially when you try to live each moment to the fullest and tap into your moments of pleasure. Unfortunately, we all sometimes get snagged by bad habits, negative talk, worrying about the future, or dwelling on the past. Some of us torture ourselves with negative self-talk related to work, diet, or exercise, all in the name of living longer. By developing a sense of irony (another form of humor), we can begin to appreciate some of our own absurdities. For instance, isn't it ironic to make life miserable just to have more of it? The life you work so hard to extend is worth living only when you learn to enjoy and appreciate all of its aspects.

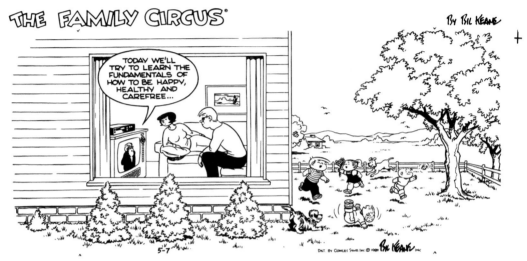

Reprinted with special permission of King Features Syndicate, Inc.

Preventing hardening of the attitude

Even very young babies smile at their mothers' smiling faces. As youths we giggle freely. But many of us lose touch with these simple pleasures as we age. Getting in touch with the child within is an important step toward cultivating more humor and pleasure in your life. Zen teachings on creativity tell us the beginner's mind has many possibilities, but the expert has only a few. As children, we saw the world as a magical place where anything could happen. The next time you are frustrated, ask yourself how the five-year-old you, or even the ten-year-old you, would have managed. Remember Wordsworth's wisdom, "The child is father of the man." All you need is memory and a little imagination.

Behaviors influence feelings and thoughts

Laughter eloquently illustrates the mind/body connection. Just as thoughts trigger laughter, body postures and sensations such as tickling trigger laughter as well. As you know, body sensations or postures communicate with your thoughts and feelings just as your thoughts and feelings communicate with

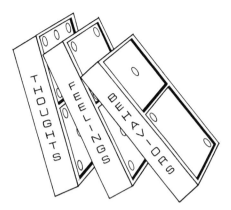

your body sensations and postures. You are a whole person, not simply a collection of isolated parts.

Do you ever find yourself worrying "I have too much to do," "I can't cope," "I'll never get all this done"? Beware. These thoughts can translate into body postures that make you look like a dead parrot or a disheveled dishrag. As your body crumples like a dishrag, your brain gets the message and begins to think, "This must be terrible, I hope it is over soon." If this happens to you, turn to the humor antidote for rejuvenation.

Take a Moment To . . .

- Stand up and repeat to yourself three times, with solemn conviction, "I have so much to do!" How do you feel? A little overwhelmed, a little drained?
- Stand up with a broad smile on your face, twirl around three times (or do a little dance), and with each twirl, say, "I have so much to do!" How do you feel now? A little better, a little energized? Are you surprised at how quickly your feelings and thoughts change to match your body postures?
- Greet each morning with a *ta-dah!* Stand in front of a mirror or a loved one and say *ta-dah!* as you fling open your arms. This proclamation lets the world know you are back! Do not underestimate the power of thoughts coupled with behaviors. A simple *ta-dah!* not only affirms your belief in you, but your belief in life as well.

A smile on your face is a light to tell people that your heart is at home.

Allen Klein, *The Healing Power of Humor*

Most of us think that facial expression is the outward manifestation of emotions and thoughts. The reverse is true as well, however. As you now know, a smile is mood-altering. It is uplifting as a gift either from a stranger or a friend, or to yourself. If you are not in the habit of smiling, practice, until the act becomes as automatic as wearing your seat belt. Every time you pass a mirror or find yourself needing a mental break, smile.

> Humor is a drug which it's the fashion to abuse.
> Sir William S. Gilbert, *His Excellency:*
> *The Played-Out Humorist*

Take a Moment To . . .

Experience the power of your thoughts combined with behaviors. Clench your fist and pound it on the table several times as you squint your eyes and tighten your lips. Now continue these behaviors and say out loud, "I'm angry, really angry! I've had it!" Shortly, you will begin to adopt uncomfortable feelings to match. As an antidote, smile gently, sit back comfortably, and say to yourself, "I'm really happy, very very happy."

Harnessing humor to change behaviors

To increase humor in your life, act the part. The old saw "Fake it till you make it" has validity here. We know an easily expressed smile fosters a positive attitude and increases our ability to see the amusing, humorous side of things. Other behaviors known to promote the development of humor include:

- reading and collecting cartoons
- seeing funny movies
- writing down jokes you enjoy
- seeing a comedian perform
- spending time with those you enjoy and find uplifting

Consult that child within on what you enjoyed as a child. If you loved the swings, go to a local playground and let loose. What about gathering a few friends together to create a scavenger hunt? Did you enjoy playing ball, ball games, swimming, skating, skiing, playing in the snow . . . water. . . ? If your childhood years lacked fun and pleasure, it is never too late to build these experiences into your life and to reap all the benefits that ensue. All you need to do is nurture that part of you that thrives on wonder and excitement by exploring the vast and rich opportunities of life.

Internal jogging

How do you feel after a good belly laugh? The late Norman Cousins posited a relationship between the remission of his illness and the laughter he enjoyed from humorous videos. He called these healing processes *internal jogging*.

Take a Moment To . . .

Experiment with the Anatomy of a Laugh

1. Place both hands on your belly.
2. Lift your eyebrows; this helps you look tall and thin (ha ha, this is a joke).
3. Smile until your molars show.
4. Add sound by saying "ha ha ha."
5. Add movement by gently rolling your head up and down.

Enjoy! Rx: At least three times a day.

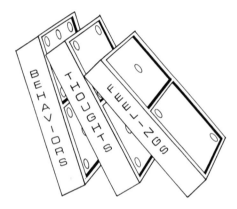

Feelings influence thoughts and behaviors

This is the most subtle relationship in this triad of thoughts, feelings, and behaviors. Because feelings are frequently less tangible for us than are thoughts or behaviors, they can persist unchallenged. If our feelings are negative, over time they can seem insurmountable. Therefore, building experiences for positive feelings and memories is an essential ingredient for developing optimism and humor.

Take a Moment To . . .

Congratulate yourself for learning more and making a commitment to personal growth. Take a few minutes right now to value and honor yourself. Next ask yourself how that compares to the feelings associated with criticizing yourself.

Once you identify feeling good about yourself, examine your thoughts. Are they positive? Are you holding your body differently? Perhaps you are sitting up straight or smiling. Feelings are as effective at altering behaviors and thoughts as thoughts are at altering behaviors and feelings. Change either thoughts, feeling, or behaviors, and the other two will change as well.

Recall three episodes from your life that felt wonderful or humorous. (Of course you can do this!) Perhaps you can recall a childhood playmate or the feeling of pride after a well-earned compliment.

_____

_____

_____

Once you have reexperienced the emotions, observe your body posture. What expression is on your face? Are your thoughts positive?

Harnessing humor to change feelings

Three important don'ts in life are

1. Don't take yourself too seriously.
2. Don't set perfectionist standards for yourself.
3. Don't overidentify with one facet of your life.

The truth is that most of us are pretty funny (especially when we are trying not to be), imperfect, and multifaceted. When we commit one of the above, we set ourselves up for failure. If you learn to lighten up and pull away from these don'ts, you are more likely to experience greater pleasure in your life. If you slip and find yourself doing one of the don'ts, see if you can picture its adverse effects and correct the frame. For instance, if you realize you are overidentifying with one aspect of your life, see yourself as a buffet rather than a single hors d'oeuvre.

As Warren S. Poland, M.D., writes,

> "The gift of laughter" . . . refers to a capacity for sympathetic laughter at oneself and one's place in the world. . . . Humor . . . requires a self-respecting modesty based on underlying self strength and simultaneous recognition of and regard for others.

Correcting the frame: "Seeing the muse in youse"

The Perfectionist   Company was coming for dinner the next day. To prepare, Mary went into a cleaning frenzy. She cleaned, polished, scented, dusted, and tidied everything in sight. If her house looked perfect, then everybody would consider her perfect: the perfect mother, perfect housewife, perfect hostess. She even cleaned under the toilet to the point where she could see her own reflection because . . . you never know. What is it you don't know? Who knows! Suddenly gazing up at the bowl, it dawned on her, "How important *is* this?" A little *humor insight* exposed the absurdity of her behavior: "This is ridiculous. One thing I do know, no one this short is coming to dinner!" Enjoying a good laugh on herself, she imagined escorting her guests on a tour of the house to show off everything she had cleaned. All would duly respond with frequent *oohs* and *aahs*. At the end of the tour, they would be invited to lie down on the bathroom floor to gaze up at the glistening bowl as she took her bow.

With the benefit of a humor insight, Mary dropped her perfectionism long enough to relax and enjoy her guests. But how was she able to come to this humor insight? It turns out that developing humor insight is as simple as observing thoughts as we elicit the relaxation response, and very similar. Mary was able to step out of herself to witness the absurdity of her behavior. Just as we learn to witness our thoughts with nonjudgmental awareness as we elicit the relaxation response, we need to witness ourselves with the same nonjudgmental awareness when we are stressed. This openness allows us to see ourselves in the context of the "big picture" called life.

> Humor is a wonderful gift for living with our imperfection; it is the synapse between the perfection we seek and the imperfection we have.
>
> Joel Goodman, creator and director of the Humor Project,
> Saratoga Springs, New York

Real-life roles

Many of us have played the following roles or encountered others portraying them. Also included are a few humorous strategies proven to buffer the negative impact of these roles. Remember, presence of mind is needed to respond in the moment, and practice helps.

The Martyr   Martyrs are the people who always offer to help if anything needs to be done. What they want is irrelevant; they do not believe in their own intrinsic value—they feel valued through self-sacrifice. At times, however, self-sacrifice becomes too costly and leaves them feeling victimized, but being out of touch with their own self-worth prevents them from asking for help or recognition, which causes further feelings of victimization.

In dealing with martyrs, the best strategy is to exaggerate their tendency to disregard their own self-worth.

> MARTYR: I don't like carrot cake, but I know you do, so I baked one for you.
> HUMOR RESPONSE: Thanks, you're right. I love carrot cake. And it's only right you neglect your needs for mine.

Captain Hook   Captain Hooks thrive on chaos and try to hook you into fear and anxiety. Like Peter Pan's Captain Hook they're always trying to get you into the mouth of the crocodile.

In dealing with Captain Hooks, the best strategy is to jump in and agree.

CAPTAIN HOOK: Isn't that dress a little tight on you?
HUMOR RESPONSE: Yes, and I have one smaller at home.
CAPTAIN HOOK: I heard Harry's getting a promotion next week. Now if my memory serves me, aren't you suppose to be the one up for a promotion?
HUMOR RESPONSE: Harry's getting a promotion? That's great! Just the other day I was thinking, when's Harry going to get that promotion?
CAPTAIN HOOK: Now don't take this the wrong way, but your sister thinks you're a bad mother.
HUMOR RESPONSE: Well, she's never been wrong. I'll give her my children.

Attila the Hun   Attilas have to build their own self-esteem by putting all others down. They build themselves up by stacking others under their feet. In dealing with Attilas, the best strategy is to exaggerate.

ATTILA THE HUN: If it wasn't for me, nothing would be done right. I'm surrounded by incompetents. It's a good thing I'm here—these people can't be trusted to carry out even the simplest order.
HUMOR RESPONSE: Thank God for you. If it weren't for you, where would we all be? My guess is probably under a rock somewhere.
ATTILA THE HUN: You look great. If you only lost another five pounds, you'd look perfect.
HUMOR RESPONSE: Thank you. I'm honored by your insult.

Imagery and humor

Imagery is a useful tool to alleviate anxiety-producing situations and to replace feelings of helplessness. Whenever you confront a particular stressor, create an image in your mind to combat its threatening aspects. For example, many of us fear speaking in public. A simple strategy to overcome this is imagining your audience in outlandish hats or other humorous garb; thinking of audience members as comical combats their threatening aspects. Another way to use imagery is to focus on whatever produced the anxiety rather than on yourself. When you are the target of a poisonous comment, focus on the speaker rather than your pain; imagine him brewing up a vat of poison or wearing a ridiculous costume. When such a shift in focus is successful, you will instantly feel less anxious because you have chosen not to take the source of the anxiety too seriously. Woody Allen uses the same strategy to deal with anxiety about dying:

It's not that I'm afraid to die. I just don't want to be there when it happens.

Woody Allen, *Without Feathers*

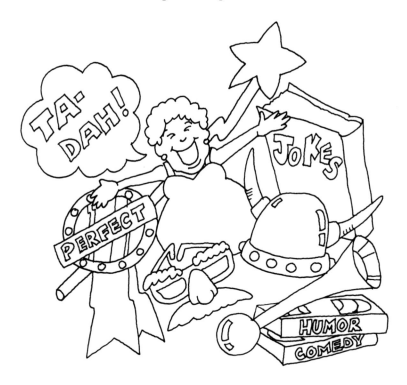

CREATE A HUMOR SURVIVAL KIT

Creating your own humor survival kit is a labor of fun. Props are invaluable to the workings of humor because they (1) facilitate visual humor (use a Viking helmet to represent stubbornness); (2) decrease inhibitions by allowing you to hide behind them (wear Groucho glasses); (3) enhance exaggeration (have a ball and chain for moments when you feel overburdened); and (4) help you exploit literal interpretations (bang a gavel whenever you feel the need to pronounce a judgment). Here are a few other suggestions to enhance your use of humor and help keep you young at heart:

- Groucho glasses: with a big nose, bushy mustache, and eyebrows
- A medal for perfection
- A red cape to escort others through your perfect house
- A Viking helmet for when you encounter or become Attila the Hun
- Books of humor and comedy
- Funny videos
- List the people and events that have brought you joy. Write down all your blessings. Review your list daily to maintain a sense that pleasure and joy are real. Reviewing this list immediately after you elicit the relaxation response will accelerate changes in your outlook.

- Try to be absorbed in the moment. Remember, humor comes when you are fully present and aware. You have to show up to see the humor.
- Exercise your imagination frequently. Stay in touch with the child within. Adopt an attitude of playfulness. Keep your mind open to silly, irreverent, iconoclastic thoughts.
- Find a space to create a humor corner at home and at work. Have a basket of silly apparel that you don while fixing dinner, talking with a friend, mowing the lawn . . .
- Don't get caught up in being funny. A sense of humor sees fun in everyday experiences. It is more important to have fun than to be funny.
- When your thoughts are negative, put on your Groucho glasses, look in a mirror, and ask yourself, "How serious is this?"
- Have a staff laugh or family fun night. Gather co-workers or family and share some funny events around your own behavior. Own up to your own humanness. This helps people connect in a common ah-ha! Remember, don't take yourself too seriously.
- On the occasion of her fiftieth birthday, at a staff celebration a social worker quipped, "I may be the oldest in the group, but I am certainly not the most mature."
- Celebrate life. Stop writing your "to do" list long enough to *ta-dah!*

> You can't help getting older, but you don't have to get old.
> George Burns, "60 Minutes"

Have you begun to understand and feel more in control of your feelings, your thoughts, your behaviors? Are you *committed* to having more fun? When you examine your daily lifestyle, are you *challenged* to incorporate a positive attitude? As you probably recognize, control, commitment, and challenge are the key ingredients of the stress-hardy personality introduced in Chapter 10, "Managing Stress." Applying these key ingredients toward developing a positive attitude and seeking humorous experiences is likely to enhance the quality of your life. And remember:

> Always Leave Them Laughing When You Say Goodbye.
> George M. Cohan, from *Mother Goose*

Margaret Baim, M.S., R.N.
Loretta LaRoche, B.A.

HUMOR
HEALTH COMMITMENT

Long-Term Goal: _____

_____

Signature

_____

_____

Witness

Expected Date of Reaching Goal: _____

Short-Term Goals	*Comments (supports, rewards, etc.)*

CHAPTER 15

SAMPLE
HUMOR
HEALTH COMMITMENT

Long-Term Goal:
  To build more optimism and humor into my life

_____ Signature

_____ Witness

Expected Date of Reaching Goal: _____

Readiness to Change	Short-Term Goals	Comments (supports, rewards, etc.)
Never considered change; need information.	1. Read humor chapter in *The Wellness Book*. 2. Carry out the exercises in the humor chapter.	
Considered change, but not yet committed.	1. Read Norman Cousins's *Anatomy of an Illness*. 2. Observe the attitudes (explanatory style) of two friends and two relatives for three weeks to see if more positive attitudes relate to more successful coping.	
Desire change; need motivation.	1. Smile at least five times a day and to at least three people each day. Observe this response. 2. Send a friend who's going through a difficult time an uplifting card. Then call later for feedback.	

(continued)

Readiness to Change	Short-Term Goals	Comments (supports, rewards, etc.)
Attempting change; need structure, support, and skills.	1. Read Allen Klein's book, *The Gift of Humor*, and practice at least one strategy from this book or from the humor chapter each week. 2. Share something positive with mate or significant other each day.	
Change made; need reinforcement.	1. Think of all the people I enjoy being with and assess their sense of humor and optimism. 2. Spend time with an optimistic friend.	
Change made, slipping back into bad habits, need renewed motivation and support.	1. Spend a day being completely negative and assess my mood and effect on others. 2. Go out to view a positive, uplifting performance, i.e., a play, movie, or comedian.	

PART 5

SPECIALTIES

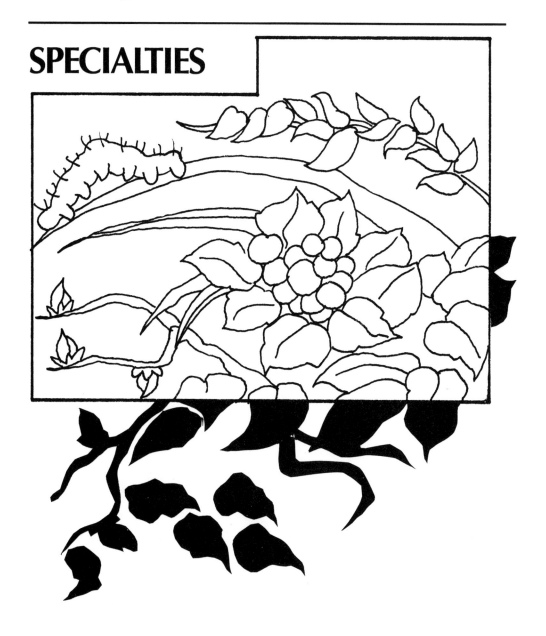

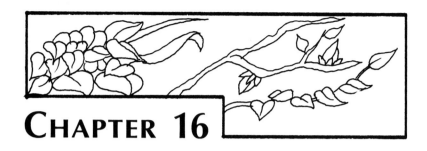

CHAPTER 16

IMPROVING YOUR SLEEP

Sleep is a state in which a great part of every life is
passed. . . . Yet of this change so frequent, so great, so
general, and so necessary, no searcher has yet found
either the efficient or final cause; or can tell by
what power the mind and body are thus chained down in
irresistible stupefaction; or what benefits the animal
receives from this alternate suspension of its active
powers. . . . And once in four and twenty hours, the gay
and the gloomy, the witty and the dull, the clamorous
and the silent, the busy and the idle, are all
overpowered by the gentle tyrant, and all lie down in
the equality of sleep.

Samuel Johnson, *The Idler*

In this chapter you will explore

- basic facts about sleep
- self-help techniques for improving your sleep
- developing a sense of control over your sleep

Most individuals suffer occasional sleepless nights or periods of poor
sleep during stressful life events such as job or home difficulties, pregnancy, a
wedding, an illness, or a death. For some, occasional sleeping problems can
evolve into chronic insomnia. Over one hundred million Americans are estimated to have occasional sleep problems, and about one in six have chronic
insomnia and consider it a serious problem.

Fortunately, a significant amount of research devoted to sleep and insomnia over the past twenty-five years has uncovered many things you can do to

improve your sleep. In fact, because of side effects from sleep medications, behavioral techniques are now considered the most effective form of treatment for chronic insomnia.

Our program incorporates a number of clinically-proven behavioral techniques for managing insomnia. Our research suggests that this program results in significant improvements in sleep in about 75 percent of our patients. To obtain these benefits, however, it is necessary to practice these techniques in the sequential, stepwise manner in which they are presented.

Each set of techniques requires about one to two weeks of practice before they begin to affect your sleep consistently. Once you are practicing one set of techniques consistently, begin to practice the next set.

Overcoming insomnia cannot be done quickly. Too many people abandon a behavioral technique after two or three nights if it doesn't produce an immediate change in their sleep. Our behavioral self-help program requires time, patience, and persistence. Furthermore, although the changes resulting from behavioral interventions may be slower than those produced by medication, they are more enduring and effective. If you are persistent and use these techniques regularly over a ten-week period, you should significantly improve your sleep.

To facilitate these improvements, keep a daily Sleep Diary during this self-help program. See the Sleep Diary form at the end of this chapter; it will take about one minute to complete each morning when you wake up. At the end of each week, review your entries to determine more objectively your sleep patterns. Sleep diaries also help you to assess your progress and are an excellent form of self-reinforcement.

WHAT IS INSOMNIA?

There is no standard definition of insomnia, since the amount of sleep required for feeling rested varies widely among individuals. Some feel rested with four hours of sleep while others require ten. According to Dr. Patricia Lacks, at Washington University in St. Louis, an arbitrary definition of insomnia may include any of the following:

a. sleep-onset insomnia: difficulty falling asleep defined by an average of at least thirty minutes per night to fall asleep
b. sleep-maintenance insomnia: difficulty staying asleep as defined by an average awake time after falling asleep totaling more than thirty minutes per night, or early morning awakening before the desired wake-up time with an inability to fall back asleep
c. poor quality of sleep

You may have one or a combination of these types of insomnia. Insomnia can result in daytime fatigue, impaired performance, and mood disturbance. For a diagnosis of insomnia, you must exhibit at least one of the sleep-disturbance patterns and at least one of the effects that carry over into your day. Even if you experience only one of these elements, you can benefit from behavioral techniques.

Insomnia can be caused by stress or other behavioral factors such as unrealistic sleep expectations, inappropriate scheduling of sleep, trying too hard to sleep, consuming caffeine, inadequate exercise, and a number of other behavioral factors. Insomnia can also be caused by depression, a medical problem, or alcohol or drug use. Before beginning this self-help program, get a complete physical history and medical examination from your physician. The techniques discussed in this chapter are not appropriate for insomnia caused by depression, alcohol or drug use, or a medical condition.

Take a Moment To . . .

Reflect on your sleep pattern. Do you

- have difficulty falling asleep?
- have difficulty staying asleep?
- feel your sleep is of poor quality?
- have a combination of these types of sleep patterns?

If yes, reflect on behaviors that may influence your sleep pattern. Do you

- worry or feel anxious at bedtime?
- try too hard to sleep?
- consume caffeine or smoke near bedtime?
- spend too much time in bed?
- get too little exercise?
- have an inconsistent sleep schedule?

Read on to learn strategies to change these and other behaviors which may negatively affect your sleep.

BASIC FACTS ABOUT SLEEP

Sleep is divided into five stages. Stage 1, the lightest stage, marks the transition from wakefulness to sleep; if awakened during Stage 1, you would probably report being awake. Stage 2 sleep is the first "true" sleep stage, a "light" sleep from which you can easily be awakened. Stages 3 and 4 sleep are called *delta* sleep and are the deepest stages of sleep; it is very difficult to be awakened from delta sleep. In Stage 5, rapid eye movement (REM) sleep, or dream sleep, your eyes move horizontally and vertically because you look around while you dream; virtually all dreaming occurs during REM sleep. You are more likely to awaken during REM sleep than delta sleep because REM is a "lighter" stage of sleep.

During normal, good, restful sleep, you progress from Stage 1 to Stage 4, then back to Stage 2, and then to REM sleep in about ninety minutes. The typical sleeper will go through four to six of these cycles per night. However, during the first part of the night, delta cycles (Stages 3 and 4) are longer and REM cycles are very short. As the night progresses, delta cycles become shorter and the length of REM cycles increase. Thus, we obtain most of our deep sleep during the first half of the night and most of our dream sleep during the second half. It is normal to wake up several times during the night but not remember this the next morning.

The eight-hour myth

The belief that everyone must sleep eight hours a night is a myth. According to Dr. Peter Hauri, at the Mayo Clinic in Rochester, Minnesota, adults average about seven to seven-and-one-half hours of sleep per night, and many individuals function effectively with four to six hours of sleep. In fact, 20 percent of the population (slightly more in men) sleep less than six hours per night.

Many people worry needlessly about not sleeping eight hours. If you sleep only five hours a night but are not sleepy or fatigued the next day, you may be trying to sleep more than you really need. Dr. Edward Stepanski and his team of researchers at the Henry Ford Hospital in Detroit, Michigan, and the Grandview Hospital in Dayton, Ohio, have shown that poor sleepers are not usually sleepier during the day than good sleepers. Another significant fact is that sleep changes with age. Not only does total sleep time decrease (to an average of about six-and-one-half hours during old age), but deep sleep decreases and light sleep increases, making it more common to have problems sleeping as we get older.

The effects of sleep loss

The effects of sleep loss are subject to a number of popular misconceptions. Contrary to popular belief, the human nervous system has a remarkable tolerance for sleep loss, at least on a temporary basis. As Dr. Hauri notes, one night of total sleep deprivation makes healthy young volunteers sleepy, but has remarkably little effect on their day's performance. Even extended sleeplessness has little effect on abilities—it simply makes you feel extremely sleepy. (One volunteer stayed awake for eleven days and showed no major effects on physical or psychological functions!) Even after extended sleeplessness, two to three nights of extended sleep returns volunteers to normal.

Dr. Claudio Stampi, at the Institute for Circadian Physiology in Boston, Massachusetts, observes that most individuals can maintain their usual performance with 60-to-70 percent of their normal sleep. If you are an eight-hour sleeper, this means your performance at work will not suffer significantly if you get four and one-half to five and one-half hours of sleep. In fact, a study, conducted by Drs. Jeffrey Sugerman, John Stern, and James Walsh, at the

Deaconess Hospital and Washington University in St. Louis, Missouri, found that individuals suffering from insomnia perform as well on tests of mental performance as good sleepers.

Finally, people who have difficulty sleeping often overestimate the time it takes to fall asleep and underestimate total sleep time. You may, in fact, be getting more sleep than you think!

Since performance is not usually significantly affected after sleep loss, what are its consequences? For moderate sleep loss, the major effects are irritability and fatigue. These feelings are often due to our appraisals about loss of sleep. Consider how differently we regard sleep loss due to late-night socializing, travel, or entertainment compared to sleep loss due to insomnia. Tossing and turning all night in bed is frustrating and aggravating; we appraise it as stressful, and it adversely affects our mood the following day.

For moderate sleep loss, the *perception* is as important as the amount lost. So, don't be afraid of insomnia. The less you fear insomnia and the less you appraise sleep loss as stressful, the better you will sleep and the better you will feel the next day.

Take a Moment To . . .

Assess your reaction to sleep loss. Are you overly concerned about getting eight hours of sleep?

Do you panic about sleep loss?

Do you get angry and frustrated when you cannot sleep?

Do you tell yourself you will be unable to function the next day?

Now that you understand some basic facts about sleep and insomnia, let us turn to the first set of behavioral techniques to improve your sleep. These are called *sleep hygiene,* referring to the daytime and before-sleep behaviors that affect sleep.

IMPROVING DAYTIME AND BEFORE-SLEEP BEHAVIORS

Practice these steps daily.

Step 1. Under the supervision of a physician, gradually eliminate the habitual use of sleeping pills. The effects achieved by most sleep medications are only temporary, since they lose their effectiveness after two to four weeks of continued use. They also decrease delta sleep and dream sleep, so that while you may fall asleep faster, your sleep will be of poorer quality. Besides disrupting sleep, sleep medications are usually not eliminated from the body by morning and produce a "hangover" effect which can decrease daytime alertness and impair thinking. People also tend to develop tolerance for the medication and need increasingly larger doses. Additionally, psychological or physical dependence can develop if the medication is used for an extended period. Finally, when you stop using them, many sleep medications result in a temporary "rebound" insomnia which can be worse than the initial insomnia! So, if you must take a sleeping pill, limit yourself to one per week.

Christine's Experience

Christine, a twenty-eight-year-old housewife, came to our program complaining of difficulty falling asleep, daytime fatigue, and irritability. Although she took sleeping medication nightly for over three months, she often required one to three hours to fall asleep. As part of her treatment program, she first gradually withdrew from her medication under the supervision of a physician. The first week she experienced some rebound insomnia, and her sleep remained poor for a second week. At that point, she began to use the behavioral techniques discussed in this chapter. Within three weeks, she was regularly falling asleep within twenty minutes. Christine also reported increased energy, less irritability, and feeling more "like her old self."

Step 2. Reduce your consumption of alcohol and caffeine. Alcohol disrupts sleep by reducing deep sleep and dream sleep; it should not be consumed within two hours of bedtime. Caffeine is a powerful stimulant and should not be consumed within six hours of bedtime. Many foods, beverages, and medications contain caffeine—learn to read the product labels carefully. Chapter 8, "Nutrition for Good Health," gives some tips on reducing caffeine consumption. If you smoke, stop. Nicotine is a stimulant, and nonsmokers fall asleep more quickly than smokers.

Step 3. Establish a regular aerobic exercise program. As suggested by Dr. Hauri, people who have difficulty sleeping tend to lead more sedentary lives than good sleepers, and we now know that physical inactivity may contribute to insomnia (by inhibiting our normal and rhythmic increases and decreases of body temperature). Regular exercise in the late afternoon or early evening eliminates this problem because it makes your body temperature rise and then fall (as you cool down). Dr. Deborah Sewitch, at the Griffin Hospital in Derby, Connecticut, observes that this aids your sleep because decreasing body temperature facilitates the onset of sleep and promotes deep sleep. However, exercise early in the morning does not affect sleep, and exercise within three hours of bedtime may stimulate you, which will make it more difficult to fall asleep. For many individuals, brisk walking in the late afternoon or early evening is sufficient to increase core body temperature. You should exercise at least three to four times per week in order to affect your sleep consistently. Chapter 7, "Move into Health," addresses exercise and can help you establish an effective exercise program.

Roberta's Experience

Roberta, a fifty-year-old housewife, came to our program complaining that she often felt sleepy and "on edge," and had difficulty coping when she slept poorly. Roberta's sleep diaries revealed that she required an average of sixty minutes to fall asleep at night. Furthermore, her nighttime awakenings averaged over ninety minutes per night. Because she did not exercise, Roberta was instructed to begin a regular aerobic exercise program. She began brisk walking every evening after dinner for thirty minutes. Within two weeks, she was falling asleep in an average of thirty minutes per night, and she reduced both the frequency and duration of her nighttime awake time by 50 percent. She also felt more rested, and her mood and daily functioning began to improve. Roberta's exercise program clearly had a significant and rapid effect on her sleep.

Step 4. Plan tomorrow's activities, complete phone calls and personal business, and review the day's events early in the evening so the two hours prior to bedtime can serve as a relaxing, wind-down period. Activities during this transition between waking and sleeping might include reading or watching television or a movie. A light carbohydrate snack during your wind-down period may help you sleep, because carbohydrates increase the production of serotonin, the brain chemical responsible for sleep.

Step 5. Make sure your sleeping environment is conducive to sleep. Minimal levels of light and sound aid sleep. For many individuals, the hum of a fan or an air conditioner or a commercially-available sound conditioner will aid sleep. Also, make sure the temperature of your bedroom is comfortable. In general, a cooler room temperature will facilitate sleep, since this will help decrease your core body temperature.

Step 6. Reduce your fluid intake after eight P.M. to help reduce any chance of waking up at night because of a full bladder.

Practice these sleep-hygiene techniques regularly until they become an integral part of your daily and before-sleep routine. This will probably require at least two weeks of daily practice.

Take a Moment To . . .

List sleep-hygiene behaviors which might interfere with your sleep pattern:

_____

_____

List steps you might find useful to improve your sleep hygiene behaviors:

_____

_____

_____

Once you have established the sleep-hygiene techniques as a regular part of your daytime and before-sleep behaviors, you are ready to practice the next set of behavioral techniques; these are called *sleep-scheduling techniques.*

SCHEDULING YOUR SLEEP

One of the most important ways to improve your sleep is to reduce your time in bed. It is common for poor sleepers to extend time in bed, especially after a restless night, in order to "catch up" on sleep. However, as Dr. Hauri notes, the more time you spend in bed, the more difficulty you will have falling asleep and the lighter and poorer your sleep will be. By reducing that time, you will be drowsier at bedtime, can consolidate and deepen your sleep, and also create a slight sleep debt that will make it easier to fall asleep and sleep more deeply the next night.

Step 1.   Reduce your time in bed to no more than six to seven hours. For most people, this means delaying bedtime by about one hour. If you become drowsy earlier in the evening, use activity to help ward off drowsiness—move around your house, socialize, do some light cleaning—anything to keep you slightly active. Spending too much time in bed is the most common mistake a person with insomnia can make. Cutting down that time is *crucial* to improving your sleep.

    Neil's Experience

Neil, a thirty-seven-year-old financial consultant, came to our program with sleep-maintenance difficulties. Although he fell asleep easily, Neil woke up regularly between two A.M. and four A.M. and often required three hours to fall back to sleep. His poor sleep was adversely affecting his mood, motivation, and job performance. As part of sleep-scheduling techniques, Neil was instructed to reduce his time in bed by delaying his bedtime by about one hour each night. Within two weeks, he reduced his nighttime awakenings significantly and was able to enjoy five hours of uninterrupted, solid sleep. By reducing time in bed, Neil's sleep improved, as did his mood and energy level.

Step 2.   Get up at about the same time every day (including weekends), even if you have a poor night's sleep. This will help to maintain a consistent circadian rhythm—the twenty-four-hour internal body rhythm or cycle—that keeps us awake during the day and asleep (usually) at night. With time, the hour that you become drowsy will become more consistent. As noted by Dr. Charles Reynolds, at the University of Pittsburgh School of Medicine in Pittsburgh, Pennsylvania, getting up at the same time each day and not "sleeping in," also promotes a slight sleep debt that will make it easier to fall asleep and sleep more deeply that night.

Step 3.   Use prior wakefulness to regulate when you get drowsy and how deeply you sleep. The longer you are awake (that is, the earlier you get up), the quicker you will fall asleep and the deeper you sleep that night. If you have an important meeting early Monday morning and want the best chance of getting to sleep at a reasonable time Sunday night, get up earlier Sunday morning.

Step 4.   Do not nap longer than one hour, especially late in the day, since naps of this length can make you less sleepy at bedtime. Naps under sixty minutes, however, may be beneficial after a sleep-deprived night, especially around three-thirty in the afternoon. According to Drs. Scott Campbell and Juergen Zulley, at the Max Planck Institute in Munich, Germany, our mood and performance decline in midafternoon due to a biological need for sleep. A short nap can satisfy that need and usually will not affect sleep-onset.

   Take a Moment To . . .

Reflect on your sleep schedule.

> What time do you usually go to bed?
> What time do you usually get up?
> How much time do you spend in bed?
> Do you nap frequently?
> Identify several strategies to improve your sleep scheduling:

_____

_____

_____

Allow yourself at least two weeks to integrate sleep-scheduling techniques into your daily routine. At the end of this period, you should be practicing both sleep-hygiene and sleep-scheduling techniques regularly.

The next behavioral technique to improve sleep is called *stimulus control*.

STIMULUS-CONTROL TRAINING

For most people, the bed and bedroom are associated with relaxation, drowsiness, and sleep. For many poor sleepers, however, the bed and bedroom have become conditioned cues for mental arousal, sleeplessness, and frustration because they are used for many activities other than sleep, including reading work-related materials, talking on the phone, worrying, and most importantly, trying too hard to sleep. Interestingly, some individuals with insomnia sleep well everywhere except their own bedroom, including other rooms in their house, in front of the television, or even in a sleep laboratory! The goal of stimulus-control training is to teach you to reassociate the bed and bedroom with relaxation, drowsiness, and sleep. Most importantly, stimulus control will teach you not to try to sleep, which is one of the biggest mistakes anyone who has difficulty sleeping can make.

Based on our research and clinical work with people who sleep poorly, we have developed a modified version of the stimulus-control technique originally developed by Dr. Richard Bootzin at Northwestern University in Evanston, Illinois.

Step 1. Use your bedroom only for pleasurable, relaxing activities and sleep. Do not use your bedroom for any stressful activities. Furthermore, do not use your bed in the evening until bedtime. The goal is to associate your bedroom and bed with relaxation and sleep only.

Step 2. Go to bed only when drowsy even if that moment comes later than your new delayed bedtime. The goal is to associate bedtime and your bed with drowsiness.

Step 3. When you are quite drowsy, get into bed and relax for fifteen to twenty minutes by reading, listening to music, or watching television until you are very drowsy. Then turn out the lights with the intention of going to sleep. If you are not asleep within twenty to twenty-five minutes, *do not try to sleep!* The harder you try, the more you will stay awake. Instead, open your eyes and read—a book-reading light works well—or watch TV until you are drowsy again, then turn out the lights to sleep again. Repeat this procedure as often as necessary. If you regularly repeat this process three or four times, you are going to bed too early.

If you are wide awake and your mind is very active, you are probably better off getting out of bed and leaving your bedroom. This is especially appropriate if you sleep well everywhere (including other rooms in your own home) except your bedroom, or if you tend to try to go back to sleep too soon when you stay in bed. Engage in quiet, relaxing activity until you begin to feel drowsy again, then return to your bedroom with the intention of going to sleep. Repeat this procedure as often as necessary until you fall asleep.

If you wake up in the middle of the night and are still awake after twenty to twenty-five minutes, open your eyes and read or watch TV until you are drowsy; then close your eyes to go to sleep. Repeat this procedure until you fall asleep. If you are wide awake and your mind is very active, you may be better off leaving your bedroom for another activity until you are drowsy. However, getting out of bed in the middle of the night is disruptive for some individuals, so try reading or watching television in bed first. Repeat this procedure as often as necessary.

Since one of the goals of stimulus-control training is to engage in a relaxing, distracting activity instead of trying to sleep when you are unable to, plan an enjoyable, relaxing activity in advance. If you have nothing to do, you will increase your frustration and aggravation. Boredom is one of the surest routes to insomnia!

Finally, remember that even if you do not sleep, but lie relaxed in bed or another room reading or watching television, you will feel more rested the following day than if you toss and turn all night.

Take a Moment To . . .

Reflect on any of your bedtime behaviors that are conditioned cues for wakefulness, mental arousal, and frustrations which interfere with your ability to sleep.

Do you use the bedroom for nonrelaxing activities?
Do you go to bed when you are not really drowsy?
Do you continue to try to sleep if you are still awake after twenty-five minutes?

After identifying these behaviors, identify strategies to help you reassociate the bed and bedtime with relaxation, drowsiness, and sleep:

_____

_____

_____

Stimulus control is one of the most effective behavioral techniques for improving sleep but also one of the more difficult to master. Many people want to go to bed before they are drowsy, and many have difficulty with not trying to sleep. At least two weeks are often needed to begin mastering stimulus-control techniques. Without consistent usage for at least two weeks, you will not learn to associate your bed and bedroom with relaxation, drowsiness, and sleep. Practice stimulus-control techniques every night!

Byron's Experience

Byron, a thirty-year-old law student, came to our program averaging about one hour per night to fall asleep; his poor sleep was adversely affecting his mood and his performance at work. He began to practice stimulus-control techniques each night, using his bedroom only for relaxing activities and sleep. Additionally, he did not go to bed until he was drowsy and did not try to sleep if he was still awake after twenty-five minutes; instead, he read until he was drowsy again. His sleep did not improve during the first week of practice, but Byron noticed some improvement during the second week. After three weeks of consistently practicing stimulus control, Byron was falling asleep in an average of twenty minutes each night and his sleep diary entries resembled the patterns of a normal sleeper! As a result of his improved sleep, Byron's mood and daytime performance also improved.

The final behavior technique to improve your sleep is the relaxation response.

DAYTIME AND BEDTIME TECHNIQUES TO ELICIT THE RELAXATION RESPONSE

Chapters 4 and 5 contain instructions for eliciting the relaxation response and present you with a variety of techniques. Practicing the relaxation response during the day can reduce the daytime physical and mental arousal that may disrupt sleep. In addition, research by Drs. Kenneth Lichstein and Thomas Rosenthal suggests that bedtime mental arousal—worrying, planning tomorrow's activities, or anxiety about falling asleep—can significantly disrupt sleep. Our research suggests that the relaxation response reduces mental arousal by producing slower brain-wave activity. Normally, you do not fall asleep when eliciting the relaxation-response because you are sitting up. However, practicing the relaxation-response instructions at bedtime while lying down can help you fall asleep. Do not attempt to use the relaxation response to fall asleep until you feel comfortable with these techniques, because trying too hard to relax may actually disrupt sleep. To prevent this from occurring, do not practice the relaxation response at bedtime until you have practiced it during the day for at least two weeks. Then try it at bedtime, after turning off the lights and closing your eyes. If you have little mental arousal at bedtime, you may not need the relaxation response at this time. However, our experience suggests that most individuals with insomnia benefit from this approach, and some find it the most helpful of the behavioral techniques.

When you begin to practice the relaxation response at bedtime, combine it with stimulus control. That is, go to bed only when drowsy, distract yourself for fifteen to twenty minutes, then use the relaxation-response instructions after you lie down, turn off the lights, and close your eyes. You may find you are drowsy enough to fall asleep before completing the relaxation-response instructions. However, if you are still awake after twenty-five minutes, do not continue to use the relaxation-response instructions; open your eyes and read or distract yourself until drowsy again. Then close your eyes and use the relaxation-response instructions again. Repeat this process until you fall asleep. If your mind is very active, you may be better off getting out of bed and going to another room until you are drowsy.

If you awaken in the middle of the night, elicit the relaxation response to help you fall back to sleep. However, if you do not fall back to sleep within twenty-five minutes, open your eyes and read or distract yourself until drowsy again. Leave the room only if you are wide awake and your mind is very active.

The key to successful relaxation-response practice at bedtime is to not try too hard. The relaxation response requires a passive approach of letting relaxation happen. As you develop this skill, your ability to reduce mental arousal at bedtime will improve.

Kim's Experience

Kim, a thirty-nine-year-old banker, had been having trouble falling asleep and staying asleep. Her poor sleep made her irritable, angry, and fatigued. After practicing the relaxation response during the day for two weeks, she found that she could use it at bedtime to fall asleep more easily. She also found that she could go back to sleep within twenty-five minutes when she woke up in the middle of the night. Kim felt that the relaxation response was the most helpful behavioral technique she had learned and she began to approach her sleep with a new sense of confidence.

MAINTAINING IMPROVEMENT

If you give yourself a few weeks to master each set of self-help techniques and practice them regularly, your sleep should improve significantly. Be tolerant of occasional sleepless nights, however, and remember that even good sleepers have nights of poor sleep. If your sleep does not improve, getting an evaluation at a sleep clinic at one of your local hospitals would probably be a good idea.

Finally, be sure to continue practicing your self-help techniques so that they become a permanent part of your daily behaviors. Follow-up data from a number of research studies suggest that people who use these behavioral techniques regularly rarely relapse into old sleeping patterns. In fact, one-year follow-ups show that improvement stays the same or increases for people who continue their sleep-healthy habits. Regular practice is worth the effort. Not only will your sleep improve, but your sense of control over your sleep will improve as well.

Gregg D. Jacobs, Ph.D.

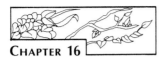

SLEEP DIARY

Name _____

Day _____

Date _____

0) What time did you go to bed last night? _____

1) How many minutes did it take you to fall asleep last night?

   _____

2) How many times did you awaken during the night? _____

3) For each occurrence listed in question 2, indicate how many minutes you were awake.

   _____

   _____

   _____

4) What is the total number of hours and minutes you slept last night?

   _____

5) What time did you wake up this morning? _____

6) What time did you get out of bed this morning? _____

7) How difficult was it for you to fall asleep last night?

1	2	3	4	5
not very difficult				extremely difficult

8) How rested did you feel this morning?

1	2	3	4	5
very re-sted				poorly re-sted

9) Rate the quality of last night's sleep.

1	2	3	4	5
excellent				very poor

10) What was your level of physical tension when you went to bed last night?

1	2	3	4	5
extremely relaxed				extremely tense

11) Rate your level of mental activity when you went to bed last night.

1	2	3	4	5
very qui-et				very active

12) How well do you think you were functioning yesterday?

1	2	3	4	5
very well				very poorly

HEALTH COMMITMENT

Long-Term Goal:

_____

_____

_____
Signature

_____
Witness

Expected Date of Reaching Goal: _____

Short-Term Goals	*Comments (supports, rewards, etc.)*

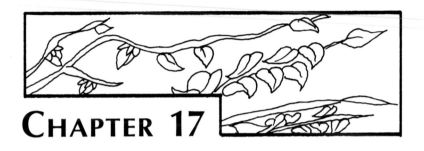

CHAPTER 17

INFERTILITY AND WOMEN'S HEALTH

In this chapter you will explore

- how to use relaxation-response and stress-management techniques during the infertility workup and treatment phases
- the infertility/stress connection
- other support options for infertile individuals and couples
- coping after a miscarriage
- coping during a high-risk pregnancy
- menopausal symptoms and how to alleviate them

Participants in our Behavioral Medicine infertility and women's health programs commonly report feeling less depressed, less anxious, less tired, more energetic, and much more in control by the end of the ten weeks. If you follow the components of our programs described in *The Wellness Book,* you are likely to notice similar changes. However, these techniques are not a substitute for medical care, but rather a complement; they are methods which you can use to help yourself feel better and optimize your medical treatment.

INFERTILITY

Although people with infertility often feel their problem is unusual, infertility is actually very common. In the United States, one out of every six couples of childbearing age has an infertility problem. This means millions of people, many of whom report that infertility is the worst experience of their lives. Undergoing an infertility workup and subsequent treatment can be very difficult—physically, psychologically, and financially.

A highly prevalent feeling of people with infertility is loss of control. Most people assume they can have children when they choose. After twenty or thirty years of assuming you would have your children when wanted, and maybe even spending time and energy trying *not* to get pregnant, realizing that you may never have a baby can be very distressing.

Most of us were taught from an early age that the harder we work at something, the more likely we are to get it. Infertility is different. How hard you work at getting pregnant or what kind of person you are is irrelevant. Because the idea of having children is so fundamental to our identity, those who have infertility can begin to feel that life is utterly unfair, that their own lives are completely out of control.

The infertility/stress connection

No study has proven that being calm causes conception. However, there *is* preliminary evidence that very high levels of emotional stress can contribute to infertility by causing fallopian tubal spasm, irregular ovulation, hormonal changes, and perhaps by decreasing sperm production. Thus, perhaps a cycle of physiological and psychological events occurs as a result of the stress of infertility. And the circle goes both ways: stress affects infertility and infertility affects stress.

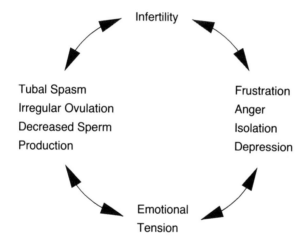

The infertility workup and treatment may cause stress that contributes to the infertility. Even if the original cause of infertility is treated, the extreme level of emotional distress may be causing other problems which sustain infertility. If so, taking concrete steps like eliciting the relaxation response, doing minis to relieve tension, and challenging negative thoughts may increase the chance of becoming pregnant. However, these approaches cannot treat organic problems like endometriosis, tubal scarring, and blockages.

So, what is the relationship between stress and infertility? We know that there is a relationship between stress and infertility, but the specific nature of the relationship is unclear. We do know that most causes of infertility (95 percent) are physical. However, since we know that infertility causes stress, it makes sense to try to alleviate that stress. At the very least, you should feel better. In our program, 34 percent of the participants conceived within six months of starting the program, a higher rate than one would expect. For example, in a study done by Drs. John Collins and Timothy Rowe, from McMaster University and the University of British Columbia, of women with unexplained infertility who did not participate in any kind of relaxation treatment program, 18 percent conceived within a six-month period. In addition to the elevated conception rates in our program, nearly 100 percent of the participants felt better. See if you can take control of the situation by helping yourself feel better.

The relaxation response can help

Once you begin to elicit the relaxation response, you may feel calmer and less anxious throughout the day, which will help you feel more in control. Enjoying life when you feel depressed, anxious, and angry much of the time is very difficult. You may remember what you felt like before you started to "try," and you may want to start feeling that way again.

Trina's Experience

> Trina, a thirty-six-year-old legal secretary, attended one of the first infertility groups. She was so depressed she cried throughout the first two sessions. At the third, she cracked a joke. She came to provide some much needed levity to the group. By the last session, other participants told her how much they appreciated her spirited wit and humor. She later reported that she had always been a very funny person, but had completely lost her sense of humor while undergoing infertility treatments. By eliciting the relaxation response daily, her anxiety level dropped, allowing the "old" Trina to reemerge.

Another advantage of eliciting the relaxation response is that it gives you time every day which is just for you. Most women going through the infertility process tend to take care of themselves last. Between trying to keep up with work, taking care of your spouse, housekeeping, and going for seemingly endless medical tests and appointments, you tend to forget about taking care of yourself. You might feel guilty about doing things just for you, such as spending an afternoon reading a novel or soaking in the tub. Many women undergoing infertility unconsciously feel they don't deserve nice things because they are angry at themselves for not getting pregnant.

All people need time for themselves. If you feel you absolutely cannot find twenty minutes every day for the relaxation response, examine your priorities. You deserve time to help yourself feel better. Look carefully at how you do spend your time and on whom. The first step in having more control over your life is to make yourself more of a priority.

Elicit the relaxation response daily to help feel less anxious and more in control throughout the day. Review chapter 5 for the basic techniques. Choose a thought, word, prayer, or phrase which is calming and meaningful to you during the experience of infertility. Do not focus on achieving conception; this can be counterproductive.

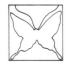

Take a Moment To . . .

Reflect on an image, thought, word, phrase, or prayer which evokes for you feelings of calm serenity.

These suggestions for using the relaxation response may be helpful:

- Elicit the relaxation response daily. Choose a time, place, and method, and begin today. Make a commitment to *your* health and well-being in this time of uncertainty in your life.
- Try eliciting the relaxation response in the doctor's waiting room.
- Elicit the relaxation response both before and after a surgical procedure. Prior to surgery, it will help reduce anxiety; afterwards, it can reduce muscle tension and pain.
- Try eliciting the relaxation response during procedures such as inseminations and "tubograms" (injection of dye into your fallopian tubes) to facilitate muscular relaxation; relaxing your abdominal and pelvic muscles will make the procedure more comfortable. After doing this, many of our patients have reported excellent results—feeling less discomfort, less anxiety, and more control over their bodies.

Penelope's Experience

Penelope, a thirty-nine-year-old computer programmer, attended the Behavioral Medicine Program for Infertility. Previously, she had had a difficult time during the egg-retrieval portion of her in-vitro fertilization (IVF) procedure. Now she listened to a relaxation-response tape with a guided imagery exercise on taking a hot bath. She fell asleep at the beginning of the procedure, literally slept throughout, and had to be awakened in the recovery room!

Using relaxation-response "minis"

"Minis" (introduced in chapter 5) can be a decided asset as you cope with infertility. The simple act of stopping and taking a breath can relieve stress and help you cope with the stress of infertility. Many patients report doing fifty to a hundred minis a day! They can be done at any time, no one need know you are doing them, and they can help diminish pain and anxiety quickly.

Try doing "minis"

- prior to and during a blood test
- prior to and during injections
- before calling the doctor's office for test results
- while waiting for a telephone call from your doctor
- when you are put on hold when calling the doctor
- when you see a pregnant woman
- when talking to a close friend and she tells you she is pregnant a third time, by accident
- before and during the insertion of an intravenous needle (IV) prior to surgery
- before using the toilet on Day 28 of your cycle
- when your mother-in-law suggests for the tenth time that you should just relax

Think of where and when else to do minis. The key is to remember to do them.

Take a Moment To . . .

Stop.
Take a deep Breath.
Reflect.
Now take another, releasing physical tension throughout your body.
Think, perhaps, of a waterfall, and as you take the breath, imagine the waterfall cascading over your mind and body, washing away anxiety and tension.
Take another breath, using the image of the waterfall. Do you feel better than when you began this mini? More relaxed? Less physical tension?

Thoughts, feelings, and emotions

As discussed in chapters 11 and 12, thoughts, feelings, and emotions influence health. Automatic thoughts, which tend to be negative in any case, can become even more automatic and negative as you go through months and years of infertility. Patients report automatic thoughts such as "I'll never get pregnant, I'll always be infertile, Why me?, I've been a good person, She doesn't deserve to have another child. What did I do wrong?" Sound familiar? Stop, Take a

Breath, and Reflect on your automatic thoughts. Challenge the thoughts that are exaggerated, distorted, or simply not true.

Become aware of how belief and expectation contribute to stress. Much of your stress may be explained by your expectation of being able to conceive at your discretion. When this does not occur, you feel internal conflict (stress), usually manifested by feelings of loss of control over your choices, your body, and your life. As you begin to reflect on and challenge your automatic thoughts, you may notice the emergence of certain irrational (exaggerated) beliefs and/or cognitive distortions such as all-or-nothing thinking or over-generalization. In this case, failure to conceive in one twenty-eight-day cycle becomes "I'll never conceive" and then overgeneralized to being a "failure" in life. Recognize these patterns and challenge them.

Sally's Experience

Sally, a twenty-nine-year-old artist, realized she was constantly thinking she would never have a baby, she would always be infertile. After learning about automatic thoughts, Sally began to focus on what her mind was actually saying:

> I did not get pregnant again last month.
> This treatment is not working.
> It is never going to work.
> IVF will be a waste of time and money.
> I am never going to get pregnant.
> I will be miserable and lonely for the rest of my life . . .

She realized her mind was racing ahead, not allowing her to take things one step at a time. When she recognized her automatic thoughts, she was able to Stop, Breathe, Reflect, and logically appraise her situation. She saw she would not enter an IVF program if she *knew* she would always be infertile. She was able to restructure her negative thoughts into the realization that she did not know what lay in her future. IVF was a logical next step, and she knew that she and her husband would start discussing adoption when they both felt ready.

Look at what your thoughts are saying to you. See if you can challenge them and turn them into a more positive alternative which you believe in your heart to be true.

Every woman having difficulty conceiving has been told at least once "Just relax and you'll get pregnant," "You're working too hard at it," "Go on vacation," "Just have a glass of wine," or "Adopt, then you'll get pregnant right away." Not only are these statements offensive, hurtful, and guilt-producing, they are not true. Following the suggestions in this book will not guarantee conception. The main reason for you to use our techniques is that infertility can be a very difficult experience. Most women with infertility feel anxious and depressed. We have found that the women who go through our program feel significantly less anxious, depressed, angry, and tired; they feel they have more control over their lives and can lead a more normal life. A basic goal of our program is to help people stop living in twenty-eight-day cycles and to start getting more enjoyment out of their lives.

Several group participants decided to stop focusing their lives around the possibility of getting pregnant and to pursue their own goals. One realized that she stayed with a job she hated because the hours were flexible and accommodated her infertility treatment. She applied for and was awarded a promotion, found she could still pursue treatment, but was much happier in the process.

Kristen's Experience

Kristen was a thirty-three-year-old physician with a four-year history of infertility. She found herself being angry, furious, and feeling out of control most of the time. Through eliciting the relaxation response and utilizing cognitive strategies to uncover and challenge her automatic thoughts, she began to realize that a good deal of her anger had nothing whatsoever to do with her difficulty conceiving.

She was the daughter and niece of physicians, and most of her family was medically-oriented. She reported feeling unhappy and pressured by her job. She had expected to enjoy being an internist, especially after the rigors of medical school and residency, but during the session on affirmations, she realized she had gone to medical school only because of family expectations.

Although she had never before stopped to think about it, her work was not fulfilling, and she actually felt resentful of her family's influence over her decision-making. She recognized that these feelings contributed significantly to her general feelings of anger and being out of control.

Over the next few weeks, Kristen spent a great deal of time appraising and reflecting on what she actually wanted to do. She saw a career counselor (direct action), talked at length with her husband (social support), took long, thoughtful walks (relaxation/distraction), and listed the pros and cons of switching careers. After careful thought, and with her husband's support, Kristen resigned from her job and enrolled in a professional cooking school, which fulfilled a lifelong dream of becoming a chef.

She later reported to the group that she was experiencing a sense of peace and fulfillment that she never thought possible. She still had to cope with the frustration of being infertile, but now that she had taken control over a very important part of her life, the uncertainties of infertility were easier to tolerate.

Stop now and reflect on your automatic thoughts and beliefs as they might relate to your experience with infertility.

Take a Moment To . . .

Stop.

Take a Breath.
• Release physical tension.

Reflect.
• What is going on here?
• What are my automatic thoughts and exaggerated beliefs?
• Why am I anxious or distressed? Am I allowing the problems to get out of perspective?
• Will worrying help? What is the worst that can happen?

Choose.
• What can I do, what coping techniques would work here?
• Should I consider my emotional response separately from the practical problem?
• Am I avoiding the best solution because it will be difficult for me? What is possible?
• What do I want to do?

Now, do it!

What else you can do for yourself

Infertility can occupy not only your time, energy, and money, but also exert control over your body. Many women experiencing infertility tend to either forget about their bodies or else focus on controlling all aspects of their lives. Some feel their lives are so regulated by infertility treatments that they rebel with unhealthy habits such as smoking, drinking caffeinated beverages frequently, and not exercising. Others are very careful for the second two weeks of their cycles, but indulge themselves once their period comes. Still others work very hard to maintain exemplary habits in an effort to increase the chance of conception.

In general, moderation is the answer. Because infertility arouses many feelings of deprivation, severely restrictive diets and punishing exercise regimens are neither appropriate nor productive. Approach healthy lifestyle habits with balance and perspective. Do things you enjoy and that bring you pleasure rather than frustration and deprivation. Look over the chapters on nutrition and exercise, and make choices and changes that are both healthful *and* emotionally acceptable.

How about . . .

- inviting your husband to take a long stroll in the moonlight
- taking an interesting cooking course and practicing at home one night per week
- a girls' night out to visit a comedy club
- a new activity—miniature golf, bowling, pottery, gardening, bicycling, painting, etc.
- adopting a puppy or kitten from a local shelter
- taking a deep breath and tackling a new challenge; do something you always dreamed of but were unable to try

One of the most common problems associated with infertility is a feeling of isolation. Support groups are a way to share thoughts and feelings, to gain support from others who know exactly what you are going through, as well as for you to help and support others. Resolve, Inc., a national organization for the infertile dedicated to teaching and providing information, has local chapters in most states. One service is support groups for individuals and couples, as well as pre-adoption support groups. These groups are run by experienced group leaders, and the cost is reasonable. Look in your local phone book for the number of the nearest Resolve chapter, or call the national office at (617) 623-1156.

People uncomfortable in group situations can seek support from the many well-trained therapists who are expert in helping people in similar situations. Many Resolve chapters can supply you with a list of local therapists who specialize in infertility-related issues. Also ask your physician. Many infertility specialists work closely with psychologists, social workers, and psychiatrists. Asking your physician for a referral does not signal that you have a "problem"; you are merely doing what you can to help yourself feel better. Be sure you feel comfortable with and trust the person you choose as a therapist. The first one you see may not be the best person for you. Do not hesitate to talk to several therapists before selecting the one who feels right.

Infertility is not an issue solely for the woman. It affects the couple, and it is very normal for couples to report numerous difficulties in their relationship as they experience infertility. Frequently, both parties have different feelings at different times. Seeing a therapist together may help clarify each one's aims and goals and help both support the other.

Jill's Experience

Jill, a thirty-year-old salesperson, realized that she and her husband were consistently a year apart. She had wanted to get married a year before he did, she had wanted to start a family a year before he did, she realized they might have a fertility problem a year before he, too, came to that conclusion, and she decided she wanted to apply for adoption a year before he did. She used the skills learned in the program to calm herself, which gave her husband the time he needed before he, too, felt comfortable pursuing adoption.

This situation is very common. People reach important decisions at different speeds, and times when partners are not at the same point can be troubling. Couples therapy can be very helpful in working out these decisions. The outcomes can be beneficial and sometimes surprising.

Betsy's Experience

Betsy, a twenty-eight-year-old lawyer, and her husband went together for couples counseling because they were struggling with the issue of when to attempt "high-tech" treatment after several years of infertility. Betsy wanted to move on immediately, while her husband wanted to wait to see what would happen naturally. Through counseling, Betsy came to realize that the sense of urgency was coming from family and friends, not from her or her husband. They were both young and could wait a few months. They agreed that spending time having fun together and taking a much needed vacation would meet their needs.

    After several months, when conception did not occur naturally, they both agreed to schedule an IVF cycle. Serendipitously, Betsy conceived spontaneously the month prior to the scheduled IVF cycle and went on to deliver a beautiful baby boy.

At numerous times the support of a trained therapist can help ease decision-making as well as ensuring that the needs of both members of the couple are being satisfied.

MISCARRIAGES

Although an estimated 30 percent of pregnancies end in miscarriage, coping is not easy. The main complaint of many women in our groups has been that other people are unsupportive. Many well-meaning people say things like "It wasn't meant to be," "Forget about it and try again right away," or even "Maybe you weren't meant to have children." These statements can be hurtful and do anything but help you feel better.

A miscarriage is a true loss. As soon as you learned you were pregnant, the tiny embryo may have become a person to you. You may have started to wonder what and who it would look like, whether it would be a boy or a girl, and you may have started to think about names. Thus, a miscarriage can represent the loss of your child. This is when society slights your feelings. If you had indeed lost a child, others would expect you to be in mourning and the grieving process to be lengthy. A miscarriage, however, is not generally seen in the same light. Others may expect you to get back to your usual routine immediately.

Be kind to yourself, acknowledge that you have suffered a loss. The first thing you can do is not to force yourself to feel that everything is okay. Allow yourself to mourn your loss. You should begin to feel better at some point, but if you are grieving longer than you think reasonable, seek out a trained therapist.

You can also use the techniques in *The Wellness Book* to help yourself feel better. After a miscarriage, women frequently feel depressed, guilty, anxious, and hopeless. Daily elicitation of the relaxation response can help reduce these feelings. The cognitive-restructuring exercises can help you reduce some recurrent negative thoughts. One of the most common recurrent thoughts is that you must have done something wrong—that the miscarriage was your fault.

Linda's Experience

Linda, a thirty-nine-year-old guidance counselor, miscarried in her twelfth week and was blaming herself because she and her husband had made love several days beforehand. Although her doctor reassured her that intercourse did not cause the miscarriage, Linda felt guilt and self-blame. In fact, her doctor told her that the fetus had a genetic abnormality—one of the most common causes of miscarriage. By focusing on coping and problem-solving exercises, Linda was able to realize that she had felt so out of control over her body that it was easier to blame her voluntary action, making love, than to accept the fact that genetic normality or abnormality was out of her control.

By challenging her automatic thoughts, she further recognized her pattern of blaming herself for things over which she had no influence. She was then able to grieve for her lost child without anger, and several months later she resumed trying to become pregnant.

Seeking out others who have had a miscarriage can help validate that your feelings are normal. If you can, tell several of your close friends or relatives what has happened. You are very likely to find that one of them has also had a miscarriage. Talking to someone who has been through the same experience can be very helpful (social support). She may also be able to give you coping suggestions.

Remember that friends and relatives may want to be supportive but do not know how. People who have never experienced a miscarriage may not understand all of your feelings. Indeed, even women who have had a miscarriage may not always know what to say.

Debbie's Experience

Debbie, a thirty-three-year-old insurance agent, had just had her third miscarriage and was upset with her best friend who, although she herself had had a miscarriage the year before, did not seem to understand. When Debbie began to think closely about her own feelings after her first miscarriage, she realized that the subsequent miscarriages had been even more devastating than the first one. Thus, although she had expected her friend to be sympathetic, Debbie realized that her friend's experience was indeed very different, and this reduced her anger.

You might consider using a variety of coping and problem-solving tactics, such as those listed here.

Distraction	Go out for a romantic dinner with your husband. Go to a movie. Enroll in a class—art, gardening, music, cooking.
Direct Action	Make an appointment with your physician to discuss any possible causes of your miscarriages, how soon you can try again, and what you might do to minimize the chance of another miscarriage. Stop attending baby showers if they make you uncomfortable.
Relaxation	Elicit the relaxation response daily. Do minis when needed.
Affirmation	"I can handle this." "I am doing the best that I can." "This was not my fault."
Journal Writing	Writing about your feelings can help release some of your pain.
Social Support	Seek out support from friends, family, or others who have had a miscarriage.

Having a miscarriage is wrenching, and you need time to mourn your loss. Give yourself that time, focus on accepting your feelings, do as much as you can to help yourself feel better, and consider seeking out support, either from friends or relatives or from a trained therapist.

HIGH-RISK PREGNANCY

Being pregnant can be wonderful and also very frightening. Many women with high-risk pregnancies find themselves feeling more anxious than they would like—they sleep badly, cannot concentrate, are irritable, or cannot enjoy much of their pregnancy or their lives. In fact, some women who are pregnant and at high risk report going into the bathroom countless times every day to see if they are bleeding, installing white toilet paper because colored or patterned paper may hide staining, becoming anxious if they do not feel nauseous all the time, poking their breasts frequently to make sure they are still tender, and becoming nervous if they start to feel well. These behaviors are common for someone who lives in daily fear that her fetus may be lost.

To increase stress further, many women with high-risk pregnancy worry that high anxiety levels will somehow cause premature birth. Although research results are not definitive, anxiety alone does not seem to cause premature labor. Dr. Hiam Omer and his colleagues in Israel studied premature birthrates after the Yom Kippur War, during which nearly every pregnant woman in the country had either a husband, brother, or father involved in combat. While most would assume that these circumstances would produce very high levels of stress and fear, Dr. Omer found that the percentage of premature deliveries was actually lower during and after the war than in the same period the following year. This same pattern was found in Finland during World War II.

Many women who reported high levels of anxiety markedly benefited by following the suggestions in this book. First of all, daily elicitation of the relaxation response and the use of minis can lead to overall decreases in tension and fear. In addition, since many women with a high-risk pregnancy feel out of control, these practices help by increasing feelings of control. The mini-relaxation-response exercises can help decrease anxiety on a moment-to-moment basis. For example, you can use a mini

- if you feel a cramp
- before you use the toilet
- before and during ultrasounds
- when you see your physician
- whenever a scary thought occurs
- before and during procedures such as amniocentesis

Most women with high-risk pregnancy feel cheated of the joy of normal pregnancy. They want to feel elated, to glow, to feel secure browsing in baby stores. Give yourself time. As the pregnancy progresses, your feelings may change, you may begin to feel safer. If not, the key is not to push yourself.

Many women believe that constant worry protects them from something going wrong. This is a form of magical thinking: "If I worry enough about this event, then it will not happen." Give yourself time; take each moment of your pregnancy as it comes. You may be surprised at how quickly your fears dissolve.

Patient Experience

Three women in the high-risk pregnancy group were several months apart in their pregnancies. Monica, in her first trimester, focused her concerns on having a miscarriage. Ann, in her second trimester, was beginning to realize how different her life was going to be once the baby arrived and questioned her ability to be a perfect mother. Helen, in her last trimester, focused on the challenge of labor and delivery. As time went on, Monica worried about the changes in her life, then also focused on labor. All three women eventually had normal, healthy babies and are enjoying motherhood immensely.

Worrying about your pregnancy is normal and healthy. Read *The Wellness Book* carefully. Practice the relaxation response daily, do many minis, use the cognitive-restructuring exercises, and find ways to be good to yourself. Try to stay in the moment, to be mindful, rather than allowing your mind to run away with "what ifs." Focus on what you can do today rather than on what might happen tomorrow. Do at least one nice thing for yourself each day. Think of specific coping skills. How can you distract yourself? What direct action can you take to help yourself feel better? Which relaxation technique is your favorite? What affirmations can you think of? Of course, do not do anything in this book if it is against your physician's recommendations. Read about nutrition and exercise (chapters 7 and 8). It should go without saying, however, that you should make no dramatic changes in your lifestyle (specifically, eating habits and exercise program) without consulting your physician.

Remember, you are not alone. Many thousands of women every year have high-risk pregnancies. Ask your doctor about local support groups, talk to other women in your doctor's waiting room, or ask friends and relatives to see if others have been through this. You may wish to speak to a trained therapist who specializes in supporting women through difficult pregnancies; ask your doctor for a reference.

MENOPAUSE

If you are currently experiencing symptoms of menopause, are wondering if you are about to enter your menopause, or are facing or have just had surgery which will cause menopause, you can do many things to help yourself feel better and to improve your health. The hot flash is the most commonly reported, and is often the most distressing, symptom of menopause. An estimated 75 percent of women who go through menopause report hot flashes. Another common consequence of menopause is osteoporosis.

Hot flashes are characterized by feelings of heat or warmth in the face, upper body, or the entire body, and can be accompanied by observable perspiration. They last anywhere from several minutes to an hour; they tend to be most intense during the first two years of menopause and then decrease. Many women in our groups report that hot flashes are embarrassing and inconvenient and, since they often occur at night, cause insomnia, which can lead to fatigue and irritability.

Hormone replacement therapy has been documented to relieve hot flashes as well as other symptoms of menopause, including vaginal dryness. Whether or not to start hormone replacement therapy is a very personal decision; you should discuss the pros and cons carefully with your physician. One consideration is how seriously the menopausal symptoms are affecting your life. If frequent hot flashes are consistently disturbing your sleep, your work, and the general quality of your life, tell your physician. Other considerations are your risk factors for medical conditions which can either be increased or decreased by hormone replacement therapy. Be prepared to inform your physician about any history or family history of heart disease or osteoporosis (hormone replacement therapy may decrease your risk of developing these conditions) as well as any history of uterine or breast cancer (in this case risk may be increased by hormone replacement therapy). If you and your physician decide that you will take hormone replacement therapy, be sure to see your physician regularly to ensure that the treatment is working well for you.

If, for any reason, you and your physician decide that hormone replacement therapy is not appropriate for you, you can take other steps to decrease both hot flashes and the risk of developing osteoporosis. These steps will be discussed next.

A number of factors are known to trigger hot flashes, including emotional upset, heat (a hot day, being in a warm room, being in a very warm bed), alcohol, and hot drinks or meals. Finding cool environments, removing blankets from your bed, and avoiding alcohol and large hot meals can help you feel significantly more comfortable. In addition, since stress can exacerbate hot flashes, daily elicitation of the relaxation response is likely to decrease both the frequency and the duration of each flash. Several research projects have shown that women who practice a daily relaxation-response technique have fewer hot flashes; in one study, relaxation-response treatment led to a 60 percent reduction in the frequency of hot flashes.

Marjorie's Experience

Marjorie, fifty-two, was in her second year of menopause and had hot flashes every few hours, day and night. A teacher, she was frustrated because she had difficulty concentrating during a hot flash. In addition, she reported that she often had a hot flash when her class became unruly, which only compounded the problem. During the second session of the Menopause Program, Marjorie noted that although she started to have a hot flash during the relaxation-response exercise, it lasted only about 30 seconds, a fraction of the normal time.

Within several weeks, to Marjorie's delight, she was having hot flashes only a few times per day, and each one lasted less than two minutes. In addition, she was able to practice mini-relaxations whenever her class acted up and could actually prevent the onset of a hot flash.

Osteoporosis is another common physical problem which develops during and after menopause. When women go through menopause, estrogen production drops sharply. Estrogen plays a major role in maintaining bone strength through constant calcification; when estrogen levels drop, bones become more likely to break. Besides considering hormone replacement therapy, you can do many things to decrease your risk of developing osteoporosis. According to Dr. Sadja Greenwood, from the University of California Medical Center, San Francisco, these steps include

- engaging in weight-bearing exercise (for example, walking)
- increasing the amount of calcium in your diet
- decreasing use of salt
- decreasing alcohol consumption
- stopping smoking
- being careful not to eat a very high-protein diet

Discuss these suggestions with your physician prior to making any major changes in your lifestyle habits. However, it is reassuring to know that you can do numerous things, things within your control, to improve your health and decrease physical symptoms during and following menopause.

WOMEN'S HEALTH

Whether you have infertility, have had a miscarriage, are experiencing a high-risk pregnancy, are going through menopause or some other women's health problem, feelings of anxiety, depression, fear, isolation, and loss of control are common. Our suggestions may have little effect on any physical problem you have—for example, relaxation and stress-management strategies may not affect basic physical problems such as endometriosis, uterine abnormalities, estrogen decreases, and chromosomal problems—however, they do help in other very important ways. The key is that following these suggestions will help you feel better. You are not only likely to feel healthier, but also more in control because you took the responsibility for bringing about change. Whatever your physical problem, you will be able to deal with it better if you feel better about yourself. As we say in our meetings, "Just do it!"

Alice D. Domar, Ph.D.

HEALTH COMMITMENT

Long-Term Goal: _____

_____

_____
Signature

_____
Witness

Expected Date of Reaching Goal: _____

Short-Term Goals

Comments (supports, rewards, etc.)

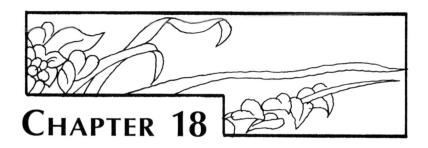

CHAPTER 18

BEHAVIORAL MEDICINE AND CANCER

> Hope is the thing with feathers
> That perches in the soul,
> And sings the tune without the words,
> And never stops at all.
>
> Emily Dickinson

In this chapter you will explore

- coping with cancer
- how to develop a healthy lifestyle
- the interaction of mental attitude and cancer
- how the immune system works
- the value of mental imagery or visualization
- how to handle your emotions
- improving the quality of your life

Living with cancer affects people profoundly. They often reevaluate who and what is important in life and what their goals are. It also raises numerous questions about how an individual can best cope with the stress of illness and stay involved in the treatment.

Any major change—be it starting a new business, gaining or losing a family member, moving to a new area, or becoming ill—interrupts our routines and requires adjustment. As we said earlier, change is stressful. A diagnosis of cancer brings its own unique stressors. This chapter suggests techniques for coping with the stress of your illness and living a full life with cancer. The first step in self-help is to become more aware of what is occurring in your life.

Becoming more aware of your physical well-being, as well as your thoughts, emotions, and beliefs, will help you gain a different perspective and see choices rather than becoming locked into only one possible solution or approach. You will be able to investigate available options, including various treatment possibilities, your participation in treatment decisions, changes in your thought patterns, readjustment of your lifestyle, and definition of your long- and short-term goals.

Becoming aware might also change some of your relationships. You can determine how much you want to share and with whom. You will discover friends who are available when you need them, but who can also stand back when you need space for yourself and want to be independent. You also might decide to change how you communicate with your family, friends, physicians, and other health-care providers.

Last but not least, this chapter can help you find a way to live a quality life with cancer. Using the techniques described throughout *The Wellness Book* can help relieve physical symptoms such as pain, sleeplessness, fatigue, and side effects of chemotherapy, as well as contribute to a sense of control and a calmer state of mind. This chapter includes specific concepts and exercises that we have found to be helpful for people living with cancer.

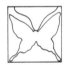 ### *Take a Moment To . . .*

Review the exercise in chapter 10, "Managing Stress," that asked you to identify which things were Important/Meaningful/Valuable to you (see pages 185–86). Your cancer most likely influenced what you wrote. Reflect on your answers; you may find that your illness has allowed you the opportunity to place renewed emphasis on those things which are important to you. You may want to do the exercise again.

This exercise can help define your long-term goals. The self-help strategies in this section should help you achieve these goals.

CANCER FACTORS

Living or working in an environment which results in exposure to a carcinogen, such as asbestos, or maintaining habits such as smoking, increases the risk of developing cancer. In addition, some preliminary evidence suggests that our mental state and behavior might affect the progress of cancer. Animal studies have shown that stress, heightened by lack of control, can increase the rate of tumor growth. Drs. Steven Greer and Maggie Watson, a psychiatrist and a psychologist at the Royal Marsden Hospital in Great Britain, have shown that patients with early breast cancer who have a positive attitude or "fighting spirit" do better than those with a less positive attitude. Dr. David Spiegel of Stanford University School of Medicine has demonstrated that patients with advanced breast cancer who participated in a group program offering support, cognitive therapy, and relaxation techniques lived longer on the average than those who did not participate in a program. Although evidence of a relationship between mental attitude and the progress of cancer is only preliminary, there is sufficient reason to examine your attitudes and become actively involved in your care. When you feel well psychologically and feel that you can cope, you will likely also have a better quality of life.

The course of cancer is influenced by many different things. Dr. Alastair Cunningham, in his workbook for cancer patients, uses the metaphor of a balance to describe the different forces affecting the outcome. On one side is the weight of the biological process of the cancer itself, on the other are medical treatment and the body's own control mechanisms, including the immune system and hormones. These factors may also be aided by self-help efforts. Such self-help approaches may increase some degree of control over the cancer, but there is no guarantee that even all three "weights" combined can outweigh the disease. Sometimes the biological processes of the cancer are too vigorous to overcome. If the disease is too strong or too advanced to alter, it often will progress.

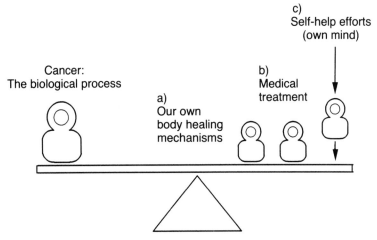

From Alastair J. Cunningham, *Helping Yourself: A Workbook for People Living With Cancer*, Canadian Cancer Society, 1989, p. 3.

Cells can become cancerous when genetic material (DNA) is damaged or changed. Through a set of complex processes, these changes result in the loss of the normal controls that regulate the growth of cells, so that they begin to multiply and spread. In fact, cells in the body probably develop genetic abnormalities quite frequently, but a variety of control mechanisms—including the body's immune system, the effects of various hormones, and perhaps the nervous system and its hormones—prevents their growing into a cancer. When the control mechanisms fail, particular cells can grow without restraint and become a cancer.

Why do we think it even possible that a mental attitude can affect cell growth? Mental attitudes or thoughts can produce physiological changes. Hundreds of billions of nerve cells in the brain become active during any mental activity and produce chemical changes. For example, in a situation perceived as dangerous or stressful, the hypothalamus, an area in the center of the brain, collects incoming "danger" messages and activates the pituitary gland, which in turn activates your adrenal glands to produce hormones that cause chemical changes in various cells and tissues. This is the fight-or-flight response discussed earlier. But in the process of bringing forth the fight-or-flight response, the immune system can become suppressed, making you less able to fight a variety of diseases, including cancer. It has also been shown that "positive messages" from your brain can increase the ability of your immune system to fight disease and thereby improve your physical and mental health.

THE BODY'S IMMUNE SYSTEM

One of the major functions of the immune system, which is among the most complicated in the body, is to defend you against cancer, infections, and other diseases. It also helps you regain health when you have an infectious illness or cancer.

The healthy immune system can discriminate between cells belonging to the body and those that are foreign and must be eliminated or destroyed. Bacteria, viruses, and abnormal cells such as cancer cells are recognizable as foreign because of surface proteins called *antigens*. After exposure to foreign antigens, the immune system reacts by producing and releasing a number of different kinds of cells and hormones to attack the foreign invader.

The immune system has two basic ways to defend the body: *cell-mediated immunity* that comes from the direct action of cells, and *humoral immunity*, which comes from antibodies. Cell-mediated immunity relies primarily on white blood cells, called *T-lymphocytes*, which act by coming into direct contact with the antigens. The T-lymphocytes release a substance (cytokine) which damages or kills the bacteria, virus, or cancer cells that carry the antigens. The major T-cells have been named killer T-cells, helper T-cells, and suppressor T-cells.

Humoral immunity relies on bodily substances called *antibodies*, which are produced by other specialized lymphocytes known as B-cells. These antibodies, traveling in the bloodstream and other body fluids, attach themselves to the antigens they encounter and act to neutralize or kill the cells containing the antigen.

Your immune system also has a memory. When exposed to an antigen, certain cells called *lymphocyte memory cells* "remember" the antigens, so that if the antigen reinvades your body, your memory cells are waiting to fight it.

Finally, your immune system is a tidy housekeeper. Scavenger cells called *macrophages* engulf or "swallow-up" the dead bacterial, viral, or cancerous cells, and carry them away to be eliminated from your body. Macrophages also play an important role in activating the immune response. At the end of this chapter, on page 335, is a more detailed description of the cells which play a role in your immune response to a foreign antigen. Additional information about the immune system is in chapter 20, "Psychoneuroimmunology and HIV Disease."

LIVING WITH CANCER

Daily hassles can become magnified when you are struggling to cope with cancer. You try to keep your balance, but even small events that remind you of your disease—a blood test or routine X-ray, an office visit, a magazine article—can set off a downward spiral. The actress Gilda Radner captured this feeling in the title of her book about her cancer, *It's Always Something*. Sometimes you feel overwhelmed by your emotions and unable to control them.

In order to gain some control, it is important to first recognize that during a crisis or illness, your emotions are often more intense than at other times. Allow yourself to acknowledge these feelings without judgment. Having feelings and emotions is perfectly all right. There are no "bad" emotions; but not acknowledging what you are feeling can interfere with your ability to cope and adapt.

We discussed the relationship of emotions to health in chapters 11 and 12, but this relationship bears repeating here, specifically as it relates to cancer. Many participants in our cancer groups express feelings of anxiety, anger, resentment, guilt, and hopelessness. Anger can mask feelings of helplessness, insecurity, disappointment, and fear. When you were diagnosed, you may initially have felt angry. Cancer was not in your life plan. It isn't fair. You have been a good person. Why now? As you adjusted to your diagnosis and treatment, you may have felt angry at the losses in your life, such as a change in body image, loss of control, and loss over life choices.

Not only are these feelings of anger understandable, they are healthy. Anger can be purposeful. It can mobilize you to change situations which are uncomfortable; it can propel you into direct action, to become more involved in your care and treatment options, to be more assertive with family and friends about what you want and need from them. What is important at this point is to acknowledge that you do indeed have feelings, to give yourself permission to have them, and to get support from family, friends, and peers to deal with your feelings constructively.

Anger that is not dealt with constructively, that has no outlet, can contribute to feelings of helplessness and lack of control. It can also, as you have read elsewhere, have physiological consequences. If your anger is constant, your body is continuously aroused by the fight-or-flight response, which can be detrimental to your general health as well as to the integrity of your immune system.

Fear and anxiety are also common for patients living with cancer. As discussed in chapter 12, "Feelings, Moods, and Attitudes," healthy fear is different from neurotic anxiety. Healthy fear is realistic; it keeps us alert and warns us of dangers. Neurotic anxiety, on the other hand, results from exaggerated, distorted thoughts with little or no basis in reality. Healthy fear can be seen as a defense mechanism that helps you remain vigilant or that prompts you to seek information important to you and to explore the options and possibilities available. Unhealthy fear can immobilize you with worry about all the "what ifs" and future events that may not occur. One negative result can become magnified a hundredfold.

Unhealthy fear and anxiety can also cause agonizing guilt over events in the past. Some patients relate being plagued by questions such as "Did I bring on my cancer by . . . ?" or "If only I had . . . everything would be different now." Unfortunately, as we are all well aware, life is uncertain. In many cases we do not know the causes of cancer. And what of those cases in which we do, such as the association between cigarette smoking and lung cancer? In such a situation, smokers must take some responsibility for their actions, but it should be put into perspective.

However, we must be clear that many factors affecting our health, including the development of cancer, are not completely within our control. We should not think of the development of illness as our "fault." A former colleague, Dr. Joan Borysenko, contrasted what she called *healthy guilt* with *unhealthy guilt*. Healthy guilt is the feeling you have after doing something "wrong" like lying, cheating, or intentionally hurting someone. Healthy guilt is characterized as remorse or regret. It can make you more aware of your motives, help you understand yourself better, and lead to changing your behavior. Unhealthy guilt results from feeling responsible for things over which you have no control, such as what you "might" or "should" have done in the past.

How can you rid yourself of unhealthy guilt? First, become aware of your feelings toward yourself; then let go of unrealistic feelings about what you should or should not have done. Forgive yourself for real or imagined transgressions, and allow yourself simply to be. If guilt is a recurrent theme for you, many exercises are recommended in the literature for both meditation and cognitive therapy. We recommend Dr. Borysenko's most recent book, listed in the References, for more specific information about dealing with guilt.

Give yourself permission to have a "bad" day once in a while. Life is challenging you to cope with and adjust to many things, some of which can be overwhelming. Recognize the limits of your capacity to cope, and be sure to replenish yourself before you reach exhaustion. Step back for a moment and reassess your resources; you will be stronger for it. Even people renowned for their strength of character become exasperated, as evidenced by this simple but eloquent statement made during a particularly difficult time in the administration of an Israeli prime minister:

I have had enough.
Golda Meir

Take a Moment To . . .

Reflect on your experience with cancer and complete this journal-writing exercise. Take some uninterrupted time to write down this experience as a way of exploring your thoughts, feelings, and emotions around your diagnosis and treatment as well as how this has interfered with your life goals. Reflect also on how your cancer experience has affected others around you. Writing down your experience is an effective way to explore difficult issues and put them behind you.

This exercise is likely to bring your thoughts, feelings, and emotions to the fore. If this makes you uncomfortable, you may want to omit this exercise or postpone it until you have appropriate support. If you choose to do this exercise, acknowledge and honor those feelings which emerge as you write. Talk about them with family, friends, or other patients. You may also want to seek out a cancer-support group or counselor.

KEEPING IT IN PERSPECTIVE

An important goal of our program is to demystify health care and empower patients to participate in their care, treatment, and healing. We encourage patients to develop a sense of personal control and wholeness as well as to acknowledge and honor their personal beliefs. However, beliefs, although important, should not be taken as absolutes, but kept in perspective to the situation. Dr. David Cella, a psychologist from the Rush Cancer Center at Presbyterian–St. Luke's Medical Center in Chicago, well known for his work in cancer, suggests that these beliefs may at times require modifiers. Some examples from Dr. Cella:

BELIEF: My health is my responsibility.
MODIFIER: I did not cause my disease.
  Considerable evidence indicates that a sense of control can lead an individual to make the changes necessary to getting well. However, given our limited knowledge of all the factors involved in the development and progression of cancer, little scientific evidence supports the view that people bring on their own cancer. It is inappropriate for patients or health-care professionals to perpetuate the idea that individuals "cause their cancer."
BELIEF: My doctor and I are partners.
MODIFIER: We both have things to learn.
  Communication between patient and physician is essential. It is a two-way street. Patients should inform their physicians of their understanding, beliefs, and expectations about their disease and treatment.

Physicians should make clear what is known and unknown about current treatment or approaches, as well as their attitudes toward care.
BELIEF: Cancer is an opportunity.
MODIFIER: I don't have to be grateful for that opportunity; I didn't need it.

As discussed earlier, a serious illness such as cancer can provide an opportunity to reassess goals and priorities. While this is often beneficial Dr. Cella points out that there is certainly no need for gratitude here.

Our concern must be to live while we're alive . . . to release our inner selves from the spiritual death that comes with living behind a facade designed to conform to external definitions of who and what we are.

Elisabeth Kübler-Ross

GETTING INVOLVED—MAKING A DIFFERENCE

In our eight-week Behavioral Medicine Cancer Program we involve our patients in planning and carrying out their treatment as well as participating in the decision-making process. We have found that using the techniques and approaches described throughout *The Wellness Book*—values clarification, goal-setting, understanding the mind-body model for health, exercise, nutrition, cognitive therapy, and humor—can help relieve physical symptoms such as pain, nausea and vomiting, sleeplessness and fatigue, as well as contribute to a sense of control and calmer state of mind. The most important point is for you to get involved, make the investment, and do the work. It *will* make a difference.

While most of the content and many of the exercises presented in previous chapters can be applied to your situation, a few areas deserve caution. Carefully review chapters 6 and 7 on exercise and body awareness prior to embarking on an exercise program. Exercise is appropriate unless you have specific physical problems. The critical concept is to listen to your body. If you are fatigued, you may need to decrease the pace or duration of an exercise or activity. Exercise serves a very therapeutic function in the treatment of cancer: not only does it keep your body conditioned, it can help counteract depression and boost your self-esteem. You may be unable to do as much as you did earlier in your life, but the key is to accept what is now, and to maximize this situation. Get up and get dressed every day. Go outside for a stroll/walk/jog/run (whatever is appropriate to your desires and physical abilities). Observe the weather, the scenery, the subtle changes of the season. Bring along a friend and revel in what you *can* do. As with any exercise program, keep your physician informed about what you would like to do and solicit suggestions about what is the most appropriate level for you.

Healthy nutrition is another fundamental component of any treatment plan for cancer. Chapter 8, "Nutrition for Good Health," presented the general principles for a healthy diet as well as general dietary recommendations for cancer prevention. If you feel well, untroubled by symptoms from your illness or treatment, chapter 8 offers the most specific information for you. If, however, you are experiencing symptoms due to your illness or treatment, chapter 19, "Healthy Eating to Prevent Undernutrition," provides specific information for strategies to prevent undernutrition and weight loss.

In the clinic we have been particularly successful in alleviating nausea and vomiting associated with chemotherapy. Eliciting the relaxation response before, during, and after the chemotherapy is one of the most effective behavioral ways to prevent nausea. If you experience nausea, elicit a "mini" and breathe mindfully until the wave of nausea passes. If you experience nausea *and* vomiting, alert your physician. In addition to the behavioral intervention just described, many new medicines are now available to treat nausea.

In some cases, the nausea and vomiting associated with chemotherapy can become a learned, conditioned response, referred to as *anticipatory nausea and vomiting*. The theory is as follows: nausea and vomiting after chemotherapy can condition you to expect the same next time; after three or four unpleasant experiences, just thinking about chemotherapy might make you nauseated. Then, things associated with the chemotherapy such as your clothes, the room, the smell, the physician or nurse, can begin to elicit the symptom.

If you develop this anticipatory symptom, you can do many things behaviorally to avoid nausea. First, look at how you can change the experience. Wear different clothes each time, take a different route to the treatment, sit in a different seat in the waiting area, and choose a different bed. A frequent suggestion is to take an orange with you to smell in order to block the odors of the clinic.

Next think about ways to relax and distract yourself, because anxiety increases the symptom. Elicit the relaxation response before, during, and after the treatment. It may be useful to listen to a relaxation tape evoking any image you find peaceful and calming.

You might also consider reframing the chemotherapy as a friend and ally—something your body needs to stay well or become well—rather than a toxicant or poison. Visualize this ally circulating through your body, bringing the necessary powerful ingredient to fight the cancer cells. Adopt the affirmation each morning that chemotherapy is friend not foe.

Plan to celebrate after your chemotherapy instead of setting the day aside to be sick. Reward yourself each time with whatever brings you pleasure. Take with you dry crackers, toast, or other food which you have found helpful in preventing the nausea. Arrange to see a funny movie that day with friends who are important to you. The point is to use your relaxation skills and behavioral skills to change the experience so that nausea does not become a learned, anticipated response.

Janet's Experience

Janet, a forty-two-year-old office worker and single parent, was diagnosed as having cancer of the breast. After a portion of her breast was removed, along with some lymph nodes in her axilla (armpit), she had six weeks of radiation therapy. Because two of the lymph nodes in her axilla were found to contain cancer cells, she was to receive a six-month course of chemotherapy, with treatment given every twenty-eight days. Following her first chemotherapy treatment, she experienced considerable nausea and vomiting for several days.

After this first treatment Janet joined the Behavioral Medicine Program for Cancer Patients and learned to elicit the relaxation response regularly. She was also instructed in behavioral and cognitive skills to prevent nausea. She found it helpful to elicit the relaxation response before, during, and after the chemotherapy. Before the treatment, Janet used an image of the sea, with waves lapping at the shore, as her focus. During the treatment, she focused on the chemotherapy as a powerful healing potion circulating to all parts of her body, neutralizing the cancer cells.

She arranged to have a friend take care of her child on the day of her treatment, and planned a special treat for him. She made plans for herself, labeling each treatment a milestone in her therapy and treating it accordingly. She found that dressing up for the chemotherapy gave her a more positive perspective, and in this way she was ready to have friends over later for dinner. It was not easy, but Janet found herself better able to cope with the side effects of her treatment. She invited good friends who she knew would not be uncomfortable if she did get sick, but amazingly enough, she was never nauseated after starting her new plan.

She also found that allowing herself quiet time after the treatment to elicit the relaxation response, using a spiritual focus, was important to her ability not only to decrease the symptom of nausea and vomiting, but to maintain her overall ability to cope with her illness and keep things in perspective.

IMAGERY AND VISUALIZATION

During the past twenty years, considerable research on stress and its effect on animal and human immune systems has shown, in general, that stress, especially stress outside one's control, may decrease the effectiveness of the immune system. In contrast to these findings, elicitation of the relaxation response and its combination with certain imagery exercises may increase the effectiveness of the immune system.

During the past ten years, additional research has been carried out on how the mind and the immune system communicate with each other. This field, called *psychoneuroimmunology* (PNI), is discussed further in chapter 20, "Psychoneuroimmunology and HIV Disease." One technique of interest to researchers in psychoneuroimmunology is mental imagery.

Mental imagery, or visualization, was introduced in chapter 5, "Eliciting the Relaxation Response." For example, if you describe your living room, you may see it in your mind, or if asked for directions, you may traverse the route in your head. Our fears and anxieties are often associated with visual expectations of what can or will happen. When you say you are "looking forward" to something, you imply "fore-seeing" the event. Many of our thoughts consist of visual images—memories, daydreams, hopes for the future. So, why do we discuss visualization or imagery as something unusual if we do it naturally, without really noticing it? Because, like focusing on breathing to elicit the relaxation response, imagery can be used as a specific therapeutic strategy. As a method to elicit the relaxation response, imagery can be useful, for example, before unpleasant or frightening procedures or during treatment.

Take a Moment To . . .

Imagine a lemon. Visualize it carefully, notice its color, texture, and shape. Now peel it, then separate it carefully into sections. Feel and smell the sections. Imagine eating a piece of the lemon just as you would a piece of orange. Carefully put a piece of the lemon into your mouth. Taste it. Smell it. Feel the texture. What changes do you notice in your mouth? You may find yourself salivating or puckering up from the sour taste.

Drs. Carl and Stephanie Simonton, and Jeanne Achterberg, while at the Cancer Counseling and Research Center in Fort Worth, Texas, began using the power of imagery—which you just experienced with the lemon—in cancer treatment. They wanted to determine if imagining the body's immune defenses as strong and successful could assist a patient in fighting his or her cancer. They asked their patients to draw (with colored crayons) pictures of their cancer, their treatment, and their immune system. Some patients made fairly realistic drawings of cancerous cells, the body's immune cells, and treatments such as chemotherapy or radiation. Others drew symbolic figures such as dragons (the cancer cells) and white knights (the body's immune system). The results from this study suggested that patients with images of a strong defense that dealt effectively with the intruding cancer had a greater probability of remission or slowed progression of the cancer two months after the drawings were made.

However intriguing these findings, they require a great deal more rigorous scientific investigation before we can confidently say that imagery plays a role in the regression of illness.

In our Behavioral Medicine Cancer Program we have chosen to use imagery as one technique to complement our program and traditional cancer treatment. We use it as a technique to elicit the relaxation response and to help patients gain insight into their feelings, fears, and expectations. We do not focus on imagery as a way to halt progression or promote regression of cancer. We simply do not know enough at this stage of imagery research to say if or how it works with disease.

Peter's Experience

Peter, a seventy-year-old with leukemia, was undergoing chemotherapy when he joined our program. He imagined and drew the treatment as weak and disconnected from himself and his disease; he seemed to have no confidence in it whatsoever. When he realized the implication of his drawing, he became very upset, and, with the support of the group, decided to discuss his doubts with his doctor. His physician was able to give Peter enough information to increase his confidence in the chemotherapy and to help him realize that it was the best treatment option for him.

If your imagery reveals doubts, use this information constructively, as Peter did. Choose the type of imagery that works best for you. You might imagine a safe place where you see yourself as cancer-free, or visualize your body fighting the cancer cells, or visualize the chemotherapy medication as doing its job.

Rose's Experience

Rose, a very active woman in her fifties, devised her own image to elicit the relaxation response. She imagined a boxing match between her white cells and her cancer cells, during which she cheered and shouted, "White cells fight, white cells fight!" The white cells always won. This image became so strong for her that she actually acted it out, jumping out of bed each morning to shadowbox while chanting, "White cells fight, white cells fight!" This became her daily affirmation.

Rose is a woman with a solid faith in God, a strong will to live, and a "fighting spirit." She has had breast cancer for many years, had two mastectomies at different times, and radiation and chemotherapy treatments. Last year she had a transplant of her own bone marrow after high-dose chemotherapy when she had another recurrence. She was discharged from the hospital after only twelve days, which is unusually fast, and recuperated well. She felt that her boxing image had a great deal to do with giving her a fighting chance.

Take a Moment To . . .

Elicit the relaxation response. Imagine yourself in a special, safe place. When you are calmly centered, let an image come to mind that represents your cancer or any symptoms that bother you. If you are currently in remission, do not imagine cancer cells being present; instead focus on any trouble spots you might have—symptoms, pain, things that don't feel right. Accept whatever image comes, however strange or mysterious—it's okay, let it be.

Allow the image to become clearer. You might see cells that have become abnormal, or organs that look diseased, or the whole body in need of repair and healing. You may see symbolic representations of the processes occurring in your body. Whatever image occurs, accept it and observe it carefully and in detail.

Now visualize your own defenses. Remember, your body is wonderfully designed with built-in protective devices. Imagine your defenses in any way that feels right to you—as cells battling cells, white knights fighting invaders, animals or Pac-Men eating diseased tissue, sun rays healing damaged tissues, or healing energy. Visualize your defenses as strong, numerous, and powerful, helping to restore you to health.

Add your chemotherapy, radiation therapy, or other treatment to this picture. See them as your allies, powerful friends in your fight against the cancer.

Finally, visualize yourself in good health. You might see a beam of light scouring through your whole body, restoring it to harmony and health. Imagine yourself in a place of peace and natural beauty, feeling totally healthy. Keep that picture in your mind. Take a few deep breaths. Slowly return your thoughts to the place where you are sitting.

If you found an image that might be helpful to you, describe it here.

_____

_____

_____

_____

_____

If this exercise raised questions or doubts for you, note them here, and be sure to follow up and get the appropriate information from your health-care practitioner.

_____

_____

_____

_____

_____

If imagery feels comfortable and useful to you, you might consider making it a part of your daily routine.

We have found that the techniques described in this chapter improve the quality of life for individuals living with cancer. Evaluations from participants in our programs have shown less depression and anxiety as well as an increased sense of control or fighting spirit. In addition, they report that using these techniques can significantly decrease the nausea and vomiting resulting from chemotherapy and also help to manage pain more effectively, improvements that were highly valued.

A most eloquent summary of the benefits of the techniques discussed in this chapter comes from one of our critically ill patients:

> It has been interesting to me to notice that as my outer (physical) condition has worsened, my inner (spiritual) condition has become stronger. I have become convinced that healing is a journey, not a sudden happening. It isn't that the physical doesn't matter. Of course it does. The amount of pain in a day, an hour, certainly affects the quality of one's life and one's ability to cope with that life and one's capacity for enjoying that life. But the inner attitude toward what is happening affects how one feels about life. If that attitude is one of bitterness and despair, then pain comes as a cruel blow from life or punishment from God. If the attitude is one of faith and hope, then pain is certainly real, but it doesn't carry the other burdens of the cruelty of God and the unfairness of life. I think a positive attitude can reduce the pain. Meditation and relaxation can certainly soften its grasp.

Ursula Brandt, Ph.D.
Leo Stolbach, M.D.

IMMUNE RESPONSE TO A FOREIGN ANTIGEN

Macrophages are derived from white blood cells called monocytes. They serve as scavenger cells and "swallow up" invaders. They specialize in "cleaning up" debris. For example, if a cancer cell has been killed, macrophages will swallow up the dead cell and remove its skeleton. When they swallow the antigen on the surface of the bacterium, virus, or cancerous cell, they send a message that a foreigner is invading the body. This signal attracts T-cells to the area and starts the immune response aimed at neutralizing or killing invading organisms or cells.

T-cells are derived from stem (immature) cells produced in the bone marrow, and then transported by the blood to the thymus (a small gland in the upper part of the chest), where they are transformed into mature T-cells. These mature T-cells travel throughout the body by way of the bloodstream and other body fluids, destroying or damaging cells containing foreign antigens. They also further regulate the immune response. T-cells are further categorized as:

a. Helper T-cells, activated by Interleukin (IL-1) released by macrophages that have identified a foreign antigen. Helper T-cells carry the message that an invader is present to T-lymphocytes throughout the body. When activated, helper T-cells release Interleukin 2 (IL-2), which stimulates various T-cells to multiply. They also release a B-cell growth factor (BCGF) which causes B-cells to multiply (see below).

b. Killer T-cells are recruited and activated by the IL-2 released by helper T-cells. When previously exposed to a specific foreign antigen and then reactivated, they will kill cancer cells, bacteria, or other cells, containing that specific antigen.

c. Suppressor T-cells can slow down or stop the action of activated B-cells and T-cells once an infection or cancer has been eliminated.

d. Lymphokine activated killer cells (LAK cells), activated by IL-2, can recognize and kill cancer cells without previous exposure to a cancer antigen.

B-cells are lymphocytes found in the lymph nodes and the spleen, having migrated there from the bone marrow. When activated they produce proteins, called antibodies, which can travel to all parts of the body. B-cells are activated by exposure to a foreign antigen and a B-cell differentiating factor (BCDF) produced by helper T-cells. The antibody produced by B-cells can neutralize, damage, or kill cells containing the foreign antigen that originally caused the antibody to be made.

Memory cells are B- or T-lymphocytes activated by exposure to a foreign antigen. Memory cells remain in the body for years and can recognize a new attack by an organism or cell to which they have previously been exposed. They respond rapidly by instructing the immune system to produce appropriate antibodies and killer T-cells. Long-term immunity from vaccination or previous exposure to certain infections relies on memory cells.

HEALTH COMMITMENT

Long-Term Goal:

_____

_____ Signature

_____

_____ Witness

Expected Date of Reaching Goal: _____

Short-Term Goals	Comments (supports, rewards, etc.)

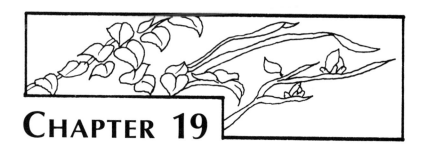

CHAPTER 19

EATING HEALTHFULLY TO PREVENT UNDERNUTRITION

Oh, better, no doubt, is a dinner of herbs,
When season'd by love, which no rancor disturbs,
And sweeten'd by all that is sweetest in life,
Than turbot, bisque, ortolans, eaten in strife.

Owen Meredith, *Lucille*

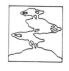

In this chapter you will explore

- ways to maintain your weight
- the many important roles of food in healing
- specific strategies to help you overcome some of the eating problems that can occur with illness

Chapter 8, "Nutrition for Good Health," described the basics of healthy nutrition and suggested ways to create a more healthful diet for yourself. If your illness is in remission or you are not currently experiencing symptoms or problems, follow the general guidelines for healthy eating already presented in chapter 8. If, however, you are currently feeling ill or suffering from side effects of your treatment, you may need to alter these basic recommendations in order to prevent weight loss and poor nutrition.

This chapter will be important as you begin to learn how best to incorporate some of these nutritional ideals into your specific needs. Do not underestimate the importance of healthy eating and balancing your nutritional intake among the four food groups (outlined in detail in chapter 8), but also remember that these are only guidelines and you will need to work with your dietitian and other health-care providers to create a food plan that meets your individual needs. Consult with them regularly.

A Registered Dietitian is a food and nutrition expert who can help you improve your diet and nutritional status. You can find one by asking your physician for a referral, or by calling the dietetics department of your local hospital or state dietetic association.

FOOD: A SOURCE OF STRENGTH

Food is an important ingredient in any active treatment plan for health promotion as well as in prevention or treatment of illness. When people are ill, they often experience changes in moods and feelings, isolate themselves from friends or family, or change long-standing patterns of behavior, including exercise patterns. All of these changes, important in and of themselves, can also affect your attitude toward food. When you feel down, depressed, or blue, you may find your eating patterns changing significantly. Isolating yourself after being accustomed to eating with others, at home or going out, may change your food intake. Consider these other aspects of your life when you develop strategies for enhancing your food intake.

Healthy eating while coping with illness—cancer or human immuno-deficiency virus (HIV) infection—means choosing foods you can tolerate and which nourish, strengthen, and contribute to the healing process. It also means examining the roles of certain foods or the patterns of eating that have nurtured you to this point. Does chicken soup have certain connotations for you? Many families consider it a panacea to heal any sickness. Every family has its own traditions about foods that soothe, heal, and comfort. Family rituals may associate food with a comforting social experience. Recall the good experiences you have had with food, which can be important building blocks in healing or coping with an illness. Capitalize on these experiences as you begin to eat a diet that will help either to maintain or rebuild your strength.

EATING WELL WHEN YOU DON'T FEEL WELL

The most problematic issue facing many patients who are coping with illness and the side effects of treatment is to maintain weight. Weight loss is usually due either to a loss of appetite or poor digestion of food, accompanied by poor absorption of nutrients. Weight loss and malnutrition can often be prevented or successfully reversed by a cooperative combination of nutritional strategies, self-help strategies, and medical treatment.

When you don't feel like eating . . .

To understand why you may not feel like eating, think back to having the flu or a common cold. With the flu or a cold, you probably noticed a decrease in your appetite. The body has enough readily available stored energy to fight the illness for the first few days. But after a few days, these reserves run low and must be replenished. If your appetite does not return and you don't begin to eat a nutritious diet to fulfill your daily requirements, your body begins to use fat and muscle tissue to provide the energy it needs to fight the illness. When muscle and fat stores are used for too long without being replenished, you will begin to lose weight and feel weak. The weaker you feel, the less you eat. And thus the cycle becomes self-perpetuating.

A lack of appetite can make maintaining a healthy and balanced diet difficult over the long run, leading to malnutrition. Malnutrition is a problem because it compromises your ability to fight infection and build the necessary strength for the healing process. You can use many strategies to help maintain your weight. Consider these suggestions:

- Give food a chance. Remember, what sounds unappealing today may sound good tomorrow. Try different foods and have an open attitude. Experiment with herbs and seasonings. You may find that your preferences change and that some flavorings actually help your digestion and make you feel better while others may upset your system. Experiment with this.
- Ambience can make a tremendous difference. Set the table attractively—consider flowers, candles, a bright tablecloth. Eat with friends and family. Play your favorite music at dinnertime. For a change, go out to a favorite restaurant.
- Eat small meals often. Keeps snacks handy for nibbling. Go with your cravings. During the "not hungry" times, rely on foods you really love. Eat foods that make you feel good emotionally; try comfort foods such as chicken soup, hot or cold cereal, ice cream, macaroni and cheese, french toast. Think of some of your own special favorite foods.
- Develop a system of rewards. Once you have planned your menu for the day, based on what you want or feel you should eat, identify a meaningful reward and contract with yourself to eat your meal and then collect the reward. Your reward might be a movie (rented or in a theater), buying a favorite magazine and reading it cover to cover, or a long-distance telephone call to someone special.
- Try eliciting the relaxation response before eating.
- Have milk shakes and commercial liquid supplements instead of just a glass of milk. Supplement your diet with foods higher in fat and calories that are not necessarily prudent at other times, but which help increase calories now. For example, add sour cream, margarine, butter, and mayonnaise to foods. More specific suggestions for adding daily calories and protein are listed at the end of this chapter.

Meredith's Experience

Meredith, a forty-seven-year-old with a diagnosis of uterine cancer who participated in the Behavioral Medicine Cancer Program, related that she had had some difficulty maintaining her food intake during her medical treatment. She was usually an energetic, active, social person, but, during her course of chemotherapy, found that she not only lost her appetite, but also lost interest in eating with friends, either going out or eating in. As she ate less and felt weaker, she isolated herself more and began to feel depressed. This, in turn, decreased her food intake further.

Upon recognizing this pattern, Meredith decided to make each mealtime an enjoyable experience and set about doing this with real zeal. She decorated her table, chose foods of long-standing meaning to her, and made a commitment with herself to invite friends in twice a week, whether she felt like it or not. Each time she felt herself becoming discouraged, she took a deep breath and reflected on what was really important to her. Fairly quickly, Meredith found that these strategies helped her significantly improve her food intake, and she began to feel a bit stronger day by day.

To supplement or not to supplement

We know that deficiencies of certain nutrients can alter immune function and may worsen the rate of recovery after surgery or infection. It is not at all clear, however, that supplementing an already well-balanced diet with additional vitamins, minerals, and trace elements improves resistance to infection or prevents the progression or recurrence of disease. In fact, consuming too much of some trace elements, vitamins, or minerals that the body requires only in small amounts may adversely affect your health. In some instances, taking large amounts of one nutrient can interfere with the absorption of another. For example, many people take zinc tablets because zinc deficiency has been found to effect immune function adversely. However, in 1979, Dr. Ananda S. Prasad and colleagues of Wayne State University School of Medicine reported that taking zinc in amounts greater than the minimum daily requirement of about 15mg can result in a deficiency of copper, another essential nutrient. Likewise, since a deficiency of the trace element selenium has been associated with certain types of cancer, many people take selenium supplements. In fact, however, selenium deficiency is quite rare in industrialized societies; deficiencies and associated cancers are found in societies without access to a variety of foods from different sources. Furthermore, according to Dr. R. K. Chandra, in the British journal *The Lancet*, excess selenium may actually impair immune function.

Large doses of certain vitamins, such as vitamins A and D, are known to be dangerous. High doses of other vitamins are also unadvisable. Vitamin B$_6$ (*pyridoxine*) can cause permanent sensory nerve damage. Niacin, in even moderate doses, can cause potentially serious inflammation of the liver or hepatitis. Vitamin C can cause bladder or kidney stones consisting of oxalic acid, or iron overload in susceptible individuals. Excess vitamin C also can decrease the kidney's ability to clear some chemotherapy medications such as methotrexate from your body.

We believe patients should take no individual nutrient supplements unless they have first worked to improve intake of these nutrients in their diet. Any supplements to your diet should be initiated under the direction of a dietitian and the physician overseeing your treatment. On the other hand, taking a daily multivitamin/mineral supplement, with amounts not exceeding 150 percent of the U.S. recommended dietary allowance, is generally harmless.

UNPROVEN METHODS OF CANCER MANAGEMENT

A great many dietary programs claim to improve resistance to disease and immune function and have recently been loudly and prominently promoted. Many of these programs are based on complicated and often illogical meal schedules and food combinations. Others rely on unknown, untested, or potentially harmful mineral supplements, or are themselves deficient in some essential nutrients. Most claims are unsubstantiated.

The difficulty with many of these diets is that they are simply inadequate to meet your specific needs for rebuilding and maintaining the strength necessary for healing. To fulfill your individual requirements, the diet may need adjustment. For example, the American Dietetic Association regards vegetarian diets as generally healthful and nutritionally adequate when appropriately planned; however, for those with special needs, whose nutrient requirements are especially high—due to growth, lactation, recovery from illness—careful planning is necessary to ensure adequate intakes of calories, protein, and vitamins B$_{12}$ and D. It is imperative that you work closely with your dietitian and physician to be certain that any dietary plan you pursue is adequately balanced to meet your special needs.

Macrobiotic diets, consisting largely of cooked vegetables and whole grains, are among the most popular unconventional approaches used by cancer patients. The concept of macrobiotics extends beyond diet alone and encompasses a philosophy of life supportive of approaching health in a holistic way by emphasizing mind/body interaction and the creation of a balanced, more harmonious relationship with the environment. Macrobiotic diets were developed not primarily as a treatment for cancer, but as a general lifestyle option and preventive measure against cancer, with their low-fat, high-fiber food plan.

However, in the last ten years or so, macrobiotics has become the most popular unconventional approach used by cancer patients to treat their illness. In 1988 the American Cancer Society published its finding that no objective evidence demonstrates that adherence to any macrobiotic diet helps in the treatment of cancer in human beings. Lacking such evidence, the American Cancer Society strongly urged individuals with cancer not to use a strict macrobiotic diet. In fact, their conclusions were that macrobiotic diets, when strictly adhered to, are low in certain vitamins, total calories, and protein, and can result in extreme weight loss which can weaken the body and complicate disease.

In the 1990 congressional report from the Office of Technology Assessment on unconventional cancer treatments, the efficacy of macrobiotic diets was again looked at quite carefully. This latest report, which takes into account the overall lifestyle as well as the philosophical and spiritual goals of the macrobiotic diet, again cautions of the possible adverse effects of strict adherence to the diet for cancer patients. It seems to suggest, however, that if the overall philosophy of macrobiotics is appealing, you may be able to supplement the diet to correct its deficiencies. If you plan to do this, be sure to work closely with your physician and dietitian as well as your macrobiotic practitioner.

THE VALUE OF BECOMING INVOLVED

As someone living with illness, making dietary changes or defining a nutritional plan to help nourish and replenish your strength can offer a degree of control over your life, health, and treatment. This can be enormously important when medical examinations, tests, medicines, and chemotherapy are being planned and administered according to a predetermined schedule and with what may seem to be complete disregard for your preferences.

Begin to get involved in as many ways as possible. Insist on being part of the decision-making regarding your treatment. Many areas of your treatment are beyond your control; take control whenever possible. Your diet is an excellent area for your involvement. For instance, when implementing your overall food plan, you know best which foods you find interesting, palatable, and desirable. Work with your dietitian and physician to develop a nutritional plan and to define strategies that will enable you to maintain a well-balanced diet. Use your past experiences with food as a resource.

Looking at diet as one area of treatment over which you can exercise some control offers many advantages. For one, it sends a clear and strong message that you want to be an active participant in your treatment. Research has shown that active participation—a sense of control—can make a difference in slowing disease. In one series of studies carried out in 1982 by Dr. Madelon Visintainer and colleagues in the Department of Psychology of the University of Pennsylvania, two groups of animals with transplanted tumors were given intermittent, mild, but uncomfortable electric shock. One group of animals could turn off the current by pressing a bar; the second group had no way to avoid the shock. The implanted tumors in the second group grew faster and larger than those in the group able to turn off the shock. Interestingly, the tumor growth rate in a third group of animals (which were not given electric shock) fell between that of the other two groups, suggesting that the challenge of the shock was in some way, as yet unclear, beneficial in stimulating tumor rejection.

By taking responsibility for your food plan, you can feel empowered, increasing your role in your care and helping to build the partnership between you and your clinician which can be so important in the healing process.

Eating defensively: Buffering your immune system

During the course of your illness, when your immune defenses may be compromised either because of your illness or the treatments for it, strict adherence to principles of hygienic food preparation is critical to avoid introducing bacteria from food sources into your system. Follow these general guidelines when you prepare food:

- Wash all fruits and vegetables thoroughly. Keep a vegetable brush handy for easy scrubbing.
- When preparing meat, cut raw chicken or meat on a surface which can be cleaned thoroughly. Wash hands, utensils, and cutting surface with soap and hot water after handling meat. Bacteria, particularly salmonella, can be transferred via your hands to your mouth and to other foods.
- Don't eat raw meat, fish, shellfish, or oysters. Sushi is out.
- Discard any raw eggs with cracked shells. Always refrigerate eggs as soon as you get them home, and serve immediately after cooking.
- Prepare eggs with care. Undercooked eggs can harbor salmonella. Boiled eggs must be hard-boiled until the yolks are thickened; cook for at least seven minutes. Avoid soft or medium-boiled eggs. Fried eggs should be cooked until the whites are opaque and the yolks thickened, not runny.
- Don't eat raw eggs; avoid items made with raw eggs. Common examples are caesar-salad dressing, eggnog, hollandaise sauce, and homemade mayonnaise (commercially prepared mayonnaise is safe because it is made with pasteurized eggs).
- When purchasing meats or other perishables, take them home and refrigerate immediately.
- Be sure to cook beef, pork, poultry, and fish thoroughly. This is critical in destroying the organisms and bacteria carried in these foods. When eating out, choose foods which have been prepared or cooked thoroughly rather than foods which are served raw.

COPING WITH SPECIFIC PROBLEMS

Nausea and vomiting

Medical treatments such as chemotherapy and antibiotic treatment can cause nausea and vomiting. This, in turn, can make food less appetizing. Many self-help approaches as well as medical treatments alleviate nausea and vomiting. Medications called *antiemetics* may help during acute episodes; discuss these with your physician if you feel they would help you. Behavioral therapies, especially the elicitation of the relaxation response, can reduce symptoms of nausea associated with chemotherapy. Prior to mealtime, you may want to elicit the relaxation response and visualize an image that evokes feelings of calm to make your stomach feel settled, and not nauseous. If you feel a wave of nausea while eating, put down your fork, stop for a minute, take a few deep breaths to reproduce this feeling of calm, and allow the wave of nausea to pass. If you suffer from anticipatory nausea and vomiting, that is, feeling nauseous in anticipation of the treatment, you may want to refer to chapter 18, "Behavioral Medicine and Cancer," for more information on using the relaxation response to reduce this symptom.

Experiment with the following strategies—intended only as guidelines—which may help decrease nausea, especially at mealtimes.

- Eat dry foods, such as toast or crackers.
- Avoid greasy foods, fried foods, or foods high in fat; these often seem to make nausea worse.
- Clear, cool beverages are recommended. Popsicles and gelatin often help.
- Avoid food odors that are unpleasant to you.
- Take advantage of times when you are not feeling nauseous—feed yourself well then.
- Avoid spicy or pungent foods and foods with strong aromas.
- Avoid very sweet foods.
- Do not lie down immediately after eating.

Harold's Experience

Harold, a sixty-seven-year-old college professor, enrolled in the Behavioral Medicine Cancer Program. He was diagnosed with lymphoma and was undergoing a course of chemotherapy. Extreme nausea was interfering with his ability to eat, contributing to weight loss and depletion of his strength and energy reserve. Working with his clinicians in the program, he decided on three strategies: eliciting the relaxation response, changing how he viewed his chemotherapy, and choosing and preparing foods that were palatable and most conducive to his being able to tolerate them.

The first step was to consider his symptom of nausea and vomiting. Harold realized that as soon as he arrived at the hospital for chemotherapy and was confronted by the sights, sounds, and smells of the clinic, he instantly began to feel nauseous. He had developed a conditioned response based on his first few experiences with chemotherapy. He worked with exercises for visualization and elicitation of the relaxation response to help decondition his anticipatory response to chemotherapy. He created an image of the treatment as an ally in his fight against cancer; the chemotherapy became his friend. As he sat in the chair during the procedure, he thought of this ally circulating throughout his body, bolstering his own innate healing capacities. When he left the hospital, he allowed himself a couple of hours to readjust, then he would eat a meal—prepared ahead of time—in celebration of completing that day's chemotherapy. His particular favorites were a clear miso soup and orange sherbet. Alternatively, he would arrange to dine with a friend after the chemotherapy and worked to keep the conversation off the subject of his illness. Over time, he was able to control his pre-treatment nausea and vomiting, and the nausea that accompanied his post-treatment meals began to subside substantially. He felt empowered and successful because the strategies involved him as a primary participant in the plan. Harold was pleased to note that he was able to maintain his weight as he proceeded through his treatment.

Maldigestion and malabsorption

Both maldigestion and malabsorption can occur when the body is under stress or with certain medical conditions. *Maldigestion* means that foods are only partially broken down in the small intestine, making it impossible for the body to extract all the nutrients the food provides. If this occurs, you may notice particles of undigested foods in your stool. *Malabsorption* means that the nutrients from food which has been digested are not absorbed into the body. This condition can cause persistent diarrhea. By preventing essential nutrients from being taken into the body, both conditions result in weight loss and can cause vitamin and mineral deficiencies. These dietary strategies may help in managing maldigestion and malabsorption:

- Eat frequent, low-fat, low-lactose meals to help reduce diarrhea.
- Increase your intake of yogurt with an active culture (this will be noted on the label). This may replenish beneficial bacteria in your intestinal tract. Yogurt is often well tolerated—even by those who are lactose intolerant.
- Increase your intake of fluids. Have fruit juice, popsicles, gelatin, water, and broth frequently.
- To replace lost potassium, choose bananas, orange juice, tomatoes, potatoes, and meat.
- Try decreasing the amount of fiber in your diet. Foods like peas,

beans, raw fruits and vegetables, corn, onions, popcorn, and whole-grain products sometimes irritate the intestines, especially when diarrhea is present.
- Avoid beverages and foods that contain caffeine. Common sources are coffee, tea, colas, and chocolate.
- Try eating cooked fruits and vegetables, mashed potatoes, bananas, and applesauce.

Anyone who develops persistent or frequent diarrhea, or who finds undigested food in the stool for longer than a few days, should consult his or her physician as soon as possible.

Difficulty swallowing

People coping with symptoms of cancer or HIV infection sometimes avoid food if chewing and swallowing become painful. Depending on the cause, certain strategies can reduce the intensity of these problems and allow you to develop and maintain a more healthy schedule of meals. Consult with your physician to help determine the cause and with your dietitian to develop a nutritional plan. Inflammation of the mouth, called *stomatitis*, can be caused by infection or some medications used for treatment of HIV infection or cancer; it can make chewing and swallowing painful. If this is a problem for you, ask your physician to prescribe a local anesthetic such as viscous Xylocaine. To make chewing and swallowing as easy as possible, try

- eating bland, nonacidic foods
- eating small, frequent meals
- choosing soft or pureed foods, liquid supplements, or other nutritious liquids to ease swallowing
- choosing clear, cool beverages or frozen desserts such as popsicles, gelatin, or sherbet
- using sauces and gravies to make foods more liquid and therefore easier to swallow
- avoiding spicy foods
- keeping your mouth as clean as possible by following your physician's recommendations for oral hygiene.

Charlie's Experience

Charlie, a twenty-seven-year-old computer programmer diagnosed as HIV-positive, developed candida esophagitis (a fungal infection of the esophagus). Swallowing solid foods became difficult and painful for him. His doctor started a course of medication for his esophagitis, and his dietitian recommended a high-calorie liquid supplement. Charlie experimented and found that he preferred the supplement cold. By taking the supplement regularly, he avoided losing any weight whatsoever during the four weeks of treatment that cleared up his esophagitis.

For individuals with difficulty swallowing, anticipating another painful meal can cause increased tension and anxiety. Eliciting the relaxation response regularly can significantly reduce this factor. In addition, addressing some of the cognitive elements or negative thoughts that occur in anticipation of a painful experience can also markedly decrease the effects of pain on eating. This is illustrated in the case which follows.

Edith's Experience

Edith is a vibrant, seventy-year-old with esophageal cancer which was successfully treated surgically. Several months after surgery, she began to find swallowing painful and had lost some weight shortly before entering the Behavioral Medicine Cancer Program. Her physician found no apparent recurrence of the cancer, but she continued to experience pain, which her doctor attributed to spasm of the muscles of her esophagus. The more difficulty she experienced swallowing, the more she tensed up before eating, which intensified the pain.

She was taught to elicit the relaxation response daily. She also learned to use a mini-relaxation-response exercise before each meal to bring forth the physiology of the relaxation response. The muscular relaxation this achieved decreased her anticipatory muscular tension and contributed to a significant decrease in her level of pain.

Edith recognized her pattern of dreading every meal for fear of the pain it would bring. To address this, she decided to use her newly learned cognitive skills to reframe the experience. She relabeled mealtime a challenge, rather than a painful experience, and began to put her energies into carefully choosing foods that she liked and that would minimize her pain. For example, she enlisted her blender in making strawberry milk shakes, which she had always loved in the past. Within four weeks, she began to experience relief from her pain and slowly began to regain the weight she had lost.

Shortness of breath

Prolonged shortness of breath may occur with pulmonary infections or certain types of cancers, particularly lung cancer. As you probably well know, feeling short of breath can be exhausting. You will need to reserve your strength for mealtime in order to consume the calories necessary to preserve your strength and energy. Organize your activities carefully so that your meals are not rushed and plan your day so that you are well rested prior to meals. If you use supplemental oxygen, consider using a nasal cannula (small tube) since having to stop eating and use an oxygen mask can be disruptive and frustrating. Liquid supplements may be more practical in this situation. Eating several small, frequent meals may also be easier than trying to have three normal-size meals. Keep your goal in mind: to maintain your weight and strength by consuming enough calories. Consider your particular symptoms and energy capacity, and work with your dietitian to create a workable plan. Arrange a network of friends to call on when you may feel particularly short of breath or depleted in energy. Perhaps they could cook for you to relieve the burden on either you or your family, or they might join you for a meal, making it more pleasurable. Remember that atmosphere helps, so make the table pleasing and get yourself dressed for each meal. These subtle suggestions can profoundly affect your appetite, particularly during periods of feeling somewhat depleted in morale and energy.

BE PROACTIVE

When coping with illnesses that cause undernutrition, a healthy, well-planned diet can help maximize your potential for healing and health. Maintaining adequate nutrient intake and preventing weight loss are particularly important and probably contribute more to maintaining health and ensuring a desirable quality of life than we had previously thought.

Remember that "balance in all things is best," including your diet. Listen carefully to what your body is telling you about your diet. Develop your awareness of the complex interactions between the foods you eat and your sense of well-being. Try eating mindfully, conscious that while food itself is important, your approach to food and eating may be equally important. (Review chapter 5 on mindfulness.) If certain foods seem to disagree with you, try eliminating them and see what happens.

As you experiment and develop strategies that put your self-awareness skills to work, it is important that you work in conjunction with your dietitian to ensure that all nutrients and essential ingredients are included in your personal diet plan. Although you may feel beset by the problem of eating well while feeling ill, in many ways this situation offers you an opportunity—the opportunity to explore new ways of eating, connect with old traditions and beliefs about food, and reconnect with friends and the aesthetics of eating. You may gain new insights into the role you want food to play in your life.

Judith Linsey Palken, M.S., R.D.
Alan E. Shackelford, M.D.

Suggestions for Getting Enough Calories and Protein Even If You Don't Feel Like It

- Snack frequently, about every two hours. High-protein tidbits include small pieces of poultry, meat, or tuna on bread. (If a whole sandwich seems overwhelming, try half a sandwich.) Or choose a hard-boiled egg, a small yogurt, a cube of your favorite cheese, or a serving of three-bean salad.
- Other good snacks for boosting calories and/or protein are dried fruits and nuts (raisins and walnuts are a delicious, munchable combination), toast with peanut butter, cereal with milk, custard, pudding.
- Add margarine, sour cream, mayonnaise, honey, and molasses to foods to boost calories further.
- "Enhance" your hot cereal—add chopped nuts, bits of dried fruit, margarine.
- Add gravies, sauces, and canned creamed soups to poultry, fish, vegetables, potatoes, and pasta.
- Avoid nutritionally empty liquids such as soda, coffee, tea, or water. Nutritious liquids like milk, fruit juice, milk shakes, or liquid supplements provide more calories and nutrients.
- Use powdered milk (nonfat dried milk) to fortify other foods. Double the nutritional value of your regular milk by stirring in several heaping teaspoonfuls of powdered milk. You can also stir powdered milk into soups, sauces, scrambled eggs, cocoa, casseroles, milk shakes, yogurt, and even peanut butter.
- Commercially prepared nutritional supplements can be a convenient way to add value to your diet. Available in many pharmacies, these supplements come in liquid and powdered form, in a variety of flavors. Ask your doctor or dietitian if you need such a supplement, and if so, which brand would be best for you.
- If you use a liquid supplement, feel free to create your own "new, improved" version. Blend them with fresh or canned fruit, ice cream, frozen yogurt, or chocolate or strawberry syrup.

For further information, send for *Eating Hints,* a booklet of recipes and tips for better nutrition during cancer treatment, published by the U.S. Department of Health and Human Services, Public Health Service, and National Institutes of Health (NIH Publication No. 91-2079). Write to:

Office of Cancer Communications
National Cancer Institute
Building 31, Room 10A 24
Bethesda, Maryland 20892

HEALTH COMMITMENT

Long-Term Goal:

_____

_____

_____

Signature

_____

Witness

Expected Date of Reaching Goal: _____

Short-Term Goals	*Comments (supports, rewards, etc.)*

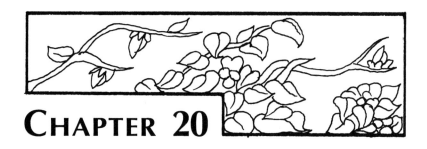

CHAPTER 20

PSYCHONEUROIMMUNOLOGY AND HIV DISEASE

I am not an optimist, because I am not sure that everything ends well. Nor am I a pessimist, because I am not sure that everything ends badly. I just carry hope in my heart. Hope is a feeling that life and work have a meaning. You either have it or you don't, regardless of the state of the world that surrounds you.

Life without hope is an empty, boring, and useless life. I cannot imagine that I could strive for something if I did not carry hope in me. I am thankful to God for this gift. It is as big a gift as life itself.

Vaclav Havel, Czech playwright and President

In this chapter you will explore

- the immune system
- the field of psychoneuroimmunology (PNI)
- the relationship between emotions and immune functioning
- human immunodeficiency virus (HIV) and its effect upon the immune system
- components of our Behavioral Medicine Program for HIV-Related Illnesses

Since ancient times, from Hippocrates to Galen to Dr. Paul Dudley White, astute clinicians have sensed the effect of psychological and social factors on the health and illness patterns of patients. The pioneering stress research of Dr. Hans Selye has shown that stress can damage our health and impair the healing process. Recent advances in our understanding of immunology and the psychophysiology of stress have combined to yield further knowledge of the role of emotional factors in physical disease. This has given rise over the past decade to the developing interdisciplinary field of *psychoneuroimmunology* (PNI), which is concerned with the complex interrelationships between stress, emotions, the nervous system, immunological function, and disease.

THE IMMUNE SYSTEM

The immune system consists of a number of organs—the thymus gland, spleen, lymph nodes, and bone marrow—as well as blood cells that circulate between these organs and throughout the body. The primary functions of the immune system are to maintain health and promote healing by defending the body against foreign invaders such as bacteria, viruses, and fungi; and to protect us from abnormal cells like those of cancer.

One kind of blood cells, the T-lymphocytes, are particularly important in defending against viruses, bacteria, and fungi. The major T-cells are identified as helper T-cells, killer T-cells, and suppressor T-cells. Other lymphocytes called B-cells produce antibodies which travel through the blood stream searching out invading foreign viruses.

The nervous system influences immune functioning directly through connecting nerves to the spleen, lymph nodes, and thymus, which are all part of the immune system. In addition, the nervous system indirectly influences the immune system through hormones. For example, stress initiates the fight-or-flight response, which triggers areas of the brain (specifically the hypothalamus and pituitary) to release hormones. The pituitary gland secretes adreno-corticotropic hormone (ACTH), which stimulates a portion of the adrenal gland to release cortisol. Simultaneously, stress leads to increased arousal of another branch of the nervous system, the sympathetic nervous system (SNS). The SNS stimulates a different portion of the adrenal gland to release cortisol, epinephrine (adrenaline) and norepinephrine (noradrenaline) into the bloodstream. Current evidence indicates that cortisol and adrenaline compromise immune-cell functioning by interfering with the ability of T-cells and B-cells to divide and multiply.

The interaction between the immune process and the nervous system is obviously exceedingly complex, but it may be viewed in a simplified fashion. If you are experiencing emotion, such as fear or anger, the disturbing thoughts enter the cerebral cortex of your brain. In response, the cerebral cortex sends messages to the hypothalamus, which, in turn, stimulates your pituitary gland to release hormones that travel through your bloodstream to the adrenal glands. They begin secreting cortisol along with epinephrine and nor-epinephrine, all of which have an effect upon the ability of your body's T-cells and B-cells to divide. It means that stress and your emotions can affect your immune system. (You can read more about the immune system in chapter 18, "Behavioral Medicine and Cancer.")

PSYCHONEUROIMMUNOLOGY (PNI) RESEARCH

Commonplace stress can affect immune functioning. In a series of studies, Drs. Janice Kiecolt-Glaser and Ron Glaser, at Ohio State University College of

Medicine, compared the immune systems of medical students during final exams to the baseline of one month before exams. During exams, natural killer T-cells activity decreased. Moreover, the lonelier students had more suppression of natural killer T-cell activity than the less lonely students. Exam stress has also been associated with a decrease in T-lymphocytes and the body's production of interferon (another important component of the immune system).

Why are these data important? Despite their long histories of test-taking and exams, the medical students experienced them as stressful enough to result in compromises in their immune functioning. The heightened distress of the exam period is probably comparable to that resulting from other commonplace events, such as times of frenzied activity or profound emotional adjustments. Could similar decreases in immune functioning accompany these ordinary life occasions as well?

Other research in the field of PNI addresses these possibilities. Because marital disruption, through either divorce or death, appears to be one of the most stressful of life events, Drs. Kiecolt-Glaser and Glaser also investigated immune functioning in a group of recently separated and divorced women. The women who had been separated one year or less had poorer immune functioning than did a group of demographically-matched married women. Moreover, both shorter separation periods and continued contact with the ex-spouse were associated with greater depression and poorer immune functioning. Similar data were obtained in a study of divorced men.

Other data from diverse populations—bereaved spouses, caregivers of people with severe, long-term illnesses, people in unhappy marriages—also suggest that stress can adversely influence immunity. Therefore, the question was asked whether stress-reduction might have a positive effect on immune functioning. In other words, by reducing stress, can we improve immune functioning?

Going back to the medical students, Drs. Kiecolt-Glaser and Glaser randomly assigned half of the students to a relaxation-response group and half to a control group. They found that more frequent elicitation of the relaxation response was related to higher levels of helper T-lymphocytes during exams.

As we age, our immune systems become less effective. Drs. Kiecolt-Glaser and Glaser also explored the possibility of boosting immune functioning in elderly adults by teaching them relaxation-response techniques. They recruited a group of elderly residents of a nursing home and randomly assigned them to one of three groups: relaxation training, social contact, or no intervention. After one month, the subjects in the relaxation-response group experienced a significantly heightened immune response compared to baseline. No changes in immune functioning were found in the social-contact or no-intervention groups.

In another PNI study, Dr. James Pennebaker, at Southern Methodist University in Dallas, and, again, Drs. Kiecolt-Glaser and Glaser found that when volunteers spent twenty minutes on four successive days writing about their most traumatic experiences and their feelings about them, their level of

T-lymphocytes was significantly boosted. They had fewer visits to the student health clinic and higher grade-point averages the following semester. The investigators claim that various types of self-disclosure of traumatic events can bring about direct and cost-effective improvements in health.

At the University of Pittsburgh, Dr. Sandra Levy studied thirty cancer patients in remission as they went through an eight-week course in relaxation and cognitive therapy that focused on altering negative beliefs and being more optimistic about life. Patients who took the course had more active natural killer cells. At the Pittsburgh Cancer Institute, Dr. Levy also studied thirty-six women being tested at the National Institutes of Health for recurrent breast cancer. Patients who had been free of illness longer before their recurrence, who expressed more joy at the baseline psychological testing, who were predicted to live longer when initially seen by their physicians, and who had fewer areas of metastases tended to live longer than others in the sample. This study demonstrated that several factors, behavioral as well as biological, are important in looking at long-term survivors.

Dr. Jay Weiss, in a series of experiments with laboratory rats at Duke University, showed that mild electrical stimulation enhances immune functioning 20-to-30 percent. Dr. Weiss's findings support the notion that not all stress is bad for the immune system. Perhaps the excitement of a full and meaningful life, termed *eustress* by Dr. Hans Selye, is necessary to strengthen immunity.

From these PNI studies, it appears that distressing psychosocial events which elicit feelings of helplessness and hopelessness can affect immune functioning, and that strategies which reduce stress may give the immune system a boost.

> There is an energy in us which makes things happen when the paths
> of other persons touch ours and we have to be there and let it
> happen. When the time of our particular sunset comes, our thing,
> our accomplishment, won't really matter a great deal. But the clarity
> and care with which we have loved others will speak with vitality of
> the great gift of life we have been for each other.
>
> Monks of Weston Priory, Weston, Vermont

HIV DISEASE AND THE IMMUNE SYSTEM

Historically the disorders HIV (human immunodeficiency virus), AIDS (acquired immune deficiency syndrome), and ARC (AIDS related complex) were thought to be somewhat distinct. We now believe that HIV disease (HIV-positive) is a condition that ranges from no symptoms to the serious condition of AIDS. In this chapter when we refer to HIV disease or HIV infection, we are referring to the continuum of this illness.

The immune system is comprised of various parts that work together in a highly synchronized fashion. It involves the coordinated action of different immune cells that serve to identify, attack, and scavenge foreign particles and infected cells. As we have noted, one of the major cell types is the T-lymphocyte. This set of cells includes helper T-cells, killer T-cells, and suppressor T-cells. The helper T-cell—also know as the T_4 cell—is considered to be the quarterback of the immune system because it coordinates all of the interdependent parts into an effective machine. (See chapter 18 for more on the immune system.)

The human immunodeficiency virus—HIV—is insidious because it has a special affinity for T_4 cells. By destroying T_4—the quarterback—the HIV overpowers the ability of the immune system to fight disease. When the immune system is sufficiently compromised, a person may begin to experience serious infections and other symptoms which can lead to AIDS (acquired immune deficiency syndrome).

Without a functioning immune system, the person becomes vulnerable to foreign substances such as bacteria, protozoa, fungi, and other viruses and malignancies which may cause life-threatening illness. Because HIV infection has an asymptomatic phase that can last ten to fifteen years, and because several treatments are now available, some researchers in the field believe that HIV infection can be viewed as a chronic disease that is manageable.

The relation between emotions, immune functioning, and disease progression in people infected with human immunodeficiency virus is not yet understood. Since stress as well as psychological and behavioral variables are associated with adverse changes in immune functioning, stress may contribute to HIV-disease progression. Researchers are examining behavioral and cognitive interventions such as aerobic exercise, elicitation of the relaxation response, and stress-management strategies which may enhance immune functioning and perhaps slow disease progression.

For example, Drs. Michael Antoni, Neil Schneiderman, and Arthur LaPerriere, at the University of Miami School of Medicine, have investigated the effect of two interventions on immune parameters in a group of asymptomatic men infected with HIV. In separate ten-week programs, aerobic exercise and progressive muscle relaxation (a technique that elicits the relaxation response) resulted in an increase in T_4-lymphocytes. The researchers concluded that these interventions may act as stress buffers, and suggested that such boosting of immune functioning could possibly slow down the progressive deterioration of T-cells.

OUR HIV-POSITIVE PROGRAM

> To live is to suffer, to survive is to find meaning in the suffering. The ability to see something good in adversity is the central trait needed by all of us.
>
> Victor Frankl, M.D., *Man's Search for Meaning*

Being diagnosed as HIV-positive is very frightening. Many people become depressed and hopeless, others experience extreme anxiety, while others feel angry and enraged. Because this diagnosis is so stressful, behavioral interventions should be available for HIV-positive individuals as early as possible.

Our eleven-week clinic program for HIV-positive individuals is designed to help people *live with* their diagnosis and to see it as a doorway to growth and self-development rather than as a death sentence. We offer a combination of relaxation techniques, yoga exercises, nutrition information, cognitive restructuring, and interpersonal skills training which enables people to modify or eliminate the powerful psychological responses that accompany this diagnosis. Participants learn to deal with stress; cope with the uncertainties and ups and downs of the disease; communicate with families, friends, and acquaintances about their diagnosis; develop healthy lifestyles; and continue to lead positive and meaningful lives. Believe it or not, we even find humor about AIDS. Because of the group setting, participants also benefit from the group's support and sharing of medical information.

The goal of the program is to decrease some of the symptoms associated with HIV-disease; there are two major components:

1. ***Elicitation of the relaxation response.*** We teach various relaxation techniques to quiet the body and the mind, and perhaps counteract the stress-induced reactions in immune functioning. Participants learn about how stress affects us physically, emotionally, cognitively, and behaviorally. We focus on the psychoneuroimmunology research demonstrating the injurious effects of stress upon the immune system.

2. ***Development or enhancement of characteristics of long-term survivors of HIV infection.*** Dr. George Solomon, a pioneer in the field of psychoneuroimmunology at the University of California in Los Angeles, and Dr. Lydia Temoshok, a psychologist at Walter Reed Army Medical Center, have been following HIV-positive individuals for a number of years. Dr. Temoshok reports that long-term survivors seem to share eight specific characteristics. They

   - "are realistic and accept the AIDS diagnosis, but do not take it as a death sentence"
   - "have a fighting spirit and refuse to be helpless/hopeless.
   - "have changed lifestyles"
   - "are assertive and have the ability to get out of stressful and unproductive situations"
   - "are tuned in to their own psychological and physical needs and take care of themselves"
   - are able to "talk openly about their illness"
   - "have a sense of personal responsibility for their health and look at their treating physician as a collaborator"
   - "are altruistically involved with other persons with AIDS"

Our program facilitates learning how to develop and strengthen these characteristics. Many of our participants are long-term survivors of HIV, coping well five to ten years after diagnosis. Many have undergone numerous opportunistic infections yet continue to have a tremendous fighting spirit and will to live.

For each of the eleven weeks of our program, there is a different focus of discussion and new skills to be learned.

As mentioned in earlier chapters, the first step is to learn about mind/ body interactions and to recognize how stress affects us physically, emotionally, cognitively, and behaviorally. Participants begin monitoring stress in their lives and how it manifests itself (the stress warning signs). It's also important for the group to learn about the psychoneuroimmunology research previously described—to know that stress can have a detrimental effect upon the immune system and that by reducing stress through eliciting the relaxation response, one's immune system may stay healthier. We practice various types of relaxation techniques in each session.

We invite the participants' significant others to the first session so they can learn firsthand what we do, and so they will be supportive of the activities and changes the participant will be experiencing.

At the next session, we practice yoga exercises as another way to elicit the relaxation response. We do exercises of specific benefit to this group, for example, exercises to "open up" the chest for anyone with pneumocystitis or respiratory problems. We also do exercises that massage the gastrointestinal area, for leg pains due to neuropathy, and to stimulate the lymphatic system. Many participants cannot do aerobic exercises because of fatigue and lack of energy, so yoga is an effective way to keep the body flexible and stretched. Participants learn about diaphragmatic breathing and using deep breathing as a mini-relaxation response.

Our third session focuses on nutrition—how to eat to stay healthy and to keep one's weight up (the material covered in chapter 19, "Healthy Eating with Cancer or HIV Infection"). We show the film *Eating Defensively*, which teaches how to prepare food safely and what foods to avoid. We also spend time talking about adjunctive therapies such as acupuncture, massage, herbal medicines, etc. Most participants seek out other techniques to augment what modern medicine has to offer.

The concept of stress-hardiness is an important component of all our programs, as you have seen. Anyone with a chronic health problem wants to feel in control, needs to be committed to certain things in order to have meaning in each day, and wants to look at the condition as a challenge, feeling that he or she can still grow and develop rather than feeling helpless and hopeless. Victor Frankl, a Viennese psychiatrist, writes about his experiences in a Nazi concentration camp, in his book *Man's Search for Meaning*. He describes how those with a purpose for living were able to withstand torture or starvation, while those without purpose, goals, or positive self-direction died quickly. While a prisoner, Frankl planned lectures he would give and the books he would write once he was free.

In a writing exercise, participants focus on what they want to be committed to by setting short-term (next week) and long-term (next year, or five to ten years from now) goals for themselves in eight areas: career or education, relationships, creative things, play, health, material objects, spirituality, and as a volunteer.

Take a Moment To . . .

Review your responses to the exercise in chapter 10, "What is Important/ Meaningful/Valuable to You" (page 185–86). Most likely your illness influenced your answers significantly. Take a moment again and ask yourself if you are really doing what you want to be doing.

We spend time talking about these goals and priorities throughout the program, and it is very gratifying to see the participants attaining their goals. At this point we give participants an assignment for every day for the rest of their lives: "News and Goods," that is, do something new or good for yourself every day. It need not be a big deal—perhaps treating yourself to a bubble bath instead of a fast shower, or eating an exquisite piece of chocolate, or calling a friend that you have not spoken to in a long time. The small pleasures make each day a little special.

Many participants come to the HIV program feeling very anxious, depressed, or angry. Because the natural tendency is to stay fixed in one of these powerful mood-states, the cognitive-restructuring component of our programs is one of the most important techniques we teach. Participants begin to recognize a connection between their thoughts and their moods, how some of their thoughts are exaggerated or distorted, or that they are jumping to conclusions. By challenging their negative automatic thoughts and replacing them with more positive statements, they gain a great deal of control over their emotions. We see participants coming to the sessions in a more positive, hopeful frame of mind. (Chapters 11 through 15 cover cognitive restructuring in more detail.) At the end of this session, we share everyone's "News and Goods" from the previous week.

We call this group's session on communication "Talking about Talking." We discuss "Who needs to know about my diagnosis? What do I say to other people?" (This might include family, as some participants have not yet told their parents or siblings about their HIV status.) For many, the session is an opportunity to hear others' experiences in telling family, friends, or employers. We also talk about communicating with health-care providers—how to get the care and information that you need.

Based on the findings of Drs. Pennebaker, Kiecolt-Glaser, and Glaser that writing about traumatic events brings health benefits, the group explores emotions in a writing exercise. For twenty minutes, participants write about the most powerful emotions around being HIV-positive. For some, the diagnosis might be the traumatic event; for others, telling their parents might be the most emotional time. The group then discusses the feelings and issues they wrote about in order to process them and perhaps get a different perspective.

 Take a Moment To . . .

Reflect on your experience with HIV. Writing for twenty uninterrupted minutes to explore your thoughts, feelings, and emotions around your diagnosis and treatment, as well as how this has interfered with your life goals, may be helpful. Reflect also on how being HIV-positive has affected others around you. Writing about your experiences is a powerful way of exploring difficult issues and putting them behind you.

This exercise is likely to bring thoughts, feelings, and emotions to mind that may make you uncomfortable. You may want to omit this exercise or postpone it until you have the appropriate support. If you elect to do this exercise, be sure to acknowledge and honor the feelings that emerge. Talk about them with family, friends, or other patients. You may also want to seek out a support group or counselor.

We think anyone with HIV disease needs a basic understanding of how the immune system works. We show slides of the immune cells, explain their function, and describe which parts of the immune system seem to be affected by HIV. With this background, we practice visual imagery. The participants imagine what their T_4 cells look like, where they are in their bodies, the treatment they are receiving, what the virus looks like, and where it is. In any way that seems persuasive to them, they imagine their bodies making more T_4 cells and see these cells working together with their medications to eliminate the virus. If they want, they can draw a picture of their visualization. We consider visual imagery another "tool in the toolbox." More specific information on how to use imagery is in chapter 18, "Behavioral Medicine and Cancer."

Because HIV can be transmitted sexually, we talk about safer sex, including the issues of intimacy, sexuality, and connectedness. Common topics raised in the group are: "Is anyone ever going to love me again? Where do I go to meet someone? When do I reveal my HIV status? How do I deal with the rejection if he (or she) leaves?"

A big issue for anyone with a chronic health condition is how to cope with uncertainty, how to handle the "bumps in the road" without being over-whelmed with fear and anxiety. We do an interactive exercise in which everyone contributes ideas about how to protect yourself in times of uncertainty. We plan what we call "certains." We ask, "What physical self-care habits do you have in place that will help you deal with uncertainty?" The certains may include any relaxation technique, any type of physical exercise, a warm bath, a good meal, massage, etc. We ask, "Who are your supports?" The answers may be friends, a lover, family members, health-care providers, therapists, spiritual counselors, pets, etc. Then we ask, "What attitudes and beliefs do you have to help you cope with the ups and downs?" From our cognitive-restructuring exercise come suggestions such as "I can handle this," "It's okay to ask for help," "HIV = Hope Is Victory."

Our last session is about humor; it is a very effective coping strategy, and it makes us feel good. We share jokes and stories, we wear costumes, we watch funny movies—we laugh for two whole hours. We also talk about how to stay motivated to use the strategies and techniques learned once the program is over.

The program is rich and full. Besides the skills we teach, we share a great deal of information about physicians, medications, vitamins, support services, insurance, living wills, health-care proxies, reading materials . . . whatever is of concern and interest to someone who is HIV-positive.

Edges

When we walk to the edge of all the light we have
and take a step into the darkness of the unknown,
we must believe one of two things will happen—
there will be something SOLID for us to stand on
or we will be taught how to fly.

Patrick Overton

J.D.'s Experience

J.D., a thirty-two-year-old actor, had a long history of asthma and could not tolerate aerosolized pentamidine, a treatment to prevent pneu-mocystis. Each time he was treated with pentamidine, he would have an asthma attack lasting for days, and he feared he would die. In order to be eligible for DDI, an antiviral medication, however, he had to be receiving aerosolized pentamidine. DDI was his only hope, since his body was no longer responding to the other antiviral, AZT. J.D. found that if he listened to his relaxation tape just before an aerosolized pentamidine treatment, he could tolerate the medication and would not develop an asthma attack. This then enabled him to receive the antiviral that he desperately needed.

Preliminary data from our own pilot study have shown that our participants experience a significant reduction in anxiety, depression, obsessive/compulsive thinking, somatization, and stress levels. Almost every participant reports improved sleep, and some experience increased appetite and weight gain. In fact, one woman, who had lost her appetite and was very thin, gained ten pounds during the program.

Participants find that eliciting the relaxation response increases their tolerance of leg pains due to neuropathy, relieves nausea and vomiting side effects of medication, and enables them to tolerate medical procedures in a more calm and controlled way. Most significantly, participants consistently rate themselves as feeling more healthy after completing the program.

Ann Webster, Ph.D.

HEALTH COMMITMENT

Long-Term Goal:

_____

_____
Signature

_____

_____
Witness

Expected Date of Reaching Goal: _____

Short-Term Goals	*Comments (supports, rewards, etc.)*

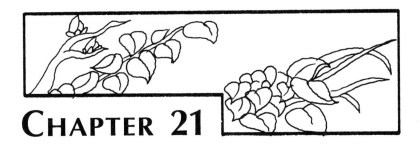

CHAPTER 21

CARDIOVASCULAR DISEASE: THE HEART OF THE MATTER

A merry heart doeth good like a medicine.

Proverbs 17:22

In this chapter you will explore

- risk factors that can lead to cardiovascular disease
- specific ways in which the mind and heart are connected
- basic facts about the cardiovascular system and cardiovascular disease
- self-help strategies to modify your cardiovascular risk factors and improve your cardiovascular health

For centuries we have acknowledged the interaction of the heart, mind, and emotions through language, literature, and art. Consider the commonplace expressions "with all my heart," "coldhearted," "heartfelt," "cold hands, warm heart," and "heart to heart." In medicine as well, descriptions of the connection between the mind and heart abound. In 1790, Sir John Hunter, an eighteenth-century English surgeon who provided some of the earliest clinical descriptions of angina pectoris, noted the link between conflict with his colleagues and his "chest pains." He wrote:

> The first attack of these complaints was produced by an affection of the mind, and every further return of any consequence arose from the same cause; although bodily exercise and distention of the stomach brought on slighter affections, it still required the mind to be affected to render them severe.

This description bespeaks an early assumption of the mind/body (bio-psychosocial) model for health as it relates to cardiology. Given the state of current knowledge, we cannot judge the relative importance of either mind or body in the development and treatment of heart disease, but we can acknowledge that this relationship exists and needs to be considered in any discussion of cardiovascular disease.

In 1990 the National Center for Health Statistics reported that diseases of the cardiovascular system are the number one cause of death in the United States, accounting for approximately 42 percent (or two out of five) of all deaths. Although the problem has declined over the past twenty years, many men and women still suffer from angina, heart attacks, strokes, and peripheral vascular disease. Improvements in technology such as mobile advanced life-support units, cardiac-care units, medications that can dissolve blood clots to prevent heart damage, angioplasty, and surgical techniques have contributed greatly to the decline in cardiovascular deaths. Of equal importance (but with less fanfare), research published in the *New England Journal of Medicine* by Pamela Sytkowski, Ph.D., and William B. Kannel, M.D., from the Framingham Heart Study, suggests that the lowered incidence of death from cardiovascular disease is for the most part due to the reduction of cardiovascular risk factors, that is, primary prevention and changes in lifestyle by people like yourself. Prevention of cardiovascular disease largely centers on an individual changing his or her health and lifestyle behaviors and lowering the known risk factors for developing heart disease.

This chapter discusses both the prevention and treatment of cardiovascular disease, including what you can do to contribute to your cardiovascular health.

CARDIAC RISK FACTORS

The concept of identifying risk factors to predict the development of cardiovascular disease grew out of the landmark Framingham Heart Study, which began in 1948 and still continues today. The researchers followed the health of 5,209 men and women from Framingham, Massachusetts. Every two years the study subjects had examinations which included health histories, physical examinations, electrocardiograms (EKGs), blood tests, and psychological questionnaires. The information was stored and analyzed over time to see what factors—either demographic, biological, and/or psychological—predicted the development of cardiovascular disease. The predictive factors have come to be known as *cardiac risk factors* (or cardiovascular risk factors).

The knowledge that certain factors increase a person's risk for developing cardiovascular disease has dramatically altered health practices in the United States and in the world.

Although cardiac risk factors may be thought of as falling into different categories (biological, psychological, and social), each risk factor is strongly influenced by the presence of other risk factors, and the development of risk factors can be influenced by a variety of mind/body variables.

Cardiac Risk Factors

Biological:
- hypertension (high blood pressure)
- hyperlipidemia (high cholesterol and other fats)
- smoking
- obesity
- sedentary lifestyle (no exercise)
- diabetes
- genetics (heredity)
- age
- gender
- race

Psychological:
- coronary-prone behavior patterns
- stress

Social:
- lack of social support

While it is impossible to guarantee how long anyone will live based on cardiac risk factors, we know that having one or more increases the chance of developing cardiovascular disease. Conversely, having fewer decreases the chance of developing disease. Cardiac risk factors also act synergistically. They are interconnected and strongly influence each other. The presence of one increases the influence of other risk factors.

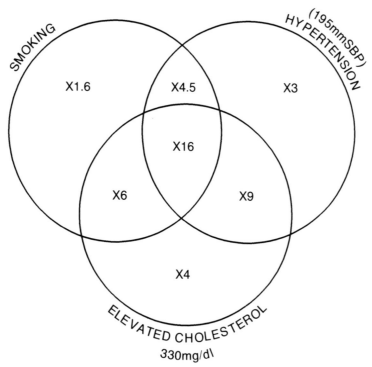

From Giuseppe Mancia, M.D., Milan, Italy, "Opening Remarks: The Need to Manage Risk Factors of Coronary Heart Disease," *American Heart Journal* 115, no. 1, pt. 2 (January 1988): 240.

The diagram shows a smoker has 1.6 times the risk of developing coronary heart disease as compared to a nonsmoker. Someone with high blood pressure has three times the risk as someone with normal blood pressure. A person with elevated cholesterol has four times the risk as someone with normal cholesterol. If, however, an individual smokes, and also has high blood pressure and elevated cholesterol, the risk for developing coronary heart disease increases to *sixteen times* that of the individual without these risk factors.

 ### John's Experience

John, forty-eight years old and a successful salesman for a major national corporation, enjoys his work but finds it busy and stressful at times. He enrolled in our Hypertension Program to address his work stress and its impact on his blood pressure. His intake evaluation noted he had high blood pressure, was more than 30 percent over ideal body weight, and had elevated blood cholesterol levels.

Being more than 20 to 30 percent over ideal body weight is a risk factor for developing cardiac disease. In addition, increased weight can cause increased cholesterol and blood-pressure levels. These three risk factors in combination increased his risk for a heart attack more than tenfold.

The development of certain risk factors such as obesity is influenced by a variety of mind/body variables, each important to consider when attempting to modify these risk factors. In addition to heredity and metabolism, a person's weight may be influenced by a number of lifestyle factors. Being a successful salesman required John to travel a great deal. On the road and on the run, John found that fast foods—albeit high in fats, calories, and sodium—accommodated his hectic schedule. His fast-paced lifestyle also interfered with his ability to exercise regularly and contributed to his inability to effectively manage his stress, which, in turn, can affect blood pressure.

We reminded John that foods high in fat and calories, as well as irregular exercise and stress, contribute not only to being overweight; but also to elevations in cholesterol. Further, eating is affected by moods and emotions. Lack of social support, being lonely, and eating alone can cause some people to overeat, or to choose their foods unwisely. When stressed, many people consume increased amounts of food and fat. Stress can also act directly to elevate blood pressure and cholesterol. With time, John recognized that his lifestyle was having a direct, adverse effect on his risk factors.

As John progressed through the Hypertension Program he was able to prioritize his goals and create a balance in his life which allowed for both healthy lifestyle behaviors and a successful career. He made a commitment to eating a heart-healthy diet and to exercising regularly. Through regular elicitation of the relaxation response in combination with cognitive strategies, he was able to manage his stress more effectively.

This combination of efforts yielded positive results for him. Over the course of twelve weeks he lost fifteen pounds, lowered his cholesterol by 10 percent, and reduced his blood pressure approximately 7-to-10 mm Hg, thereby significantly reducing his risk for developing cardiovascular disease.

John's case illustrates how risk factors are usually neither isolated nor the result of a single behavior or factor. Certainly being overweight is a risk factor for developing cardiovascular disease, but we can see that many interconnected dimensions contribute to the problem. Thus when looking for a way to reduce any one cardiovascular risk factor, we must consider the whole person and his or her biological, psychological, and social dimensions.

BIOLOGICAL FACTORS

Hypertension (high blood pressure)

When the heart contracts to pump blood out of its chambers, pressure is exerted against the walls of the arteries of the body. This force is called *blood pressure* and can be measured. The unit of measure for blood pressure is *millimeters of mercury* and is usually abbreviated *mm Hg*. The measurement yields two numbers: the *systolic blood pressure* (top number) and the *diastolic blood pressure* (bottom number). Systolic blood pressure is the amount of pressure the heart generates when it contracts and pushes blood out into the blood vessels to circulate throughout the body. Diastolic blood pressure is the amount of pressure in the arteries when the heart is relaxed and refilling with blood.

Consistent elevation in blood pressure, called *hypertension*, creates more strain on arteries and contributes to the development of atherosclerosis (the buildup of deposits called plaque in the arteries). Hypertension is diagnosed by averaging three or more readings, taken on three or more occasions. The Joint National Committee on the Detection, Evaluation and Treatment of High Blood Pressure categorizes blood pressure readings as follows:

BLOOD PRESSURE CLASSIFICATIONS IN ADULTS

Diastolic Blood Pressure (bottom number)

Range in mm Hg	Category
115 and over	Severe hypertension
105–114	Moderate hypertension
90–104	Mild hypertension
85–89	High normal blood pressure
84 and under	Normal blood pressure

Systolic Blood Pressure (top number), when the diastolic blood pressure is less than 90

Range in mm Hg	Category
160 and over	Systolic hypertension
140–159	Borderline systolic hypertension
139 and under	Normal blood pressure

Most high blood pressure is classified as *primary* or *essential hypertension*, meaning that the exact reason for the elevation is not known. Research indicates, however, that more forceful heartbeats—as, for example, caused by stress or additional fluid in the body (which may result from a high-salt diet)—or an increased stiffness of the arteries of the body with age are possible causes contributing to primary hypertension.

Under normal circumstances, in order to meet the body's requirement for oxygen and nutrients, blood pressure rises in response to physical exertion. This ability to respond to the need for more blood flow is important to the optimal functioning of the body. Similarly, in response to psychological stress, blood pressure increases temporarily as part of the flight-or-fight response.

Many medical scientists have speculated that repeated or prolonged exposure to stress might result in sustained increases in blood pressure, which in turn, can cause stress-related hypertension. A recent series of research reports has highlighted the importance of stress-related blood-pressure elevations. Even if such reactions do not lead to sustained elevations of blood pressure, they may be important. Consider the case of Mary.

Mary's Experience

Mary, a thirty-year-old computer programmer, had not been to a doctor since she had a painful injection at age fourteen. At age twenty-four, she needed a company physical examination.

Waiting for her blood pressure to be measured was anxiety-provoking. When the doctor inflated the blood-pressure cuff, Mary felt herself tense up. The look of concern on the doctor's face increased her anxiety. He told her to try and relax because her pressure was "a little high." Mary immediately interpreted this to mean she had hypertension. Try as she might, she could not relax, and whenever the doctor took her pressure it was high.

Her doctor considered medication to keep her blood pressure under control, but elected to wait because Mary had no other cardiac risk factors. He felt that some of the elevation in her blood pressure could be attributed to her nervousness at her visits. He ordered a twenty-four-hour blood-pressure monitor, which automatically measures and records the blood pressure every half hour throughout the day. The results from this device revealed that the only place where Mary's blood pressure was elevated was at the doctor's office.

The phenomenon Mary experienced is referred to as "white coat" hypertension and is a good example of mind/body influences on blood pressure. Dr. Thomas Pickering and his colleagues of the Cardiovascular Center at the New York Hospital-Cornell University Medical Center have shown that one out of five people with borderline high blood pressure may in fact have white coat hypertension. In their study of 292 patients who first had their blood pressure measured in a clinic by a doctor, then by a technician, and finally by an automatic twenty-four-hour ambulatory blood-pressure monitor, the doctor's reading was consistently highest. Those with white coat hypertension were more apt to be women, have a shorter history of high blood pressure, weigh less, and be younger than those who had consistently high blood pressure.

A variety of nondrug approaches helps to lower high blood pressure: exercise, weight loss, curtailing alcohol consumption, eliciting the relaxation response, stress management, and reducing salt in the diet of people who are salt-sensitive. A study conducted by members of our clinic—Eileen M. Stuart, John Deckro, Jane Leserman, Herbert Benson—found that individuals who utilized these interventions were able to lower their blood pressure and, in 80 percent of cases, reduce their need for blood-pressure medication. Studying these same individuals three to five years later, we were pleased to find that they had maintained these lower blood pressures over time without an increase in their medication.

Depending on the degree of elevation in blood pressure and the presence of other cardiac risk factors, medications may be required to treat high blood pressure. These fall into several different categories. Diuretics work primarily by increasing the amount of urine passed from the body and thereby decreasing the amount of fluid in the body. Diuretics include Hydrochlorothiazide, Lasix, and Moduretic. Beta-blockers, such as propranolol metoprolol and atenolol, cause the heart to beat more slowly and less forcefully, thus decreasing the pressure in the arteries. Calcium channel-blockers (e.g., nifedipine, diltiazem, and verapamil) also decrease the work of the heart and additionally relax blood vessels. Ace inhibitors are drugs which cause both the relaxation of blood vessels and a slight increase in urine production; enalapril and captopril fall into this category. Another class of blood-pressure medication that relaxes the blood vessels of the body is called vasodilators. Hydralazine and minoxidil are examples of this type of medicine. Finally, some medications, such as methyldopa and prazosin, act in part on the nerve impulses in the brain that help to cause increases in blood pressure.

Hyperlipidemia (elevated cholesterol)

An elevated cholesterol level is a major risk factor for cardiovascular disease. Cholesterol is a fat-like, waxy substance produced in your liver and also derived from certain foods. Carried through the bloodstream, it is critical to your body's functioning as an important component of your cellular membranes and various hormones, as well as to the production of vitamin D. Cholesterol, however, is also one of the main ingredients found in atherosclerotic *plaque* (a build-up of deposits on the walls of the arteries). High cholesterol contributes to the development of these plaques. One cause of high cholesterol is lifestyle: an excess dietary intake of cholesterol and saturated fats combined with too little activity.

A recent study by Drs. Gregory Burke, Michael Sprafka, and others from the Minnesota Heart Survey, showed that cholesterol declined in their study population, and that most of the reduction in cholesterol resulted from lifestyle changes such as diet and exercise.

In addition to dietary factors, stress hormones or adrenaline (epinephrine), released into the bloodstream can also increase the amount of cholesterol produced by the body. Scott Grundy, M.D., of the Baylor University College of Medicine, found that cholesterol levels in medical students increased 25 percent when measured during final exams, compared to measurements taken during the middle of the semester. Drs. Michael Cooper of the Kaiser-Permanente Medical Center in Oakland, California, and Maurice Aygen of the University of Tel Aviv Sackler School of Medicine, instructed a group of twelve patients with high cholesterol in a technique which elicits the relaxation response. After thirteen months, their cholesterol had dropped an average of 29 mg/dl, from 254 to 225. A comparison group of patients showed no change.

Three components to cholesterol need to be considered: *total* cholesterol, *HDL*-cholesterol (high-density lipoprotein), and *LDL*-cholesterol (low-density lipoprotein). Cholesterol is carried through the bloodstream by substances called lipoproteins. Cholesterol carried by HDL, often called "good" cholesterol, is transported to the liver and then enters the intestines for elimination from the body. Cholesterol carried by LDL is often called "bad" cholesterol since it can be deposited as plaque in the arteries.

CLASSIFICATION OF CHOLESTEROL IN ADULTS

Total Cholesterol

Blood Level (mg/dl)	Risk Level
240 and over	high
200–239	borderline
under 200	desirable

LDL Cholesterol

Blood Level (mg/dl)	Risk Level
160 and over	high
130–159	borderline
under 130	desirable

HDL Cholesterol

Blood Level (mg/dl)	Risk Level
35 and over	desirable
under 35	high

A desirable ratio of total cholesterol to HDL should be equal to or less than 3.5 for women, and 4.5 for men. For more information on cholesterol and how to manage it in your diet, see chapter 23, "Eating for the Health of Your Heart."

Although most patients will be able to lower their cholesterol through lifestyle changes, people with a genetic (hereditary) tendency toward high cholesterol levels are likely to need medication to keep cholesterol within the recommended range. Drugs to lower cholesterol fall into three categories: 1. Bile acid sequestrants, medications that increase the excretion of cholesterol into the intestines and subsequently out of the body, thus lowering cholesterol levels. Cholestryamine and colestipol are examples. Nicotinic acid is a bile sequestrant that works particularly well to decrease very high levels of triglycerides, another type of lipoprotein in the blood, and may also raise HDL (good) cholesterol. 2. Fibric acid derivatives work to lower high triglycerides and raise HDL-cholesterol, thus favorably modifying the lipid profile. Gemfibrozil is a fibric acid derivative. 3. HMG CoA Reductase Inhibitors are medications which interfere with the body's production of cholesterol by blocking an enzyme in the liver and thus decrease cholesterol. Even when taking any of these lipid-lowering medications, you should continue to modify your lifestyle, for example, by eating a heart-healthy, low-fat, low-cholesterol diet as outlined in chapter 23.

Smoking

Smoking any number of cigarettes per day is a major risk factor for developing cardiovascular disease. Smoking affects the body in a variety of ways.

Cigarette smoke contains carbon monoxide, which interferes with the blood's ability to transport oxygen. This in turn causes your heart rate to accelerate and your blood pressure to rise; it can also interfere with the ability of your heart muscle to pump effectively.

Cigarette smoking can lower the level of "good" or protective HDL-cholesterol. People who smoke have about a 12 percent lower HDL-cholesterol than people who do not smoke. People who smoke are also more likely to form blood clots quicker than people who do not smoke, placing the smoker at increased risk for a stroke or heart attack.

If you smoke, one of the most important things you can do to improve your health is to stop. No matter how long or how much you have smoked, your health begins to improve as soon as you quit. Dr. Judith Ockene, of the University of Massachusetts Medical Center, has demonstrated that when individuals stopped smoking, the risk of developing heart disease decreased 64 percent within three years. In a similar study, Dr. Lynn Rosenberg, of the Boston University Medical Center, reported on women who stopped smoking. Within three years after stopping smoking, their risk for developing heart disease was the same as that of a nonsmoker. Strategies to facilitate smoking cessation are located in Appendix A at the end of this chapter.

Obesity

Being overweight is a risk factor for cardiovascular disease. The actual definition of *overweight* varies considerably in the literature. Most experts agree that being more than 20-to-30 percent over your ideal body weight places you at risk for developing cardiovascular disease. In addition to its independent risk, excess weight can also accelerate the development of cardiovascular disease by contributing to the development of high blood pressure and high cholesterol. That is, if you are overweight, you are also more likely to have elevated blood pressure and cholesterol.

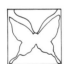

Take a Moment To . . .

Find out if you are more than 20 percent above your ideal body weight.

1. Calculate your ideal body weight (IBW).

   Women: Start with 100 pounds for the first five feet. Then add five pounds for each additional inch.

   Men: Start with 106 pounds for the first five feet. Then add six pounds for each additional inch.

   Record your ideal body weight _____ lbs.
                                    IBW

2. Record your actual weight _____ lbs.

3. Calculate the number which is 20 percent above *your* ideal body weight.

Multiply IBW × 1.2 = 20 percent above your IBW.

$$\frac{\quad\quad}{\text{IBW}} \times 1.2 = \underline{\quad\quad} \text{ lbs.}$$

Is your actual weight more than 20 percent over your ideal body weight (calculated in Step 2)? If so, to reduce your cardiac risk you need to lose weight, and chapters 8, 9, and 23 on nutrition will be important for you.

Sedentary lifestyle

Lack of regular exercise is associated with increased risk for developing cardiovascular disease. Regular exercise helps to control weight, raise the level of HDL-cholesterol, decrease blood pressure, and reduce psychological stress.

Under the direction of Dr. Ralph Paffenbarger, of the Stanford University School of Medicine, the long-term health and habits of 16,936 Harvard graduates, who entered college between 1916 and 1950, were assessed and examined for their relationship to length of life. Those alumni who reported regular exercise, such as walking, sports, or climbing stairs, outlived their more sedentary peers. Furthermore, death rates declined in proportion to the amount of exercise reported. Those individuals who every week walked nine or more miles, climbed 350 to 1049 stairs, or played three or more hours of light sports had the lowest death rates. Even when the presence of such cardiac risk factors such as cigarette smoking, hypertension, early parental death, and being overweight were figured into the analysis, alumni who exercised lived longer than those with similar risk factors who did not exercise.

The good news about exercise is it is not necessary to be an Olympic athlete. A recent study by Dr. Steven Blair and associates, at the Institute for Aerobics Research in Dallas, found the greatest gain in health in people who went from doing no exercise to doing a little exercise on a regular basis. Just getting off the couch and walking around the block regularly can lower your cardiovascular risk. Chapter 22, "Heart Disease and Diabetes: Exercise Is for You, Too," provides specific information on exercise and heart disease.

Diabetes

Diabetes, a condition characterized by continuous and high levels of sugar or glucose in the blood, is known to be a risk factor for developing cardiovascular disease. People with diabetes suffer from heart disease, strokes, and peripheral vascular disease at an earlier age than people with normal blood sugars.

Diabetes increases the risk for developing cardiovascular disease in a number of ways. It is theorized that the high levels of blood sugar may damage the inner lining of blood vessels, which in turn leads to increased plaque buildup in the arteries. Diabetes may also contribute to elevations in high blood pressure and cholesterol, although how is not entirely clear.

Managing your other cardiac risk factors and controlling your blood sugar are important contributors to reducing your risk if you have diabetes.

Genetics (heredity)

Our genes, or heredity, sometimes called "family history," play an important role in the development of cardiovascular disease. People with a primary relative—that is, a parent, grandparent, or sibling—who suffered from heart disease or a stroke before they were seventy years old are at increased risk for developing cardiovascular disease themselves.

Age

Increasing age has been shown to be a risk factor for cardiovascular disease. Coronary heart disease is relatively rare in people of either sex under the age of thirty. For men, the rates of illness and death begin to rise at around age forty-five. For women, the rates of cardiovascular disease begin to increase after menopause, at about age fifty-five.

Gender

Being male is a known cardiac risk factor. Scientists believe that the female hormones (estrogen and progesterone) play a protective role in slowing the accumulation of plaque in the coronary arteries. After women go through menopause, however, and the relative amount of these hormones decreases, the rate of cardiovascular disease increases to nearly equal to the rate for men.

Race

Race is also a risk factor for cardiovascular disease. Black people have rates of cardiovascular disease two to three times higher than individuals with similar risk factors of other races. The reason for this is unclear. Some researchers suggest that black individuals may have inherited biochemical differences that account for this higher rate of disease. Other scientists believe the harmful effects of the stress connected with being a minority in a white-dominated culture, or factors such as ethnic dietary preferences which are high in sodium and saturated fat, may be why blacks suffer from increased cardiovascular disease.

PSYCHOLOGICAL FACTORS

Coronary-prone behavior pattern

Although coronary-prone behavior is thought to be a relatively new problem, Sir William Osler, a noted researcher at Johns Hopkins, wrote on the causes of chest pain as early as 1897:

In the worry and strain of modern life, arterial degeneration is not only very common but develops often at a relatively early age. For this I believe that the high pressure at which men live and the habit of working the machine to its maximum capacity are responsible rather than the excesses in eating and drinking.

In the late 1950s, Drs. Meyer Friedman and Ray Rosenman, two cardiologists at Mount Zion Hospital in San Francisco, began pioneer research to document coronary-prone behaviors, which they called *Type A Behavior.* Type A personalities are characteristically time urgent (feeling unremitting pressure to get things done quickly), competitive, and hard driving. With time, it became apparent that all people exhibiting these behaviors did not develop heart disease at the same rate.

Research continues on how to identify which features of coronary-prone behavior most accurately predict the development of heart disease. Redford Williams, M.D., director of the Behavioral Medicine Research Center at Duke University Medical Center, has conducted a series of studies which has increasingly focused on anger and hostility as the critical component of coronary-prone behavior patterns. Dr. Williams and his associates have documented that cynical beliefs, frequent angry feelings, and acting out those angry feelings aggressively toward others, predict coronary heart disease to a high degree. Studying alumni, they found that Duke freshmen who scored high on a scale for hostility at age nineteen were more likely to have developed heart disease by age forty-two.

Dr. Friedman and nurse researcher Dianne Ulmer went on to refine the Type A hypothesis to include hyperaggressiveness, explosive speech patterns, and free-floating hostility—that is, "a permanently indwelling anger that shows itself with ever-greater frequency in response to increasingly trivial happenings."

Williams and his coworkers have conducted a number of experiments to discover the mechanisms in the body responsible for the increased heart disease associated with coronary-prone behavior. They identified individuals with high and low hostility scores who were then subjected to challenging mental problems and, at times, intentionally harassed while working on solutions. Antagonistic environmental stressors appear to cause a very strong activation of the fight-or-flight response in individuals with high hostility scores. When challenged by something perceived as antagonistic, they had higher blood pressures than people with low hostility scores. It also took longer for their blood pressure to come back down to normal. In addition to stimulation of the fight-or-flight response, individuals with high hostility scores showed a smaller response of the parasympathetic nervous system, which can slow down the arousal of the fight-or-flight response. This particularly strong and prolonged response to perceived antagonism not only makes the heart work harder but also can increase a number of other cardiac risk factors.

More information on coronary-prone behaviors and specific strategies to deal with them can be found in chapters 10 through 15.

Stress

Stress, as defined in chapter 10, "Managing Stress," is the perception of a threat to either our physical or psychological self, and the perception that our resources are inadequate to cope with that threat. Stress requires the body to adjust to this perceived threat and precipitates a cascade of hormones that prepares us either for confrontation or escape: "fight or flight." Change is stressful, and evidence suggests that Americans are stressed as never before. The tranquilizer Valium is one of the three most prescribed drugs in the United States. Extensive research in animals has shown that severe or prolonged stress increases atherosclerosis. C. David Jenkins, Ph.D., from the University of Texas Health Sciences Center in Houston, found that such states as anxiety, depression, and high occupational demands were independent predictors of coronary heart disease. William Ruberman, M.D., and his associates from the Health Insurance Plan of Greater New York, researching 2,320 survivors of acute myocardial infarction, found that three years after the heart attack, those individuals with a combination of high stress and social isolation had a death rate four times that of people with low stress and strong social support.

We know that the fight-or-flight response releases a variety of hormones including adrenaline (epinephrine) and noradrenaline (norepinephrine). These hormones, in turn, can increase blood pressure and cholesterol levels and cause the blood to clot more quickly. In this way, stress not only is a cardiac risk factor in itself, but also plays a role in the development of others factors. Epinephrine may cause the arteries of the heart to constrict enough to prevent blood flow through the coronary arteries. A surge of epinephrine can cause the heart's electrical system to misfire and beat irregularly. If prolonged or severe enough, this irregular beating can cause death. Furthermore, other chemicals released by the body in response to stress affect the heart. Cortisol, which comes from the outer part of the adrenal gland, can increase blood sugar, cholesterol levels, blood pressure, and make the blood clot more quickly. Cortisol also enhances the effects of epinephrine and norepinephrine.

The mind/body interaction can be used to counteract the harmful effects of stress. Dr. Chandra Patel and her associates in London researched 192 men and women, aged thirty-five to sixty-four years, with two or more risk factors for cardiac disease such as high blood pressure, high cholesterol, and/or cigarette smoking. They divided their subjects into two groups. Both groups received advice on risk-factor reduction, but one additionally received instruction in eliciting relaxation response and cognitive behavioral stress-management techniques. At the end of four years, the group instructed in relaxation response/stress management had lower blood pressures and significantly lower rates of coronary heart disease.

SOCIAL FACTORS

Social Support

People are by nature social beings, but as society has evolved, meeting our needs for social support is becoming increasingly difficult. The extensive family and community networks available to our predecessors are disappearing. As discussed in chapter 10, research by psychologists such as Suzanne Kobasa has demonstrated that social support is an important buffer to stress and a component of stress-hardiness. A Swedish scientist, Kristina Orth-Gomer, M.D., and her associates from the National Institute for Psychosocial Health in Stockholm, have established the importance of social support in the prevention of cardiovascular disease. Orth-Gomer followed 150 middle-aged men, some of whom had coronary heart disease, others without obvious heart disease but with risk factors (high blood pressure, smoking, and high cholesterol), and still others who were healthy and without risk factors for ten years. At the end of ten years, social isolation (as indicated by a relatively low level of social activity) was as powerful a predictor of who developed cardiovascular disease as the more biological risk factors such as high blood pressure and cholesterol.

A relationship between social relationships and health has long been observed. Dr. James House and his colleagues, writing in *Science*, note that death rates are consistently higher among unmarried individuals than among married ones. Eric Cottington, B.A., and his associates from the University of Pittsburgh, examined the roles of death of a significant other, change in residence, or change in work in eighty-one women who had suffered sudden death from coronary artery disease in Allegheny County, Pennsylvania. When the victims of sudden death were compared with a group of women selected for similarity of age, race, and area of residence, it was found that the sudden-death victims were six times more likely to have undergone the death of a close person in the preceding six months than the controls.

While retirement is viewed by many as a positive occurrence, it can also represent a major disruption in the social network of an individual's life, let alone income and self-esteem. Dr. Ward Casscells and associates interviewed the wives of 568 married men who had died within twenty-four hours after the onset of symptoms from coronary heart disease. An equal number of interviews were conducted with a control group chosen from the same neighborhood and age group. When the results were compared, after adjusting the data for age and previous history of a heart attack, the relative risk of having a fatal heart attack was 1.8, or nearly twice as high, in those men who had retired when compared to those who were still working.

Dr. Dwayne Reed and co-workers from the Honolulu Heart Program surveyed the networks of social activity of 4,653 men of Japanese descent by examining their self-reports of connections to relatives, co-workers, religious, and social organizations. Each person was scored based on the amount of contact they had in each area. The prevalence of heart attacks, angina, and total coronary disease in this group was found to be inversely related to the size of the social networks. That is, the men who reported the largest social networks had the least disease.

Jack Medalie, M.D. and Uri Goldbourt, M.A., of Tel Aviv University, found in the Israeli Heart Disease Study that a wife's love and support reduced the risk of developing angina, even given the presence of other cardiac risk factors. Men who had a high anxiety level, and who felt little support and love from their spouses, experienced more angina than men who also had a high anxiety level, but who felt loved and supported by their spouses.

The mechanisms by which lack of perceived social support contributes to cardiac risk are unclear, but new research from Sweden points to some interesting areas. Dr. Annika Rosengren and her colleagues from Gothenburg University have found that social support may decease the amount of fibrinogen, a substance found in the blood which is important in blood clotting. In a study of 776 Swedish men in the city of Gothenburg, blood samples were taken and a detailed questionnaire regarding various social variables was administered. Those men who had the highest level of social activity had the lowest levels of fibrinogen, and thus should have a lower risk of a heart attack or stroke from a blood clot. Anna-Lena Unden, B.A., Dr. Kristina Orth-Gomer, and Dr. Stig Elofsson, also of Sweden, found in a study of working men and women of varying occupations that heart rates and systolic blood pressures were significantly higher, at work and at home, in persons reporting low social support at work.

These studies attest to the powerful effect of thought, feelings, and emotions on health. In this context, the suggestions in chapter 13, "Coping and Problem-Solving," for positively influencing thoughts, feelings, and emotions are particularly poignant.

Modifying Your Risk Factors: A Decision You Can Live With

> Ah, nothing is too late,
> Till the tired heart shall cease to palpitate.
>
> Longfellow, *Morituri Salutamus*

It is never to late to begin. As shown in the preceding pages, modifying your cardiac risk factors results in a distinct protective advantage. We have consistently acknowledged that change is seldom easy, but it is possible, and we have included strategies and skills to accomplish a wide range of lifestyle changes. The information in this chapter should be integrated with all the skills learned in the previous fifteen chapters of *The Wellness Book*. Chapters 22 and 23 will provide more specific information about the cardiovascular considerations regarding both exercise and diet. When you consider modifying your risk factors, the most important thing is to make a commitment to yourself to *Just do it!* Remember, this is a decision you can *live* with.

Take a Moment To . . .

Calculate your cardiac risk factors, utilizing the following questionnaire.

The Cardiac Risk Factor Questionnaire

Name _____ Date _____

CARDIAC RISK FACTOR	0 LOW	1 BELOW AVERAGE	2 AVERAGE (Or Borderline)	3 ABOVE AVERAGE	4 HIGH RISK	5 or 6 POINTS (See Box Below) DANGEROUS	SCORE COLUMN
1. CIGARETTE SMOKING	Never	None in past 1 year	Smoked in past year or under 10 a day	20 a day	30 a day	6 Points 40 or more a day	
2. FAMILY HISTORY (Parents, grandparents, brothers & sisters.)	No history of heart disease before age 75*	1 relative with heart disease 60-75	2 relatives with heart disease 60-75	1 relative with heart disease under 60	2 relatives with heart disease under 60	5 Points 3 relatives with heart disease under 60	
3. DIABETES (Parents grandparents, brothers & sisters.)	No history	1 relative	2 relatives	Diabetes in self after age 60	Diabetes in self age 20-60	6 Points Diabetes in self before 20	
4. EXERCISE Lower score by 1 if you take part in a regular aerobic program**	Intense occupational & recreational exertion	Moderate occupational & recreational exertion	Sedentary work & intense recreational exertion	Sedentary work & moderate recreational exertion	Sedentary work & light recreational	5 Points Sedentary work with no exercise	
5. BEHAVIOR CHARACTERISTICS	Always easy-going & relaxed	Easy-going & relaxed most of the time	Frequently impatient & clock watching	Persistently aggressive in work & play	Overwhelming ambition; constantly aware of time & deadlines	5 Points Hard-driving; always rushing, no relaxation; easily angered	
6. AGE & SEX	Female under 45	Male under 40	Female 45-55 Male 40-50	Female over 55	Male 50-60	5 Points Male over 60	
7. BLOOD PRESSURE SYSTOLIC	Under 120	130 (Maximum)	140 (Maximum)	160 (Maximum)	180 (Maximum)	6 ponts Over 180	
8. BLOOD PRESSURE DIASTOLIC	Under 80	85 (Maximum)	90 (Maximum)	104 (Maximum)	115 (Maximum)	6 Points Over 115	
9. TOTAL CHOLESTEROL/ HDL	Under 3.0	3.0-4.5	4.6-5.9	6.0-7.9	8.0-9.9	6 Points Over 10	
10. WEIGHT	6 lbs. or more under S.W.†	−5 to +5 of S.W.	6-20 over S.W.	21-35 over S.W.	36-50 over S.W.	5 Points 50 or more over S.W.	
11. ELECTRO-CARDIOGRAM	Normal	No point score other than 0 or 6; physician will comment if there are other abnormalities				6 Points Left ventricular hypertrophy (LVH)	
						TOTAL SCORE	

Cardiac Risk Factor Point Score Analysis

0-7	Low Risk
8-17	Below Average
18-22	Average (Borderline)
23-32	Above Average
33-42	High
Over 42	Very high (Dangerous)

†Definition of Standard Weight (S.W.): FEMALE—Height in inches above 5′×5+100. MALE—Height in inches above 5′×6+106
*Do not include a history of rheumatic heart disease or heart defect from birth.
**A regular aerobic program is defined as vigorous, sustained exercise for 20-30 minutes at least 3 days per week consisting of continuous, rhythmic movement, such as jogging or swimming.

Developed by The Executive Health Group

Now you are ready to write your Health Commitment, your plan for change.

- Identify the highest-scoring risk factor. Alternatively, pick the risk factor you feel you will be most successful in changing.
- Identify your long-term goal, being careful to make it realistic and attainable.
- Set a time for accomplishing your long-term goal.
- Identify strategies (short-term goals) to accomplish your long-term goal.
- Consider those people or things that might help or hinder you in making the change.
- Keep a chart and measure your progress. Treat yourself to rewards as you reach certain milestones.

The ultimate reward of reducing your cardiovascular risk factors is priceless: feeling well, both physically and mentally, is well worth the time and effort it takes to accomplish.

FROM RISK FACTORS TO HEART DISEASE

As you know by now, risk factors harm the body by speeding up the rate of developing atherosclerosis through the accumulation of plaque in the arteries. The plaque hinders the amount of blood that can traverse the arteries to supply the body with nutrients critical to normal functioning. When plaque builds up in one of the three major arteries that supply the heart, it is called *coronary artery disease* or *coronary atherosclerosis*. The remainder of this chapter will address those issues specific to understanding the treatment and rehabilitation of patients with coronary artery disease.

CARDIOVASCULAR ANATOMY AND PHYSIOLOGY

The heart is a pump, approximately the size of your fist, which beats about a hundred thousand times a day, moving approximately two thousand gallons of blood daily through some sixty thousand miles of blood vessels. It has four chambers, two of which are primarily reservoirs and two of which are primarily muscular pumping chambers. Four major valves allow blood to flow forward without flowing backward. The blood vessels that provide the heart with nourishment are the coronary arteries, they completely encircle the heart muscle like a crown, hence the name *coronary*. The three major coronary arteries are *right coronary artery*, *left anterior descending coronary artery*, and *left circumflex coronary artery*. They have many branches, which provide a network of blood vessels to supply all parts of the heart with oxygen-rich blood. The illustration shows clearly the position of the coronary arteries in relation to the heart muscle.

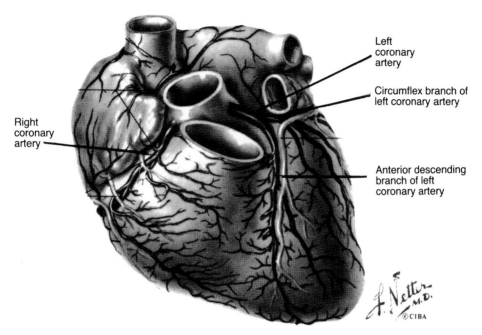

Left coronary artery

Circumflex branch of left coronary artery

Right coronary artery

Anterior descending branch of left coronary artery

To keep the heart beating regularly, an electrical nervous system with a tiny generator provides regular impulses which make the heart contract. Diseases of the heart can affect the heart muscle, the coronary arteries, the valves, or the electrical system. The most common form of heart disease is coronary artery disease.

ANGINA: THE BALANCE BETWEEN SUPPLY AND DEMAND

The heart is constantly responding to changes in the body's need for oxygen. Physical stress such as exercise and/or emotional stress are examples of conditions under which the body needs more oxygen to perform optimally. Under normal circumstances, the heart has little difficulty accommodating these changes and can increase the supply of oxygen-rich blood in response to an increased need, that is, demand.

In the presence of coronary artery disease, however, the supply of oxygen to the heart muscle is decreased because of blockage in the coronary arteries, caused either by plaque or by spasm (a sudden constriction). This decrease in supply becomes worse during times of increased demand, such as with physical exertion or emotional stress.

When demand exceeds supply, the resulting imbalance is called *ischemia*, generally defined as a lack of oxygen and nutrients caused by the lack of blood to a particular part of the body. In heart muscle, ischemia is often manifested as chest pain or chest discomfort. Such a symptom in the chest is formally called angina pectoris, but is more commonly known simply as *angina*. Sometimes, an individual with cardiac ischemia may experience no chest pain; this is known as *silent ischemia*. The electrocardiogram may change during an episode of angina or silent ischemia, but afterward returns to normal. Angina is reversible and does not damage the heart.

Understanding angina, then, depends on an understanding of the concept of supply and demand and the factors which can affect this balance. Consider activities or conditions which might increase the heart muscle's demand for blood. Aerobic exercise, heavy physical labor, a high-fat meal, stressful circumstances, and extremely cold or warm muggy temperatures all cause the heart to work harder. As the work of the heart increases, the demand for blood supply also increases. If the ability of the coronary arteries to supply increased blood to meet this increased need is compromised, due to blockage or spasm, cardiac ischemia and chest pain occur.

The Exercise Tolerance Test (ETT or stress test) is a diagnostic test which creates a situation in which this imbalance between supply and demand is likely to occur. As an individual exercises on the treadmill or bicycle, the workload of the heart increases. If his or her coronary arteries are unable to supply sufficient blood to meet the increased demand, ischemia will occur, and the person will most likely experience chest pain (angina). The electrocardiogram will change to reflect this ischemia, and thallium is often used to further assess the area of cardiac ischemia. Thallium is a radioactive substance which, when injected into the bloodstream, is carried to the heart muscle via the coronary arteries. If there is a blockage in the coronary arteries, less thallium is carried to the heart muscle, and a scan reveals those areas of the heart muscle which are not receiving an adequate supply of blood and oxygen.

While usually we are quick to identify the physical causes of ischemia, for example, exercise or exertion, scientists have shown that cardiac ischemia occurs with mental stress as well. By now you are well aware of the physical consequences of mental stress. As you activate the fight-or-flight response, the demand on the heart is increased. Researchers, including Drs. Andrew Selwyn, from Brigham and Women's Hospital in Boston, and John Deanfield, from Hammersmith Hospital in London, have demonstrated that in people with coronary heart disease, mental stress can produce a similar imbalance between supply and demand, causing the same ischemic changes in the EKG and thallium images that occur on an exercise-tolerance test. It has also been shown that the wall motion of the heart, which affects that ability of the heart to effectively pump out blood, is affected by mental stress as well as by physical exertion.

For years patients have been telling us that stress as well as overexertion is a precipitating factor in angina. To manage your angina effectively then, you need to become involved and to understand those factors which might affect the balance between supply and demand. You need to address these factors directly, modifying the way you approach them (for example, through limitation of exercise, smaller meals, and/or decreased stress).

Medications are usually prescribed in conjunction with these self-help measures. The medications also act on the principle of supply and demand. Vasodilators, such as nitroglycerine or Isordil, dilate (widen) the coronary arteries, thereby increasing the blood supply to the heart. Beta-blockers (such as propranolol, atenolol, etc.) and calcium-channel blockers (such as nifedipine, verapamil, or diltiazem) decrease the workload on the heart by slowing the heartbeat and decreasing the force of the muscle contraction. By reducing the workload, the demand is diminished.

The first thing to do if you experience angina is to stop, rest, and place a nitroglycerine tablet under your tongue. Nitroglycerine increases the blood supply to the heart and decreases demand, restoring the balance between supply and demand and preventing damage to the heart muscle. Continue taking nitroglycerine every four to five minutes until the pain is resolved. If your angina does not go away after three tablets, or if the angina is significantly different from your usual pattern, contact your physician to discuss the problem.

Eliciting the relaxation response is a beneficial adjunct to nitroglycerine in relieving angina. It acts by decreasing the demand on the heart, and if the episode of angina is precipitated by stress, it can serve to minimize the harmful effects of the fight-or-flight response. Our prescription for anginal chest pain is to: Stop, Rest, Take a Breath, take a nitroglycerine.

Overall, remember that angina is reversible and most often causes no permanent heart damage.

HEART ATTACKS AND HOW THEY OCCUR

If there is progressive narrowing of the coronary artery, or if a clot suddenly forms inside a partially blocked artery, or if severe spasm occurs, the area of heart muscle which is supplied by blood from that artery becomes starved for oxygen and nutrients. A heart attack, or *myocardial infarction*, may occur. The illustration shows a blockage in the left anterior descending coronary artery, with the resultant damage to heart muscle beyond.

Thus, in contrast to angina, a myocardial infarction results in actual damage to the heart with release of specific substances called enzymes into the blood. An elevation of these enzymes, which can be tested, is necessary for the diagnosis of a heart attack to be made. The electrocardiogram is also altered, and changes persist even after the heart heals and the acute episode is over.

The risk factors discussed previously do not fully explain why a person with coronary artery disease develops a heart attack at a particular moment. The likely explanation is that in addition to the progressive buildup of plaque, transient changes occur in the coronary blood circulation which alter the balance of supply and demand so profoundly as to cause damage to heart muscle.

For example, in the presence of partial blockages in the coronary arteries,

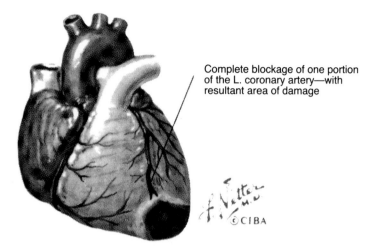

Complete blockage of one portion of the L. coronary artery—with resultant area of damage

a sudden increase in demand for oxygen and nutrients—caused by excessive exercise, emotional upset, or extreme excitement—may cause a heart attack. The exercise or emotions increase the release of adrenaline (epinephrine) and norepinephrine, which cause an abrupt increase in blood pressure and in the vigor of contraction of the heart. Furthermore, these same substances increase the clotting tendency of blood. Often these clots are at the very site of blockage in the artery so that the artery becomes even more narrowed. The situation is thus greatly worsened since blood flow may be completely blocked.

The effect is straightforward. Heart muscle which does not receive blood for a sufficiently long time becomes permanently damaged, and heart muscle cells will die. This is a heart attack, or myocardial infarction. Even with partially or completely blocked coronary arteries, a great deal of physical or psychological stress is needed to cause a heart attack or death because the rest of the circulation of the heart can compensate in most circumstances.

Dr. Jacob Haft and co-workers of the St. Michael's Medical Center in Newark, New Jersey, have conducted research which demonstrates that the occurrence of coronary atherosclerosis, coronary artery spasm, and thrombus (clot) formation are all interrelated. For example, in the presence of a large buildup of plaque, there need be only a small degree of spasm (constriction) at the same site to cause angina or a heart attack. Similarly, if 90 percent of the coronary artery is blocked by plaque, there need be only a small clot to completely block off the artery, thereby causing a heart attack.

The occurrence of heart attacks is not distributed evenly throughout the day. Dr. James Muller and his colleagues at Boston's New England Deaconess Hospital, and Brigham and Women's Hospital, have found that heart attacks are more likely to occur in the morning, specifically, within an hour or two after awakening. Obviously, the risk factors associated with heart attack, such as genetics, obesity, diet, and exercise do not suddenly change in the morning hours. There must, therefore, be a physiological explanation for why heart attacks are more likely to occur early in the day. It is theorized that platelet aggregation—the stickiness of red blood cells—varies in a way which coincides with an increase in clot formation and heart-attack frequency. Furthermore, platelet aggregation increases when levels of adrenaline (epinephrine) and noradrenaline (norepinephrine) increase. This increase in sympathetic-nervous-system activity occurs during the early part of the day, thereby coinciding with heart-attack frequency. A reasonable suggestion, therefore, is that sympathetic-nervous-system increases early in the day increase platelet stickiness (aggregation) and the tendency of the blood to clot, which in turn increase the likelihood of heart attacks. If this is indeed the case, it is interesting to speculate that the increase in adrenaline (epinephrine) and noradrenaline (norepinephrine) brought about by other types of stress might also increase the clotting of blood and thereby increase the likelihood of a heart attack.

Physical and emotional stress can also, by a similar process of nerve stimulation and release of epinephrine and norepinephrine, cause changes in the electrical system of the heart. Drs. Bernard Lown, Regis DeSilva, and their colleagues at the Brigham and Women's Hospital found that if these changes are profound, the heart's rhythm can be affected and conditions like *ventricular fibrillation*—a dangerous disruption in the heart rhythm—may occur. A great deal of physical effort and very severe or prolonged stress is needed in most instances to cause death by this means.

Stimulants, especially cocaine and amphetamines, have potent effects on the heart. They can cause constriction (narrowing) of the arteries, an increase in clot formation, and the rupture of plaque. These conditions create increased risk of heart attack, especially in young adults with no history of coronary artery disease.

MEDICAL TREATMENT OF HEART ATTACKS

There has been a great deal of public education about the usual signs of an impending heart attack such as chest, neck, jaw, or arm discomfort, nausea or vomiting, oppressive chest heaviness, or actual "crushing" chest pain. However, during the early stages of a heart attack there may be absolutely no symptoms. Sometimes the only symptom is *extreme* and *very severe* fatigue to the point of sleepiness in the middle of the day. These symptoms may continue for several hours or for days before a heart attack occurs. Most people tend to deny that these symptoms, even when pronounced, could be related to their heart, instead thinking it an attack of indigestion, since the sensation is discomfort in the lower chest with belching, nausea, and vomiting. When such symptoms are present, get to the hospital as soon as possible so that diagnostic tests and treatment may be given immediately. Have someone drive the person, or call an ambulance.

If these symptoms occur, the first thing to do is to place a nitroglycerine tablet under the tongue. Nitroglycerine increases the blood supply to the heart, limits the amount of damage to the heart muscle, and stabilizes the heart electrically. Repeat the nitroglycerine several times every four to five minutes until the person reaches a hospital. Taking several (e.g., five to ten tablets) is safe, but by then symptoms will have occurred for almost an hour and the patient should be in a hospital for treatment. Again, the relaxation response is a helpful adjunct to nitroglycerine in relieving angina pain and in minimizing the physiological consequences of stress.

At any hospital, a very standard procedure is followed for a suspected heart attack. Blood is taken to measure enzymes, an intravenous infusion is started for administering emergency medications, and an electrocardiogram is done, which may or may not yield an immediate diagnosis. In about an hour, the results of the first blood tests will be available to confirm the diagnosis, although in most cases, blood tests will need to be repeated several times.

We currently have five options for treating and preventing a heart attack:

Medications

Several classes of medications may be used to treat persons with a developing or an established heart attack. These include nitroglycerine, beta-blocking drugs, and calcium-blocking drugs, the same medicines we described when discussing angina, and the principles by which they work do not differ. In other words, the supply-demand balance is favorably altered by these medications. Antiarrhythmic medications may be used to treat irregular heartbeats. Morphine is often given to treat anxiety and pain. As discussed under the treatment of angina, eliciting the relaxation response is a beneficial adjunct to nitroglycerine in treating chest pain.

Thrombolytic therapy

If a heart attack is diagnosed within the first six hours of its occurrence, common practice in the United States, Canada, and Europe now is to give an intravenous infusion of a drug which can dissolve clots. These drugs are called *thrombolytic agents* ("clot busters") because they *lyse* (dissolve) *thrombi* (clots). Three agents are used principally today: streptokinase, tissue plasminogen activator (tPA), and APSAC.

In particular cases, these drugs cannot or should not be given. The principal risk is the development of bleeding, since blood does not clot as easily after they are administered. However, evidence today shows a significant improvement in survival after a heart attack with this treatment, and the risk of a bleeding complication is small.

Coronary angioplasty (PTCA)

In cases where a person's angina pattern changes, or if chest pain is unrelieved by rest and medication, or if there is an indication that the heart damage is worsening, cardiac catheterization may be needed. This procedure involves placing a flexible hollow tube, called a *catheter*, in an artery and vein, and advancing it into the heart chambers. Dye is then injected through the catheter to allow the coronary arteries and heart chambers to be seen on X ray and photographed on both videotape and movie film. If coronary artery blockages exist, they are visible in these pictures. In some cases, the areas of blockage can be opened to prevent the occurrence of a heart attack by a technique known as *coronary angioplasty*, more precisely called *percutaneous transluminal coronary angioplasty* (PTCA). This procedure positions a catheter with an uninflated balloon around one end at the point where the coronary artery is partially blocked. The balloon is then inflated to "squash" the plaque against the wall of the blood vessel, thereby increasing the diameter of the coronary vessel and allowing more blood to flow through the vessel. The balloon is then deflated and the catheter removed. In the case of an ongoing heart attack, successful angioplasty can prevent extension of the heart attack by increasing the amount of blood flow to the section of the heart muscle deprived of blood.

Cardiac surgery

Coronary artery bypass grafting is usually done when blockage is so severe that medication and angioplasty cannot increase the blood supply to the heart. It is usually performed to help prevent the occurrence of a heart attack, although it is sometimes used in the case of an ongoing heart attack in an attempt to avert further damage.

A vein from the leg or the left internal mammary artery—a small artery in the chest—is used to "bypass" the blocked artery so that blood can flow around the blockage and nourish the oxygen-deprived heart muscle.

Multiple-risk-factor reduction for regression of atherosclerosis

We have already discussed how lifestyle factors can affect the buildup of plaque in the arteries, as well as the incidence of spasm and the development of thrombi (clots). Now evidence is mounting that modifying cardiac risk factors may actually cause regression, that is, the progressive decline of atherosclerotic plaque in the coronary arteries.

Dr. Greg Brown and colleagues from the University of Washington School of Medicine in Seattle studied the effects of lowering LDL-cholesterol and increasing HDL-cholesterol in 162 men under sixty-two years of age who had elevated cholesterol levels, documented coronary artery disease, and a positive family history. All patients in the study were instructed to limit their daily intake of saturated fat to less than 30 percent of their total daily calories. They were then assigned to one of three treatment groups: two groups were given different intensive lipid-lowering medications and one group received a placebo. Both medication groups achieved positive results, with a significant rise in HDL-cholesterol and a significant decrease in LDL-cholesterol. The placebo group improved only slightly. In addition, intensive lipid-lowering therapy reduced the progression of coronary-artery blockages, increased the regression of coronary-artery blockages, and reduced the occurrence of subsequent coronary events. Thus, this important study showed that by intensively lowering lipids through the use of medication and diet, the progression of coronary artery disease was decreased and the occurrence of subsequent coronary events was reduced.

Dean Ornish, M.D., and his colleagues from the University of California-San Francisco School of Medicine, studied the effects of intensive dietary modification (less than 10 percent of total daily calories from fat), stress management, elicitation of the relaxation response, smoking cessation, and moderate exercise on specific measures of regression in atherosclerotic plaque. The control group was given standard advice about exercise, diet, smoking, and stress reduction, and left to make these changes on their own. With the exception of more stringent dietary requirements, the components of this study—called the Lifestyle Heart Trial—are similar to the interventions described in *The Wellness Book*.

Over the course of one year, Dr. Ornish and his co-workers were able to show that patients in the experimental group had a 91 percent reduction in the frequency of anginal symptoms, a 24.3 percent reduction in cholesterol levels, a 37.4 percent reduction in LDL, and a significant decrease in the size of the plaque in the coronary artery. The control group did not show similar favorable results. In fact, the patients got worse, with an increase in anginal symptoms, cholesterol, and LDL, as well as more plaque in the coronary artery. In addition, the researchers were able to show a dose-related effect, meaning that the greater the compliance with the interventions, the greater the evidence of regression.

This promising trial contains the first objective evidence that modifying lifestyle behaviors is possible and will progressively decrease atherosclerotic plaque in the coronary arteries. It will be important to follow the results of this trial in the years to come.

Meyer Friedman and his colleagues from San Francisco studied the feasibility of altering coronary-prone behaviors and the impact of this intervention on the subsequent recurrence rate of heart attacks. The study subjects were all men who had suffered one heart attack. Both the control and experimental groups received group cardiac counseling and were given standard advice about exercise, diet, and smoking. In addition, a comparison group received no instruction or information. The patients in the experimental group received an intensive intervention to modify their coronary-prone behavior, attending a weekly support group for one year, which incorporated principles of stress management, cognitive therapy, and eliciting the relaxation response. Over five years, the researchers found only one half the incidence of subsequent heart attacks in the group who received intervention to reduce coronary-prone behaviors, compared to the control group and the comparison group. Overall, the results of this study demonstrate that modifying coronary-prone behaviors is possible and reduces the likelihood of future cardiac events.

Cardiac rehabilitation

Following a heart attack or other adverse cardiac events, individuals should begin the process of modifying any existing cardiac risk factors. If you are recovering from a heart attack, now is the time, if you have not already started, to change any adverse lifestyle behaviors.

In addition to risk-factor reduction, recovering from a cardiac event involves two specific aspects. The first is to recondition the body slowly and carefully, and the second is to deal with the variety of emotions which invariably occur.

Chapter 22, "Heart Disease and Diabetes: Exercise Is for You, Too," deals specifically with the special considerations of beginning an exercise regimen after a cardiac event. Research has shown that in addition to modifying your risk factors, exercise at this time is important in countering the harmful effects of bed rest as well as in conditioning your heart and vascular system to become efficient, thus decreasing the demand on the heart. Therefore, beginning a graded, structured exercise program after a cardiac event is an important step.

Emotions also play an important part in the recovery from heart disease, and as they are not dealt with elsewhere in *The Wellness Book*, we will discuss them in some depth now.

HEARTFELT EMOTIONS

In the early stages of recovery from a cardiac event, people typically report feelings of fear, anxiety, and denial. Thoughts such as "Why me, why now, this can't be happening to me, not me, I'm healthy," or "This wasn't in my life plan" are frequently expressed. In addition to fear, anxiety, and denial, people often express feelings of anger and loss after a heart attack. Although they may feel confusing and threatening at the time, such feelings are common and to be expected. If is vital to take the time to acknowledge and honor these emotions. You have had a significant disruption in your health and life, and processing this is important. Eliciting the relaxation response through breath focus is an excellent way to decrease anxiety and help you balance your emotions. Talking about these feelings in the early stages of a cardiac event to family members, friends, or health-care providers has been shown to be critical in laying the groundwork for later success in modifying your cardiac risk factors and adjusting to this illness. In fact, Dr. James W. Pennebaker, a professor of psychology at Southern Methodist University in Dallas, demonstrated that people who do not express their feelings at the time of a stressful event, tend to experience more symptoms later.

Use all the strategies learned in chapters 11 through 15 to help cope successfully with the period immediately after your heart attack. Use your cognitive-restructuring strategies to help stop and challenge your automatic thoughts and exaggerated beliefs. People are often anxious immediately after a heart attack because they are unsure of what to expect. Typically, patient questions center around four "will I" questions: "Will I live?" "Will I love?" "Will I play?" "Will I work?" To understand the realistic—not exaggerated or distorted—implications of your heart condition and to deal effectively with your emotions, you need realistic answers to these questions. Talk with your physician and nurses. Ask questions until you feel you understand.

If you find yourself feeling overwhelmed by your heart disease or over-reacting to situations, Stop, Take a Breath, Reflect, and Choose how you want to respond. This is the time to use the wide variety of the coping skills you have learned. In addition to social support, cognitive restructuring, and eliciting the relaxation response, consider these strategies:

- Use direct action, become as educated as possible about your condition and what you can do to participate in your care.
- Use humor to counteract the stressful effects of this event.
- Use distraction to help you not worry and dwell on things over which you do not have control, and use direct action to influence things over which you do have control.
- Reframe the experience by looking for those opportunities which have opened up to you as a result of this illness.

In a similar context, Dr. Nancy Frasure-Smith, a sociologist at the Montreal Heart Institute, has shown that anxious patients who received social support in the post-heart-attack phase had less incidence of a second event in the twelve months following their heart attack.

 ### Take a Moment To . . .

Reflect on your experience with cardiovascular disease. Take twenty uninterrupted minutes to write about this experience as a way of exploring your thoughts, feelings, and emotions around your diagnosis and treatment as well as how this has affected your life goals. Reflect also on the impact of your illness on others around you. Consider the social supports available to you and describe them.

Writing about your experiences is a wonderfully effective way to explore difficult issues and put them behind you. This exercise is likely to bring up thoughts, feelings, and emotions. If you feel uncomfortable with that possibility, you may want to skip this exercise or postpone it until you feel comfortable with it.

If you choose to participate in this exercise, be sure to acknowledge and honor any feelings which emerge as you write. Talk about them with family, friends, or other patients. You may want to seek out a support group or counselor.

PUTTING IT ALL TOGETHER

Individuals attending our Cardiac Rehabilitation Program attend thirteen three-hour sessions, structured to teach all the skills you have been learning throughout *The Wellness Book*. In the first hour we do aerobic exercise together as a group, the goal being to attain a conditioning effect on the cardiovascular system and rid the body of physical tension. Patients have their heart rate and rhythm monitored. During the cool-down period, we teach body awareness through yoga, which reinforces the participants' ability to monitor their own symptoms and to guard carefully against overexertion. Yoga is followed by fifteen minutes of a sitting exercise to elicit the relaxation response.

After aerobic exercise, then quieting the body and the mind with yoga and eliciting the relaxation response, we do an exercise in affirmations based on the principles explained in chapter 13, "Coping and Problem-Solving." Patients are asked to make a positive statement starting with "I am." Patients typically begin with very concrete affirmations such as "I am exercising four times a week, eliciting the relaxation response each day, and eating a healthy diet." Over the weeks, their affirmations become reflective of broader life goals such as "I am relaxed," "I am bringing a balance to my life," or perhaps "I am happy and satisfied with my life." In many ways, the evolution of their affirmations bears witness to the change in their attitudes as they shift from a strict focus on extending the quantity of life toward attaining more richness and quality in their life.

Following the affirmations, we begin the lecture/discussion for the session. The topics follow a format similar to that presented in *The Wellness Book*: principles of heart disease, making a Health Commitment, the mind/body model for health, eliciting the relaxation response, exercise, heart-healthy nutrition (with emphasis on weight reduction, sodium restriction, and cholesterol reduction), cognitive restructuring, modifying coronary-prone behaviors, the healing power of humor, and adjusting to heart disease.

In addition to information and skills, patients generally gain a great deal from their interactions with one another. Sharing and mutual support are generous and facilitate the adjustment process necessary for successfully living with heart disease.

Harold's Experience

Harold, a forty-year-old lawyer, entered the Cardiac Rehabilitation Program eight weeks after suffering a mild heart attack. He recovered uneventfully without any further chest pain or complications. His cardiac catheterization showed blockages in two of the three major coronary arteries.

His cardiac risk factors included a strong family history and high cholesterol. His mother and father had high cholesterol, and both died from heart attacks—his mother at age fifty-seven, and his father at age sixty-three. Harold had been well throughout his life and considered himself a relatively healthy person. He exercised occasionally, ate moderately heart-healthy food, and attempted to keep his weight in a reasonable range. He had an active and busy professional life but currently was under great stress because he was up for a senior-partner position in his law firm. He lived with his wife and three teenage children in a local community and considered his family a source of joy and support, although he admitted to the "usual hassles of family life."

His explicit goals in entering the program were to return to his former exercise pattern, lose weight, decrease his cholesterol, learn to manage stress, and learn techniques to elicit the relaxation response.

As part of the process of entering the Cardiac Rehabilitation Program we ask patients to do the exercise introduced in chapter 2, identifying ten things that are important/meaningful/valuable to them. He came up with four: time with family, working, reading, and exercise. He expressed surprise that he could identify only four items and that one of them was work. Following this exercise, he added a new goal to his list: "To bring more balance into my life and to examine some of my Type A behaviors."

Another tool we use to open communication is to have patients draw a picture of themselves. The purpose is strictly to encourage dialogue and conversation, not to analyze the drawing. We tell them not to worry about how well they draw or what we will think, but to "just do it." The instructions are simple: draw a picture of yourself, if you have an illness draw in the illness, and if there is a treatment or cure, draw this in as well. This is Harold's picture of himself:

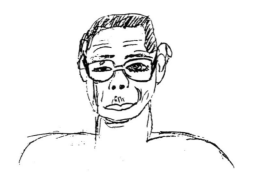

On the back he explained: "As you can see, I can't draw very well. The drawing was done in front of a mirror. Unlike having a broken leg, I don't see myself as ill. Physically I look fine, and feel fine. But inside, I'm not so good. My heart problem isn't a tangible illness, so it's difficult to believe. Very difficult." He expressed surprise at what he had drawn and described, and thus began a very helpful conversation. For the first time we were able to talk about some of his hidden fears and concerns. When asked during his history and physical about his fears, he had said only that he thought he was coping quite well with his illness. After the drawing exercise, he decided he had another goal to add to his Health Commitment, and that was to begin talking to others about his illness, as a way of making it more real to him and helping him adjust to this chronic condition more successfully.

Harold proceeded through the thirteen weeks of the program, embracing the opportunity to begin a regular exercise program and to eat a heart-healthy diet. He chose jogging as his exercise and ran three to five miles four times a week at a moderate pace. He did yoga stretches for his warm-up and cool-down. He followed a heart-healthy food plan that included limiting his intake of fat to less than 30 grams of fat per day. As the weeks went by, he began loosing weight and feeling healthier, and expressed surprise that he enjoyed what he was eating. He viewed his diet not in terms of what was off-limits, but in terms of what he could eat and enjoy. Day by day he was feeling pleased with how he was feeling and what he was accomplishing.

Over time, Harold found that his definition of "feeling healthy" had changed. He discovered that health is not simply the absence of illness, but rather encompassed a broad range of behaviors and feelings. Although he did not feel "ill" at the start of the program, as each week went by he felt better and more vigorous, and he recognized that the difference was quite apparent to him.

Through his weekly diary and participation in group discussions, he began to articulate a distinct difference in his way of handling stress. Now when he encountered stress, he was able to Stop and Take a Breath before becoming physically and mentally aroused. This left him better able to Reflect upon the stress and Choose the way in which he wanted to respond. He felt pleased about becoming less "Type A." He thought a great deal about how to cope with the stress of the impending senior-partner appointment. He decided to use both direct action (compiling the necessary documents) and reframing (viewing this as an opportunity to reflect back on how much he had accomplished over the last few years). These strategies, in combination with many minis, allowed him to feel less stress during the process. His affirmations evolved from "I am exercising, eating right, and trying to do the relaxation response" to "I feel healthy," and finally to "I look forward to the future with eagerness."

Harold had difficulty finding a method for eliciting the relaxation response. Being a "busy" person, he found it difficult to sit and just "do nothing." Although convinced it was important to his health, he could not fit this into his daily schedule. Over time, it became clear that the issue was not finding time (he found time to exercise and eat well) so much as his distaste for "doing nothing." We used physiological monitoring to show him the changes in his heart rate and blood pressure when he elicited the relaxation response, then worked to find a movement-oriented method of eliciting the relaxation response, by expanding on the yoga stretches which he used for his exercise routine. This combination of seeing the benefits for himself along with finding a technique which met his need to move helped him begin a practice he was able to sustain and benefit from.

Upon discharge from the program, Harold was delighted to find that in thirteen weeks he had lost twenty pounds, decreased his total cholesterol 85 points from 245 mg/dl to 160 mg/dl, decreased his LDL-cholesterol from 180 mg/dl to 107 mg/dl, and increased his exercise capacity by 15 percent. In addition to these objective measures, he commented on how well he felt. He had noticed feeling much more vigorous and was excited by his last affirmation, "I look forward to the future with enthusiasm." This affirmation was significant to him because previously, he was not at all sure that he had a future.

At discharge, Harold found it much easier to identify ten things that were important/meaningful/valuable to him, and was pleased that this time working was not second on his list. He felt his life was more balanced, with more time for family and self, that his career was going well, and that he was happier. When he drew his picture once again, he was surprised at how different it was from his first.

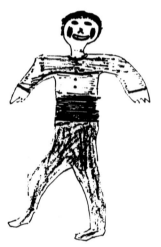

He immediately commented on the fact that he looked younger, happier, and healthier, with more color in his cheeks—although he still felt he couldn't draw. We noted he had drawn his whole body. He then described how much support he had gotten from the cardiac rehab process, and how he had come to terms with his illness by recognizing the opportunities his illness had opened up as well as the limitations it imposed upon him.

Hence, "I look forward to the future with eagerness." Harold still had coronary heart disease, but he was confident that he was doing all that he could to modify his cardiac risk factors and to live his life with meaning and purpose.

Eileen M. Stuart, R.N., M.S.
John P. Deckro, M.S., R.N.C.
Regis A. DeSilva, M.D.
Herbert Benson, M.D.

APPENDIX A
SMOKING CESSATION

To stop smoking, use this appendix in conjunction with the other behavioral changes we teach, including elicitation of the relaxation response, nutritional alterations, exercise, and cognitive restructuring. In this context of comprehensive, coordinated change, we have found the basic steps outlined in this appendix to be very useful and successful.

In 1983 Surgeon General C. Everett Koop sent a clear message to the public: Cigarette smoking is the single most preventable cause of death in the United States today. In addition to being a major risk factor for developing cardiovascular disease, smoking has also been indicted in developing the following conditions: cancer of the lung, bladder, and pancreas; bronchitis; emphysema; chronic obstructive pulmonary disease; and peripheral vascular disease. More recently, the role of passive smoke or the health risks of environmental tobacco smoke (ETS) have been studied. The Surgeon General's study concluded that the inhalation of passive smoke poses a health risk. If you smoke, the single most important thing that you can do to improve your health is to stop.

Deciding to quit

Knowing that you need to quit is only the first step. If knowledge alone was sufficient, you would never see a single nurse, physician, or other health-care provider smoking. The second step is recognizing that smoking is an addiction. Cigarettes contain chemicals, such as nicotine, that cause a physical addiction and craving for more tobacco. Nicotine acts immediately in the body to reduce pain and anxiety as well as to create a pleasurable state. In addition to the physical addiction of nicotine, smoking creates a web of behavioral addictions which must also be addressed by any program to stop smoking. Once you recognize smoking as a physical and behavioral addiction, you are better prepared to create a more realistic plan to help you successfully quit.

Start today

- Decide to quit!
- List as many reasons as you can to become a nonsmoker. Then list the advantages of continuing to smoke. Next, make the decision—do you want to quit? Making that decision yourself is important to success.
- Be careful about timing. A period of exceptionally high stress is usually not a good time to stop smoking. But don't postpone the decision indefinitely because stress is ever-present in your life. If need be, address the stress first—but keep the plan to stop smoking active in your mind.
- Consider your smoking pattern and behaviors. Write down how much you smoke, with whom, when, where, and why.

- Add up all the money you will save this year by stopping, and plan to reward yourself with a gift, or, alternatively, plan to donate this money to a cause of special interest to you.
- List the obstacles to stopping. Consider attempts you made in the past and why they were unsuccessful.
- List the supports for stopping.

Pick a date—and just do it!

- Between now and the quitting date:
  - Elicit the relaxation response each day.
  - Use positive imagery.
  - Gradually taper the number of cigarettes down to zero by the quitting date.
  - Switch brands each time you buy cigarettes.
  - Switch to a low-nicotine brand.
  - Exercise regularly.
  - Keep a piece of paper wrapped around your cigarette package to record each time you smoke one.
  - When you have a cigarette, do nothing else but smoke (this begins to disassociate smoking from common activities that you associate with smoking).

Quitting day:

- Celebrate!
- Be confident you can succeed.
- In addition to eliciting the relaxation response, use minis throughout the day whenever you have the urge.
- Ask friends and family not to offer you cigarettes nor to leave them around.
- Avoid smokers who may want you to continue.
- Get rid of all equipment associated with smoking: ashtrays, lighters, matches, cigarette boxes.
- Have low-calorie snacks around: carrot sticks, celery, fresh fruit.
- Chew gum.
- Drink plenty of water.
- Leave the table after meals and go brush your teeth.
- Increase your exercise each day.
- Be aware of high-risk situations: the second cup of coffee in the morning; after dinner; cocktails; on the telephone; driving in the car.
- Avoid the high-risk situations as much as possible at first and have distractions ready.
- Take up a new hobby to keep you distracted.

- Use your hands to knit, sew, do jigsaw puzzles, make models, use a toothpick.
- Have a support person to call on if you feel overwhelmed with the urge to smoke.
- Make a contract with a friend to donate a sizable sum of money to an organization you dislike if you start smoking again.
- Write down all the positive things you have noticed since stopping: increased taste, better smelling clothes and breath, more pocket money.

After you quit . . .

- Enjoy your success.
- Celebrate!
- Make plans to extend your success and prevent relapses. All of the information in chapters 2 and 24 can help you make a realistic plan to avoid relapsing.

The good news is that the physiological addiction to nicotine is largely gone after about a week. The first week can be difficult, but you can "ride out" the urges to smoke by routinely using some of the above steps: distractions, taking a deep breath, telling yourself NO and getting up and moving to another environment. Overcoming the behavioral addiction takes much longer, but using all our behavioral suggestions will help you be successful.

Gaining weight is a serious consideration for many people contemplating stopping smoking. Although many ex-smokers do gain from five to ten pounds when they stop, keep this in perspective. For weight gain to be as much a risk to your health as smoking, you would need to gain seventy pounds. You can also plan and work to counteract potential weight gain: eat plenty of low-calorie snacks such as carrots, plain bagels, and fresh fruit, drink more water, and increase your daily exercise.

Nicotine gum helps some individuals ease withdrawal symptoms as they stop smoking but should be used only with supervision of an experienced clinician. Others wishing to quit smoking find the support of a psychologist and/or the use of hypnosis to be extremely useful.

If you succeed in stopping, congratulate yourself and make plans to honor and acknowledge this accomplishment. If you fail on your first attempt, however, don't feel bad or guilty: quitting tobacco is very difficult. Most people who quit smoking successfully do so only after several attempts. Think of the attempt as a practice run, and write down the valuable things you have learned: when the urges to smoke were worst, what situations were most tempting, which low-calorie snacks you liked best. Incorporate what was successful for you, adjust your plan to meet the problem areas, and pick another date to stop.

Many people find the support of a group helpful in making a major lifestyle change such as giving up smoking. Hospitals sponsor smoking-cessation groups as do local branches of the American Lung Association, the American Heart Association, and the American Cancer Society. The telephone numbers of these organizations are in your local telephone directories.

Other Resources

A Lifetime of Freedom from Smoking. American Lung Association.
I Quit Kit. A Self-help Smoking Program from the American Cancer Society.
Help a Friend to Stop Smoking. American Lung Association.
Freedom from Smoking in 20 Days. American Lung Association.

HEALTH COMMITMENT

Long-Term Goal:

_____

_____

_____
Signature

_____
Witness

Expected Date of Reaching Goal: _____

Short-Term Goals	Comments (supports, rewards, etc.)

CHAPTER 22

LIVING WITH HEART DISEASE AND DIABETES: EXERCISE CAN HELP

> Health is the vital principle of bliss, and exercise, of health.
>
> James Thomson, *The Castle of Indolence*

In this chapter you will explore

- the role of exercise in living with heart disease and diabetes
- the risks and benefits of exercise for this population
- the guidelines and parameters for a safe and beneficial exercise program
- how to make sound decisions in managing an active lifestyle while living with disease
- how to take responsibility for maximizing your health through an active lifestyle

As discussed in chapter 7, "Move Into Health," an active lifestyle is important in promoting and maintaining health. The list of benefits is long: exercise can help you strengthen your cardiovascular system, lose body fat, control blood sugar, and increase strength, flexibility, and endurance. It can increase self-esteem and a sense of well-being as well as decrease stress. Through exercise you can maintain more of your youthful exuberance and function as you age gracefully.

Chapter 7 also described some of the principles involved in developing an exercise program, such as motivation, safety, and FITT: how often (F), how hard (I), how long you should exercise (T), and what type of exercise is most beneficial for you (T).

Do the benefits of exercise apply if you already have heart disease or some other metabolic dysfunction? What if you have had a heart attack, open-heart surgery, or you have had a balloon procedure to open up closed heart blood vessels? What if you are at risk for developing heart disease? Is exercise still beneficial? Is it safe for you to exercise? Is it possible to improve your ability to exercise and increase your level of physical fitness? The answer to all of these questions is yes.

HEART DISEASE

Modify your risk

Heart disease is by far the major cause of death in the United States. One risk factor for developing heart disease is a sedentary lifestyle, and that risk can be decreased by increasing activity and fitness. People who are more physically fit tend to live longer than those less fit. In addition, exercise can help modify other cardiovascular risk factors such as elevated blood pressure, high cholesterol levels, and obesity. Numerous studies have shown that regular physical activity can help lower the resting blood pressure of people with high blood pressure. Exercise can improve your cholesterol profile by increasing the HDL ("good") cholesterol and reducing the ratio of total cholesterol to HDL cholesterol. In addition, recent work by Dr. Steven Blair and co-workers at the Institute for Aerobics Research in Dallas, indicates that physically fit individuals with high blood pressure and cholesterol have a lower risk of cardiac death than unfit individuals with low blood pressure or cholesterol.

The most effective way to lose fat is to combine exercise with nutritious eating. You can lose weight simply by dieting, but often that weight includes muscle and water weight as well as fat, and further, you will tend to gain the weight back rather quickly. Exercise will help you burn fat and keep you from regaining the fat. By adding exercise to your life, you have some control over the risk factors that may lead to heart disease.

Medical supervision

Do you have a history of high blood pressure or elevated cholesterol? Do you smoke? Has anyone in your family had a heart attack at an early age? Have you been sedentary for the past couple of years? Do you have diabetes? If you answer yes to any of these questions related to risk factors for developing heart disease, it is recommended you have a complete medical evaluation, including an exercise-tolerance test, by your physician before starting your exercise program. The results of the exercise-tolerance test can be used to help diagnose any existing heart disease and establish an exercise prescription that will maximize your training effect and minimize your risk of injury.

If you have only one risk factor in your history, medical clearance may be all you need before starting an exercise program, provided you start a low level and progress slowly. However, if you have known heart disease or any other disease, or if you have multiple risk factors, begin your exercise program under the supervision of a health-care professional who specializes in exercise rehabilitation. Many hospitals and health-care facilities have programs for cardiac, pulmonary, and diabetic rehabilitation. Other programs include multiple-risk-reduction programs such as our Hypertension Clinic. The best way to determine which program is most appropriate for you is to discuss your status with your physician and investigate programs in your geographical area.

Take a Moment To . . .

Check the conditions that apply to you.

Have you been told you have
    heart problems? ____
    serious medical problems? ____
    high blood pressure? ____
    high cholesterol? ____
    diabetes? ____
    a weight problem? ____
Do you smoke? ____
Have you not exercised regularly for the past few years? ____
If you checked any of these, you should talk to your physician before
    starting an exercise program.

Benefits of exercise

Keep the faculty of effort alive in you, by a little gratuitous exercise every day.

William James, *The Principles of Psychology*

Regular aerobic physical activity has been found to play a role both in preventing the onset of heart disease and controlling its negative effects once the disease has started.

Dr. Neil Oldridge, a well-known physician-researcher in the field of exercise, analyzed ten major studies involving over four thousand heart attack patients. He found that the patients who participated in cardiac rehabilitation exercise programs had 25 percent fewer deaths from coronary artery disease. No wonder increasing physical activity is recommended for people with heart disease!

We know that exercise can improve the function of your heart and the efficiency of your cardiovascular system. When you tune up a car, the result is better performance and more miles to the gallon; similarly, when you tune up your body with exercise, it performs better, which allows you to do more work with less energy expenditure. More specifically, exercise improves your heart's ability to pump blood to your working muscles as well as your muscles' ability to extract and make use of oxygen from your blood. It works. There are people who have had heart attacks or open-heart surgery who are now running marathons. People who thought they would never be able to return to work have done so, and walk three miles a day in addition to their job. Of course, not everyone wants to run a marathon, but you can achieve your maximum desired functional capabilities and improve the quality of your life, even with the threat of risk factors and documented disease. Add to this the knowledge that exercise can help modify existing risk factors, and it becomes evident that an active lifestyle is important in preventing disease as well as living with disease.

Jack and Jill's Experience

Jack and Jill found it more and more difficult to go up the hill to fetch water. In real life they are a professional couple in their late fifties who experienced cardiovascular disease. Jack was having chest pains because of blockages in three of his coronary arteries and subsequently underwent open-heart surgery. Jill had high blood pressure and disliked the side effects of three medications she was taking. Jack entered our Cardiac Rehabilitation Program, and Jill enrolled in our Hypertension Clinic. Each took an exercise-tolerance test prior to starting the exercise component of the programs. An exercise-heart-rate range was prescribed for each, and supervision in their respective programs helped them gain confidence about judging their exertion levels.

Both were highly motivated to make changes in their lives, and their compliance produced significant results. They found they enjoyed walking, and they incorporated four to five long walks into their weekly schedule, which proved to be a great stress release from the demands of their professional lives. Due to busy work schedules, coordinating times was difficult, so each would walk alone during the week, and on weekends they would walk together. Because his exercise-walk pace was normally faster than Jill's, Jack would slow down when with her and use hand weights to help raise his heart rate to his exercise target. This allowed them to both benefit from the walk and enjoy the time together.

By the end of their three-month clinic programs, both noted significant changes. Both markedly improved their exercise capacity; they could do more work with less effort. Jack lost ten pounds and Jill lost eighteen. Jill also showed great improvement in her cholesterol profile; Jack's stayed about the same. Finally, Jill was able to stop using two of her high-blood-pressure medications, reduce the third by half, and still lower her blood pressure from 153/96 to 128/86 mm Hg. Through exercise, healthy nutrition, and stress management they were able to change their risk profiles, as well as improve their health and the quality of their lives.

Take a Moment To . . .

Review this case history and list the risk factors that were changed in part by regular physical activity.

_____

_____

_____

YOUR EXERCISE PRESCRIPTION FOR A HEALTHY HEART

Before starting an exercise program, consult with your physician as well as your exercise specialist. The long-term success of your prescription is dependent on both objective evaluation information and your subjective input. You will be doing the exercise, so it is important for the prescription to reflect your medical condition along with your personal needs, interests, and goals.

If you have heart disease and the exercise program is new for you, or if your condition has changed such that it requires medical attention, initial supervision in the progression of your exercise is recommended. Once you demonstrate an ability to exercise safely and your condition is stable, you can continue your program on your own.

Frequency

Your exercise prescription should indicate how often, how hard, and how long you exercise, as well as the type of activity you will do. Remember FITT on page 122 from chapter 7. To gain any significant cardiovascular benefit, you need to exercise at a frequency (F) of three times a week. If weight loss is a goal, you will be more successful if you exercise four to five times a week. This will help increase the number of calories you burn off and speed up the weight-loss process. However, this does not give you license to be a "couch potato" the rest of the week. Think of ways you can be active every day; every little bit helps.

Intensity

The most effective way to determine the proper exercise intensity (I) is to match your calculated exercise heart rate (based on the results of your exercise-tolerance test) with your perception of how hard you are working. Also be aware of signs and symptoms of exercise intolerance. These self-monitoring techniques provide safety cues while you exercise.

Your target heart rate—the objective measure of intensity—is based on your exercise capacity. Most individuals with heart disease can safely begin exercise at an intensity of 60-to-70 percent of maximal heart rate, as determined by an exercise-tolerance test. If the test indicates a very low exercise capacity, you might start with a heart rate of 50-to-60 percent of maximum. On the other hand, with a high exercise capacity, you could probably exercise within 60-to-80 percent of your maximal heart rate. To determine your exercise heart rate, your exercise specialist would use the formula given in chapter 7, but instead of using a general maximal heart rate (220 − age) your true maximal heart rate from the exercise-tolerance test would be used.

(maximal heart rate − resting heart rate) × % + resting heart rate = exercise heart rate

Example:

Maximal heart rate from exercise test is 160
Resting heart rate is 80 beats per minute
Intensity is 60-to-70 percent of maximum capacity

A. Subtract resting heart from maximal heart rate.

$$160 - 80 = 80$$

B. Multiply the number from Step A times both 60% (.60) and 70% (.70).

$$80 \times .60 = 48$$
$$80 \times .70 = 56$$

C. Add the numbers from Step B to resting heart rate.

$$80 + 48 = 128$$
$$80 + 56 = 136$$

The exercise heart rate range is 128 to 136 beats per minute. To check if you are within this range, stop exercising and count your pulse at your wrist or neck for 15 seconds; multiply that number by 4, giving you beats per minute.

Example:

Your pulse for the 15-second count is 33

$$33 \times 4 = 132 \text{ beats per minute}$$

This means that as you exercise, your heart rate increases to 132 beats per minute, well within the target rate of 128 to 136.

Remember, these are only guidelines. What matters most is your comfort level. Your perception of how hard you are working will indicate your need to work a little harder, stay at the comfortable challenge level, or decrease the intensity.

Your perception of how hard you are working is the subjective measure of intensity. When exercising, you want to be comfortable, yet moderately challenged. Pay attention to your breathing. You should notice a change in your breathing from rest, but you should be able to talk freely. You may feel some discomfort in the muscles you are exercising, and you may feel pleasantly fatigued. However, you should not feel pain in your muscles, nor feel an urgent need to stop the exercise. If you do, then you are working too hard.

The Borg Scale of perceived exertion, which you will recognize from chapter 7, gives a framework by which you can judge your exertion.

Borg Scale (RPT)
6
7   very, very light
8
9   very light
10
11   fairly light
12
13   somewhat hard (moderate)
14
15   hard
16
17   very hard
18
19   very, very hard
20

Adapted from G. A. V. Borg, "Psychophysical Bases of Perceived Exertion," *Medicine and Science in Sports and Medicine* 14, no. 5 (1982): 377–81.

For patients with heart disease, a perceived exertion of 11 to 13 is recommended. As you can see, the shaded area is a little wider than in the original diagram on page 000, allowing you to feel slightly less exertion. This accommodates people who may have more disease or are on more medication, and have less tolerance for exercise.

Exercising with moderate intensity will allow you to be comfortable with the activity and increase confidence in your ability to exercise. At the same time it will improve your ability to do work and decrease the exertion of your heart. It is the law of supply and demand: the purpose of training is to improve your cardiovascular system's ability to efficiently supply oxygen for your body's demands. Thus, your ability to exercise and perform daily activities becomes easier.

An awareness of your tolerance for activity is important. Not only do you need to recognize when you are working hard enough, you also need to be aware of the signs and symptoms of overexertion or intolerance of exercise, when demand exceeds supply and you are working too hard. The following are cues for overexertion: angina pectoris, which may present as chest pain, jaw pain, pain down the arms, or pain between the shoulder blades; severe shortness of breath, light-headedness, or dizziness; queasy stomach; cold, clammy feelings. If you experience any of these sensations when exercising, stop and rest. Take a nitroglycerin tablet, if this has been prescribed. If the sensations persist, call a physician. Discuss the occurrence of these symptoms with your physician or exercise specialist; your exercise prescription may need to be readjusted. The simplest way to prevent these symptoms is not to overexert yourself. For everyone, but especially people with any illness, it is important to listen to your body. Body awareness, as discussed in chapter 6, "Tuning In to Your Body, Tuning Up Your Mind," allows you to appreciate how you feel and how you react to activity. Staying active is important, but too much is simply too much.

Many people with angina pectoris take nitroglycerin tablets either before exercise to prevent chest pain or to relieve chest pain once it starts. It supplies more oxygen to the heart by dilating blood vessels of the body and heart. Be sure to discuss the use of nitroglycerin with your physician before using it, and follow his or her recommendations on achieving the best results.

Take a Moment To . . .

List the most important self-monitoring techniques during exercise, and note why they are important for your success and safety.

_____

_____

_____

_____

Time

The duration of your exercise (T, time) can vary and depends on the intensity. To gain significant cardiovascular benefits, plan to exercise aerobically for at least twenty minutes. If weight loss is a goal, thirty to forty-five minutes will produce better results. However, as mentioned before, all activity counts toward the total benefit, so if you have ten minutes to walk at lunchtime, do it. If the day is beautiful and you want to walk with a friend, slow down your normal exercise-walk pace (decrease the intensity) and enjoy the company and scenery for an hour or so (increase the duration). The more active you are throughout the week, the more fit you will be. So, plan at least three good exercise sessions each week for at least twenty to thirty minutes. Make that the core of your exercise plan and add in a variety of activities that are fun and keep you moving throughout the week.

Type

Your exercise prescription will indicate the type (T) of activity which will benefit you most. Remember, it is your prescription, so the activity should be something you want to do and have the resources and opportunity to do. The goal is to create an active lifestyle that is comfortable, enjoyable, and challenging. Aerobic exercise should make up the largest percentage of your total activity plan. As discussed in chapter 7, some aerobic choices are:

> Brisk walking, jogging, cycling (in and outdoors), rowing, swimming, cross-country skiing, stair climbing, aerobics (high and low impact), dancing

The other component of your program should include some gentle strengthening and flexibility exercises. For well-balanced fitness, calisthenics, yoga, and circuit training can be added to your aerobic exercise to improve your strength, flexibility, and endurance.

Guidelines for daily activities are also part of your exercise prescription. Every activity you do throughout the day involves a certain level of effort which can be translated into an amount of oxygen your body needs to provide the energy necessary to do that task. When you are at rest, the energy expenditure is one Metabolic Equivalent (MET) of energy. The MET level of any activity is determined by how much more energy is needed to conduct the activity than is needed at rest. For example, cleaning windows or walking three miles an hour are three to four METs, light carpentry or playing doubles tennis are four to five METs, housework is three to six METs, and bicycling ten miles an hour is five to six METs. Based on your exercise-test performance, your MET capacity can be determined, and guidelines for your daily activities can be provided in much the same way as your prescribed exercise heart rate. Within this framework you will know which tasks are safe and reasonable for you.

Regular physical exercise can improve your MET capacity. This may have significance for increasing your independence or going back to work after a heart attack. If your job requires you to do physical activity at a seven-MET level, but your exercise test indicates you can perform only at a five-to-six-MET level, you probably cannot return to that job. However, regular exercise may improve your exercise capacity from six to seven METs and allow you to resume your old job. Not only does exercise have direct health benefits, but it can also help you maintain or achieve a preferred level of vocational and leisure-time activity.

Warm-up and cool-down

Warm-up and cool-down are important exercise components, especially for people with heart disease. During your warm-up, the intensity of your exercise needs to increase slowly to allow your heart and cardiovascular system the necessary time to adjust and help supply the blood and oxygen your body needs. Even a heart that has suffered injury and vessels that are partially blocked or have lost elasticity have the capacity to accommodate to the demands of exercise, but sudden demands are not handled well. A slow increase in intensity is the best way to allow systems with compromised function to handle the demands of exercise.

Your cool-down is as important as your warm-up. Exercise gets your body's systems operating at high gear. If exercise is stopped abruptly, the balance of supply and demand is upset and you are at risk for injury. When your exercise is over, keep moving at a slower pace to allow your body time to settle back down to baseline. In our clinic programs, we have found that the end of your cool-down period is an excellent time to do yoga stretches and elicit the relaxation response.

Warm-up and cool-down are also important for your musculoskeletal system. Muscles that are comfortably stretched and flexible work more efficiently with less chance of injury. To stretch again during cool-down is advantageous because muscles often tighten with exercise. Stretching will keep

Parameters for a Healthy and Effective Exercise Program

Frequency: Three to five times per week.

Intensity: Moderate by heart rate and perceived exertion. If you have a low fitness level, start below moderate. Do what feels comfortable and work your way up to a moderate level.

Time: Twenty to thirty minutes, plus five to ten minutes each of warm-up and cool-down is a good place to start. Again, if you have a low fitness level, you may need to start with ten to fifteen minutes. Gradually increase your duration, then your intensity.

Type: Aerobic exercise is recommended as the major component of your program. However, light calisthenics and muscle toning for strength and flexibility are also important for overall conditioning. Yoga is excellent for gaining body awareness.

Anaerobic exercise such as heavy weight lifting or sprinting is not recommended for most people with heart disease. The quick rise in heart rate and blood pressure may place undue demand on your heart.

Circuit training combines both aerobic and anaerobic exercise. It has been judged safe for individuals with heart disease if done at a moderate intensity (20-to-40 percent of maximal weight lifting capacity). A program of eight to ten different exercises, eight to twelve repetitions each, will tone the major muscle groups and is a good place to start.

Take a Moment To . . .

F _____

I _____

T _____

T _____

Indicate the parameter each letter stands for, and create an exercise prescription that would be realistic for you.

EXERCISE PROGRESSION

Once your prescription is established, you feel comfortable with the exercise instructions, demonstrate an awareness of your exertion level, and your medical condition is stable, then you are encouraged to exercise independently. Progress gradually as exercise capacity improves. We do, however, recommend that you communicate with your physician regularly as your program continues, and be sure to report any signs of intolerance.

How far you can progress with your physical activity is dependent on the severity of your disease as well as your motivational level. What is important is for you to reach your maximal potential. For some that may mean having the endurance to do housework without developing chest pain; for others, being able to walk thirty minutes without becoming short of breath; and for still others, being able to run a marathon. Everyone is different, with different disabilities and potentials. The goal is to be as active as you can be and to achieve the most you can within the limits of your physical abilities.

FEAR AND DEPRESSION

After a heart attack, patients frequently talk about fear and depression. Initially they may feel fear: fear of being a "cardiac cripple," fear of doing too much, fear of having another heart attack, fear of dying. Later patients often express feelings of helplessness and hopelessness as they grieve for their former lifestyle. Facing a crisis in your life is not easy. After acknowledging these emotions and taking time to verbalize them, the key to moving on is to focus on what you can do and not what you think you cannot do. Entering a cardiac rehabilitation program and starting an exercise program are excellent ways to begin to distance yourself from these negative feelings and to make

THE FAR SIDE By GARY LARSON

THE FAR SIDE © 1987. Reprinted by permission of Chronicle Features, San Francisco, Calif.

positive changes in your lifestyle. Exercise will give you confidence in what you can do and improve your self-esteem and outlook on the future. For many people, being diagnosed with heart disease, or acknowledging the presence of a risk factor, is viewed as a second chance. It forces them to realize that they need to make changes, and in making these changes, they often feel better than they have in years, with greater energy and a renewed interest in the future.

Cap's Experience

Cap, a sixty-eight-year-old insurance broker, had a history of cardiovascular disease, including a heart attack followed several months later by the development of angina (ischemia) when he exercised. His physician decided to manage the ischemia with medication and his participation in a cardiac rehabilitation program.

Cap entered our clinic program fearful that any exercise would prompt another heart attack. His exercise tolerance test indicated that he could safely exercise at a heart rate of 85-to-90 beats per minute and do daily activities with a five-to-six MET level—for example, light carpentry, housework including vacuuming, gardening, raking leaves, fishing, walking up to 4 mph, and bicycling up to 10 mph. Under supervision in the clinic, he became more comfortable exercising and could tolerate twenty minutes on the stationary bicycle at a moderate exertion level, within his target heart rate of 85-to-90. He learned to become aware of any symptoms, to listen to his body, and to adjust his exercise intensity according to the messages received from his body. On his own, he only felt comfortable, at first, walking the distance from his office to the ferry terminal, which took fifteen minutes at a slow pace. (During the summer he lives at the beach and takes the ferry into the city for work.) As his confidence and exercise capacity increased, and his symptoms waned, he was able to increase his bicycle time in the clinic to thirty minutes. He gradually extended his route to accommodate a thirty minute, brisk walk to catch the ferry home from work. On weekends, he now takes thirty to forty-five minute walks with his wife on the beach. He feels good about his progress, no longer fears and anticipates the onset of pain, and enjoys what he is doing.

DIABETES

Diabetes is a chronic disease that affects large numbers of people at all social levels. If not properly treated, it can be life-threatening. It can increase risk of cardiovascular disease (diabetics are twice as likely to have a heart attack than are nondiabetics), damage the nervous system, and damage vital body organs such as the kidneys and eyes. Diabetics are generally diagnosed as either non-insulin dependent or insulin dependent. Non-insulin-dependent diabetics are resistant to insulin and have impaired insulin secretion. This diagnosis accounts for more than 80 percent of all diabetics and is strongly associated with obesity. Insulin-dependent diabetes accounts for 5-to-10 percent of all diabetic cases and involves a deficiency of insulin due to the destruction of the cells in the pancreas that make insulin.

The goal of treatment for all diabetics is to maintain normal blood-glucose (sugar) levels. For diabetics with non-insulin-dependent diabetes, this can often be done with diet control and exercise, but they may require the assistance of oral medications. Insulin resistance is closely tied to obesity, and often the diabetes can be controlled without medications if regular physical activity is combined with a weight-loss diet. Not only is exercise part of the treatment regime but exciting new research by public health epidemiologist Susan P. Helmrich, Ph.D., and coworkers, suggests that an increase in physical activity is effective in the *prevention* of non-insulin-dependent diabetes. In contrast, people with insulin-dependent diabetes need regular insulin injections in addition to diet management to control their glucose levels. Whereas exercise is strongly recommended in the treatment of non-insulin-dependent diabetes, the risks and benefits of exercise are in delicate balance if you have insulin-dependent diabetes.

Over time, diabetes causes changes in small blood vessels that impair good circulation. Because of this, diabetics do not have the cardiovascular potential to achieve the exercise performance levels of nondiabetics. Diabetics tend to have a lower maximal heart rate and a greater chance of developing high blood pressure. However, exercise capacity can improve with training, and diabetics can experience benefits related to overall fitness and training.

Some of the major benefits of exercise for a person with diabetes include:

- Improved use of blood sugar
- Improved use of insulin
- Decreased risk factors for heart diseases
- Decreased blood pressure
- Improved weight loss and control

Insulin-dependent diabetics can realize many of the benefits of exercise. Exercise lowers blood sugar and can be used to help reduce insulin needs, although most studies indicate that it does very little to improve long-term glucose control. Some recent evidence, however, suggests that if food consumption is controlled (no extra food on exercise days), long-term blood sugar control improves despite lowered daily insulin doses. However, the inherent behavior and function of injected insulin makes exercising more complicated. The major function of insulin is to promote glucose uptake into the body's cells. During exercise, a nondiabetic's insulin secretion decreases slightly and the concentration of the counterregulatory hormones increases. This stimulates the liver to release more glucose into the bloodstream as the muscles use the glucose as fuel to keep working. Throughout the process, normal glucose levels are maintained.

With injected insulin, however, this does not occur. Insulin levels cannot decrease with exercise and the liver is not stimulated into releasing more glucose. Meanwhile, the muscle cells continue to use the glucose they need, and blood glucose levels decrease. If the decrease is too great the result is *hypoglycemia*, a potentially dangerous situation that, left untreated, could result in a diabetic reaction or seizure. Another potential problem is *hyperglycemia*, or excess sugar in the blood, which can occur when diabetes is poorly controlled, for example, by not taking enough insulin. When insulin is insufficient to assist glucose movement into the cells, glucose remains in the blood. During exercise, the liver is stimulated to release more glucose into the blood and the blood-sugar level rises, worsening the condition. The production of toxic ketone bodies may result, a serious situation that requires medical attention.

To prevent either condition, insulin-dependent diabetics must monitor their blood sugar closely and adjust their food intake and insulin doses before and after exercise.

If you have non-insulin-dependent diabetes and use an oral agent, or perhaps even insulin, to help control your glucose levels, you must also be aware of these potential problems. However, the situation for you is not quite as complicated. Because you are still producing some insulin, exercise will have less impact on the stability of your blood-glucose levels.

Due to the microvascular changes that occur with diabetes, risk increases, as we noted, for developing cardiovascular disease as well as diseases of the eyes, kidneys, and nerves. In addition, over time, muscles and joints show signs of decreased flexibility and mobility. These conditions increase risks with exercise for those with diabetes, and therefore, a full medical and cardiac workup should be done prior to starting an exercise program. If you have been sedentary, are over thirty-five years of age, and/or have had diabetes for more than ten years, you should also have an exercise-tolerance test to rule out any heart disease that might limit your exercise potential. Then, once your exercise prescription has been determined, you can work toward attaining the benefits of a reasonable exercise program. Weighing the risks and benefits, the overall goals regarding exercise for diabetics are to:

1. incorporate activity into daily life
2. pursue an exercise program geared to your medical condition
3. exercise wisely to avoid possible complications

Do not be discouraged by the many potential problems that diabetics face when considering a regular exercise program. Once the screening process is complete and you learn to adjust your medications and diet to accommodate the increased activity, you should be able to enjoy exercise as much as anyone else. Take the time to set up your program to avoid the risks, and you will be free to experience all the healthful benefits of an active lifestyle. According to Marion Franz, R.D., M.S.,

> For most persons with insulin dependent diabetes mellitus, the cardio-vascular and psychological benefits of regular exercise *far exceed* the risks.

The key to changing your activity/exercise patterns safely is frequent blood-sugar monitoring. The only way to know how you respond to an increase in activity is to check your blood-sugar level. This should be done before you exercise, twenty to thirty minutes after you exercise, and frequently throughout the day to rule out any *lag* effect. The lag effect occurs when your muscles and liver continue to remove glucose from the blood to replenish the stores depleted during exercise. This can occur for twenty-four to forty-eight hours after exercise.

Take a Moment To . . .

Reflect on your blood-sugar measurements and how they fluctuate with exercise, activity, stress, and food. Write down your range of measurements.

_____

_____

_____

_____

EXERCISING WITH DIABETES

While blood-sugar monitoring is important, you also need to be familiar with the signs and symptoms of a hypoglycemic reaction: light-headedness, fatigue, cold sweat, tremor, double vision, skin pallor, irritability, confusion, and hunger. Most diabetics already know this information, but we want to be explicit for those who might not. Each person experiences a reaction differently, and you must be able to recognize what it feels like to you when your blood sugar is too low. If you feel a reaction coming on, stop your activity, take some quick-acting carbohydrate—fruit juice works well—and rest until you feel the symptoms resolve. If possible check your blood-sugar level to determine if it is back to normal.

If you are adding only low-level activity to your usual day, no change in your diabetes management may be necessary; checking your blood sugar will confirm this. However, if you are significantly changing your existing routine, you will be most successful if you seek assistance for your insulin and diet adjustments. Depending on the time of day you exercise, the intensity and duration of the exercise, and your blood-sugar level at the time of exercise, you may want to adjust your insulin dosages or plan to eat extra carbohydrate. Blood testing before and after exercise is the only way to know accurately how you react to physical activity and what adjustments you need to make. Working with your diabetes-management team is the best way to make the proper adjustments while adding exercise to your daily life.

Parameters for an Exercise Prescription

Frequency: At least three to five times per week; the more consistent your exercise on a day-to-day basis, the easier it will be to manage your insulin and food adjustments to keep your blood sugar more stable. Doing some exercise at the same time every day is the ideal situation for blood sugar control, but increased frequency also increases the chances for injury. Pay close attention to what your body tells you.

Intensity: Moderate by heart rate and perceived exertion. If you have a low fitness level, start at an intensity level that feels comfortable and work your way up to moderate. Twenty to thirty minutes will improve cardiovascular fitness and is a good place to start. Don't forget to add five to ten minutes each for warm-up and cool-down. If you have a low fitness level, limit initial workouts to ten to fifteen minutes, gradually increase the duration, then consider increasing intensity.

If possible, exercise after meals or snacks to improve your blood-sugar response to food.

Avoid exercising at the peak time of insulin action (be sure you know the peak action times of *your* insulin types). Eat additional carbohydrate if you exercise at your peak to offset the exercise/insulin interaction.

Type: Aerobic exercise is best for cardiovascular benefits and blood-sugar control. If you exercise frequently, cross-training will help prevent injury and relieve boredom as well as result in more total body fitness. Avoid anaerobic exercise such as strenuous calisthenics and high-intensity weight lifting. This can cause sharp increases in blood pressure and has little benefit for glucose control. However, moderate muscle toning, as mentioned in the section on heart disease, is acceptable and beneficial for strength and flexibility.

Avoid high-impact activities such as jumping and running if you are prone to neuropathy in your legs and feet or you have a history of eye disease.

Don't be discouraged by all the potential risks and restrictions associated with exercise. For those of you who have been inactive, simply increasing your walking and adding healthy pleasures to your everyday life—for example, gardening, climbing stairs, hobbies, casual bicycling—is a great way to increase your activity and begin to improve your health.

Here are some further recommendations to keep in mind as you develop your exercise plan:

- Notify your physician, ophthalmologist, and podiatrist of your intent to begin an exercise program in order to get medical clearance and for them to identify any of your specific problems.
- Be familiar with the general management of diabetes as well as the interaction of diet, exercise, and insulin. A dietician and exercise specialist familiar with diabetes management can be of valuable assistance.
- With your physician, consider reducing insulin dosages before exercise—adjustments are based on type of insulin, time of day, as well as duration and intensity of exercise.

- If you have a history of eye or kidney disease, keep your blood pressure below 180-to-200 mm Hg during exercise, and keep your exercise intensity moderate.
- Use proper footwear and inspect feet frequently to prevent potential ulcers, breakdowns, and infections. If you have peripheral neuropathy, this is crucial.
- Be sure blood sugars are consistently under 250-to-300 mg/dl and your urine tests are negative for ketones.
- Monitor your blood sugars before, twenty to thirty minutes after exercise, and frequently throughout the day to rule out the lag effect.
- Avoid injecting insulin into a muscle area that will be exercised within the next thirty minutes. Exercising injected muscle will heighten the insulin effect and increase risk of hypoglycemia.
- The overweight non-insulin-dependent diabetic should not snack. Adjustments for exercise should involve monitored manipulation of oral medications or insulin.
- Carry a fast-acting carbohydrate with you whenever you exercise, such as fruit, hard candy, jelly beans, or gum drops in case hypoglycemia develops.
- Wear some form of diabetes identification.

Be familiar with your diabetes management and how your blood sugar responds to different stimuli before starting an exercise program. Once you are comfortable with yourself and the adjustments you need, then exercise can be as beneficial and as much fun for you as for anyone else. Take the time to learn how to manage your diabetes and continue your progress toward a life in which you have more control over your health and active pleasures.

 Max's Experience

Max, a fifty-six-year-old retired policeman with heart disease and diabetes, has been insulin-dependent for fifteen years and has had a heart attack, followed by open-heart surgery. When he entered our Cardiac Rehabilitation Program, he weighed 233 pounds, was taking 5 units of regular and 30 units of NPH insulin, and could ride a bicycle for about 20 minutes before complaining of claudication pain (caused by poor circulation) in his right leg. As Max began to increase his exercise, he needed to be able to monitor not only his cardiac tolerance, but also his blood-sugar response to the increase in activity.

We had Max keep a weekly exercise diary, like the one at the end of this chapter, so he could self-monitor his tolerance and progress and provide us with data so we could help guide him with his progress. Max lost weight, decreased his insulin requirement, and increased his exercise tolerance. He remained compliant with regular exercise, and was able to decrease his insulin dosage significantly, as his weight decreased and his blood sugar remained stable.

Observe Max's progress at comparative points in the program.

	WEEK 1	WEEK 7	WEEK 13
Blood sugar	140-170	120-170	125-150
Weight	233 lbs.	223 lbs.	213 lbs.
# units insulin	30 units NPH	16 units NPH	12 units NPH
	5 units regular	2 units regular	

This is significant improvement! One month after completing the program, Max had lost a total of 36 pounds, was taking only 10 units of NPH insulin, was still riding his bicycle 5 times per week for 30 to 45 minutes with no leg pain, was checking the nutrition labels on food products, and had a smile on his face. He felt he had made some meaningful changes and was feeling wonderful.

Max' story illustrates that individuals with heart disease and diabetes can improve their health profiles. Part of that change involves an active lifestyle and regular physical activity. It is true that increased risk is associated with these diseases, and exercise can potentiate that risk. However, with education and individualized prescription parameters, exercise can be safe, healthy, and beneficial. Try keeping an exercise diary similar to Max's. A diary will help you chart your own progress and monitor your tolerance, information valuable to your health-care team for adjusting your exercise practice and health care. You need not be free of disease to begin an exercise program; in fact, exercise can help you live better with that disease. Regular exercise does not guarantee a longer life, but it will help you feel better, do better, and look better, and it will effectively improve the quality of your life.

James S. Huddleston, M.S., P.T.

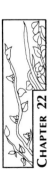

CHAPTER 22

EXERCISE DIARY

Name: _____

Date: _____

Blood sugar today is: _____
Blood pressure today is: _____
Pulse rate today is: _____

Weight: _____

	BASELINE DATA			EXERCISE							INSULIN			
											AM		PM	
Day	Wt	Pre/Post-BS	RHR	Time	Type	Duration	PHR	RPE	Symptoms		Type	Units	Type	Units
M														
TU														
W														
TH														
F														
SA														
SU														

Wt = weight
Pre/Post BS = pre-and-post-exercise blood sugar
RHR = resting heart rate
PHR = peak heart rate
RPE = rate of perceived exertion

Symptoms = fatigue, chest pain, angina, light-headedness,
dizziness, feeling faint, clammy, etc.
AM = morning
PM = evening

HEALTH COMMITMENT

Long-Term Goal: _____

_____

_____

Signature

_____

Witness

Expected Date of Reaching Goal: _____

Short-Term Goals	Comments (supports, rewards, etc.)

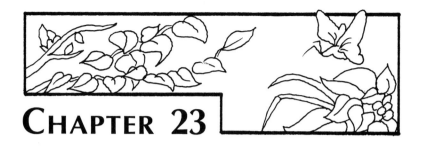

CHAPTER 23

EATING FOR THE HEALTH OF YOUR HEART

In this chapter you will explore

- dietary changes of value in the prevention and treatment of heart disease
- the desirable levels of total, HDL-, and LDL-cholesterol
- how saturated, monounsaturated, and polyunsaturated fatty acids affect serum-cholesterol levels
- what foods contain cholesterol and saturated fat, and how to limit them
- the benefits of water-soluble fiber and how to make it part of your diet
- how and why you should restrict dietary sodium

Changing eating habits, while often difficult, is important for anyone who either has cardiovascular disease or is concerned about preventing it. Adhering to the cholesterol-lowering guidelines in this chapter is particularly important if you have a high serum (blood) cholesterol level. Tell your doctor you are following a heart-healthy diet, since this is an important part of your treatment. A healthy diet, together with regular exercise, smoking cessation (if necessary), and stress reduction can help to improve your serum lipids and your cardiovascular health.

Following a heart-healthy diet need not be considered deprivation. For every food that should be avoided or limited, several others can be substituted. A willingness to try new foods and recipes is most helpful. Many people find they actually enjoy eating more healthfully, not only because of the health benefits, but because healthful food is delicious.

To begin cooking more healthfully, whether for formal dinners or for your lunch bag, consult the list of cookbooks and other resources that appears at the end of chapter 8, "Nutrition for Good Health." If you do not already have a heart-healthy cookbook, consider getting one now—the recipes as well as cooking and shopping suggestions will be invaluable.

DIET AND HEART DISEASE

Scientists have long suspected that what we eat plays a role in the development of heart disease. In early twentieth-century experiments, rabbits and monkeys were fed diets containing large amounts of cholesterol, which indeed resulted in the buildup of plaque in their arteries. Today, our knowledge of diet and heart disease goes far beyond dietary cholesterol. We now know that different types of fat affect serum cholesterol differently, dietary fiber may have an effect, and that hypertension and obesity also increase the risk of cardiac disease. But many questions regarding diet and heart disease remain unanswered. It is frustrating but true that some of our current nutritional recommendations may change as our knowledge in this field advances. The dietary advice and suggestions in this chapter are based on current research about the relationship between diet and cardiovascular disease. Stay informed as new findings are revealed.

It's easy to go wrong

Diet contributes to the epidemic of heart disease in America in several ways. The average American eats far too much fat, saturated fat, and cholesterol. This can raise serum cholesterol, blood pressure, and weight. Becoming obese increases the risk of non-insulin-dependent diabetes, and all of these factors increase the risk of heart disease.

Choosing a poor diet is understandable. All sorts of tempting and convenient foods are ready and available, and often it seems that everyone else is eating them. Have you ever said to yourself:

"Making breakfast is a bother, I'll grab coffee and a doughnut at work."

OR

"Everyone else at the luncheon is having the rich dessert, I'm really full, but I'll have one, too."

OR

"It's been a crazy week, I'll just pick up some fast food again for dinner."

Although you should keep such excuses to a minimum, eating a heart-healthy diet does not mean the end of snacks, desserts, or enjoying your meals. It does mean choosing food carefully, and most of the time, choosing healthfully.

DIET AND SERUM CHOLESTEROL

What is an ideal cholesterol level? The answer has become more precise as our knowledge of the role of cholesterol in heart disease has advanced.

Guidelines for Total Cholesterol*	
Desirable	Less than 200 mg/dl[†]
Borderline-high	200 to 239 mg/dl
High	Greater than or equal to 240 mg/dl

Fully 50 percent of American adults have cholesterol levels higher than desirable! Most could improve their cholesterol levels with dietary changes. Blaming genes from parents or grandparents may be convenient, but a high cholesterol level is not usually due to genetic factors. The major cause of hypercholesterolemia (high serum cholesterol) is lifestyle: dietary excesses combined with too little activity. As a society, we eat too much saturated fat, too much cholesterol, and carry around too much extra weight. All of these tend to elevate the cholesterol level.

"Good" and "Bad" cholesterol

To review from chapter 21, "Cardiovascular Disease," cholesterol is a fat-like, waxy substance obtained from food and also produced by your own body. Despite all the bad press, you need cholesterol for a variety of functions. You produce various hormones and vitamin D from it, and all of your cells require cholesterol in their membranes. It is not, however, essential in the diet, since your body produces more than adequate amounts. Cholesterol, which is not soluble in blood, is carried through the bloodstream on proteins called lipoproteins. Cholesterol carried on low-density lipoprotein (LDL) is called "bad" cholesterol, since it can be deposited as plaque in the coronary arteries. Cholesterol carried on high-density lipoprotein (HDL) is called "good" cholesterol, since it is carried to the liver to be excreted from the body. A high level of HDL-cholesterol is considered to be protective.

Because of the way the body handles each type, it is desirable to have a low LDL-cholesterol and a relatively high HDL-cholesterol.

---

* From the National Cholesterol Education Program, of the National Heart, Lung, and Blood Institute, 1988

† mg/dl = milligrams/deciliter

Guidelines for LDL-Cholesterol*

Desirable   Less than 130 mg/dl †
Borderline-high   130 to 159 mg/dl
High   Greater than or equal to 160 mg/dl

Guidelines for HDL-Cholesterol*

Desirable   35 to 90 mg/dl
Low   Less than 35 mg/dl

Measuring the ratio of total cholesterol to HDL-cholesterol is also useful. To obtain this number, divide your total cholesterol by your HDL-cholesterol (both must be from the same blood sample). The resulting value should be less than 3.5; a higher value indicates increased cardiac risk. If your HDL level is too low, increase it by doing regular aerobic exercise, losing weight if overweight, and, if you smoke, quitting.

Further suggestions will be given in the next few sections to help you lower your LDL-cholesterol.

HOW TO EAT LESS CHOLESTEROL

Having some cholesterol in your diet is harmless, but for many people, eating too much of it increases the level in the bloodstream.

Cholesterol is found only in foods of animal origin. Meat, poultry, fish, shellfish, eggs, and dairy products all contain cholesterol. Of all the commonly eaten cholesterol-containing foods, egg yolks and organ meats contain the most.

Plant products never contain cholesterol. They can, and often do, contain fat, which is different from cholesterol. This distinction is important because many high-fat foods made from plant products are labeled NO CHOLESTEROL or CHOLESTEROL FREE, leading many consumers to conclude that these products are good for their hearts. This may or may not be so. Vegetable oils, peanut butter, potato chips, and margarines commonly carry this claim. With the exception of a very rare brand of margarine, none of these foods ever contains animal products, so they would never contain cholesterol. But these products do contain fat. What you should evaluate is how much fat the product has, and what kind of fat it is (primarily saturated or unsaturated). As you will learn later, unsaturated fats are healthier.

The next thing to know is the amount of cholesterol recommended for a daily diet. The American Heart Association and several other health organiza-

---

* From the National Cholesterol Education Program, of the National Heart, Lung, and Blood Institute, 1988

† mg/dl = milligrams/deciliter

tions recommend a maximum of 300 milligrams of cholesterol per day. To put this number in perspective, note the amount of cholesterol in a few commonly-eaten foods:

Cholesterol Content of Common Foods (in milligrams)	
Sirloin, lean, 3 oz	76
Beef liver, 3 oz	333
Pork tenderloin, 3 oz	80
Chicken, light (white) meat, 3 oz	73
Turkey, light (white) meat, 3 oz	59
Salmon, Atlantic, 3 oz	47
Shrimp, 3 oz	130
Lobster, 3 oz	81
Clams, 3 oz	29
Scallops, 3 oz	28
Cheddar cheese, 1 oz	30
Butter, 1 teaspoon	11
Whole milk, 8 fl oz	33
Skim milk, 8 fl oz	4
Egg, 1 whole	213
Egg yolk	213
Egg white	0

You can see why egg yolks should be limited to no more than four per week, including those used in recipes. Your dietitian or doctor may advise even fewer. Keep in mind that egg whites contain no cholesterol—or fat, for that matter—and can be added to egg-containing dishes like french toast or an omelet, which will allow you to use fewer yolks. You may also want to try cholesterol-free egg substitutes, which can be bought frozen and are essentially egg white, although some brands have a little added fat.

If you never liked liver anyway, its cholesterol content is now an excellent reason to give it up. If you do like liver or other organ meats, however, eat them as an occasional treat, and limit your portion to three to five ounces.

What about shellfish? Original analyses pegged them as very high in cholesterol, and for years people on heart-healthy diets were advised to avoid all shellfish. Newer and improved methods of analysis have shown that most shellfish are quite low in cholesterol. Only shrimp is moderately high in cholesterol, but you can still eat a three-ounce serving and stay well within the 300-milligram daily limit. Lobster is comparable to beef, pork, and chicken in its cholesterol content. Mollusks—clams, oysters, mussels, scallops—are low in cholesterol and can be enjoyed often. One thing that all shellfish have in common is their very low fat content.

Fats: Good for you, bad for you

Good fat, bad fat. Why do I have to know about that?

All fats have the same number of calories, but when it comes to your heart, not all fats are equal. The two major categories are *saturated* and *unsaturated*.

Any fat or oil is a mixture of different fatty acids. If saturated fatty acids predominate, it is called *saturated fat*. Butter, for example, contains some unsaturated fatty acids, but because about 66 percent of them are saturated, we refer to butter as a highly saturated fat. If unsaturated fatty acids predominate, the fat or oil is called *unsaturated*. Unsaturated fatty acids do not raise serum cholesterol.

It is saturated fatty acids in particular that tend to raise serum cholesterol (although recent research suggests that certain saturated fatty acids do not). The ones that do raise serum cholesterol (most of them) may do this by signaling the body to manufacture fewer LDL receptors, which are needed to help transfer LDL-cholesterol to the liver for excretion.

The primary factor in raising serum cholesterol is *not* eating excess cholesterol, but consuming too much saturated fat. This is not always easily understood, since it seems contrary to logic.

 Marcia's Experience

Marcia, a fifty-year-old supervisor of state unemployment registration with a recently diagnosed high serum-cholesterol level (259 mg/dl), had read that avoiding cholesterol-containing foods would help, and that eggs are very high in cholesterol. She avoided eggs with a passion. Two months later, Marcia was surprised to find that her cholesterol level remained high. Reviewing her diet with a dietitian, she learned that despite her cholesterol intake being down, she regularly consumed foods high in saturated fat: chicken cooked and eaten with the skin on, whole-milk cheese, and powdered coffee lightener, to name a few. She learned that she could eat eggs in moderation but must reduce her saturated-fat intake. The new plan worked; two months later her cholesterol level had decreased to 211 mg per deciliter.

Which fats are saturated?

The major sources of saturated fatty acids are animal fats, butterfat, tropical oils, and heavily hydrogenated oils.

Saturated fats should be eaten sparingly, making up no more than 10 percent of your total calories. Let us look closely at ways to reduce saturated fat in your diet.

To limit saturated fat

Animal fat   To reduce the animal fat in your diet:

- In chicken and turkey, much of the fat is found in, and just under, the skin. Remove the skin and all visible fat *before* cooking.
- White meat has less fat than dark meat.
- Not all poultry flesh is low-fat. Chicken and turkey are low in fat; duck and goose are not.
- With red meat (beef, pork, and lamb), trim off-any visible fat before cooking.
- The leaner cuts of beef are sirloin, eye of round, top round, tenderloin, round tip, and top loin.
- USDA grade *Select* is the leanest, then *Choice*, then *Prime*.
- To make burgers, have one of the lean cuts of beef ground; this will be leaner than even the extra-lean meat you can buy pre-ground.
- Ground turkey makes delicious burgers. But beware! Some brands are as high in fat as ground beef. Buy either ground turkey labeled as having no more than two grams of fat per ounce, or buy plain ground turkey breast. (You may have to go to a butcher for this, but it will be *very* lean—one gram of fat per ounce.)
- When buying pork, choose the *tenderloin*—almost as lean as white-meat chicken. Other cuts of pork are not so low in fat.
- Broil, bake, grill, or roast meat on a rack to allow some of the fat to drip off.
- Your portion of meat, poultry, or fish should be about three to five ounces.
- Stretch meat by using it in casseroles, stir-fries, and other mixed dishes, with lots of vegetables.
- To reduce total fat content, instead of oil use lemon juice, flavored vinegars, wine, broth, and nonfat yogurt in marinades or for flavoring.

Butterfat   The difference in butterfat content between whole-milk products and low-fat or nonfat products is enormous. Note the difference in progressing from cream to skim milk.

Grams of Fat in One Cup Of	
Heavy cream	90.0
Light cream	46.0
Half-and-half	27.0
Evaporated milk	19.0
Whole milk	8.0
2%-fat milk	4.7
1%-fat milk	2.6
Skim milk	0.4

To reduce the butterfat in your diet:

- Use skim or 1-percent-fat milk. Do not use 2-percent-fat milk—even though it is called "low-fat," it is not much lower in fat than whole milk. One cup has more than a teaspoon of butterfat.
- Instead of butter, use margarine. You can also use fat-free spreads: jam, jelly, marmalade, honey and apple butter, and sugar-free fruit spreads.
- Choose cheeses that have five or fewer grams of fat per ounce, such as part-skim mozzarella.
- Use plain nonfat yogurt instead of sour cream or mayonnaise on potatoes, in salad dressings, and in other recipes.
- Ice cream can be extremely high in butterfat—some of the superpremium varieties have as much as 24 grams of fat per half cup! Even store brands of ice cream have at least seven grams of fat per half cup. Ice milk has less and frozen yogurt, fewer still. Sorbets, frozen fruit bars, and popsicles are also fat-free, refreshing dessert choices.
- Keep cones on hand for your frozen yogurt. They are fat-free and low in calories. Choose fresh fruit, oat flakes, and other cereals for toppings.

Tropical Oils To remember the tropical oils, think of a palm tree. The tropical oils are coconut oil, palm oil, palm kernel oil, and cocoa butter. Though you will seldom see them sold on their own, they are in many food products, such as crackers, cookies, coffee lighteners, and non-dairy whipped toppings. Cocoa butter is used in chocolate. Food manufacturers use tropical oils because they are relatively inexpensive and have a long shelf-life and a pleasing taste.

Due partly to consumer pressure for more healthful food products, some manufacturers have recently stopped using tropical oils. This does *not* mean their products are now lower in total fat content, since unsaturated oils like corn, canola, and soybean are substituted for the tropical oils. It does, however, mean that these foods now contain less saturated fat.

Consumer Beware! Tropical oils contain absolutely *no cholesterol*—they cannot, because they come from a plant. Therefore, a food full of tropical oils can have NO CHOLESTEROL splashed across its label but not mention its saturated-fat content. This is misleading; it is up to you to read the label carefully and look for the tropical oils.

A final note about foods containing tropical oils: while it is wise to avoid them, remember that most people get much more of their saturated fat from meat and whole-milk dairy products.

Hydrogenated Oils When oils are hydrogenated, hydrogen atoms are added to the fatty acids, causing some of them to become saturated. Lightly hydrogenated oils, such as those commonly used in salad dressings and crackers, are no problem since they remain far less saturated than coconut oil, lard, butter, and other saturated alternatives. Heavily hydrogenated oils become highly saturated. Vegetable shortening, commonly used for baking, is heavily hydrogenated and is best avoided. Also avoid margarines that list hydrogenated oil as the first ingredient.

Unsaturated fats: a better choice

Unsaturated fats can be either monounsaturated or polyunsaturated. They do not raise serum cholesterol—in fact, they can actually lower the cholesterol level. The monounsaturated fats seem to be better at this, since they lower only the artery-clogging LDL-cholesterol, not the protective HDL-cholesterol. Polyunsaturated fats lower the total cholesterol by lowering both the LDL and HDL levels.

Unsaturated fats have just as many *calories* as saturated fats, so use them in moderation. (For information on limiting your total daily intake of fat grams, see chapter 9, "A Sensible Approach to Weight Loss.")

Which fats are unsaturated?

Major Sources of Monounsaturated and Polyunsaturated Fats	
Monounsaturated	*Polyunsaturated*
Olive oil	Corn oil
Canola oil	Sunflower oil
Peanut oil	Safflower oil
Peanut butter	Soybean oil
Nuts	Sesame oil
Margarine	Margarine
Avocados	Mayonnaise

Yes, margarine is on both lists. Most margarines contain substantial amounts of both monounsaturated and polyunsaturated fatty acids. The key is to select one in which the first ingredient is a *liquid* oil (the second ingredient will be a hydrogenated oil—it has to be, otherwise the product cannot hold its shape). When trying to reduce your total fat intake, choose a reduced-fat margarine—these substitute water for some of the fat. Reduced-fat margarines have two or three grams of fat per teaspoon, whereas regular margarine has four.

How can mayonnaise be on any list of acceptable fats? Isn't it full of saturated fat, plus all that cholesterol from egg yolks? No! No! Mayonnaise has been overly maligned. Check the label—you'll find an unsaturated oil, usually soybean. And the cholesterol? It is barely there: one tablespoon of regular mayonnaise has only about eight milligrams of cholesterol, which is the amount in 1/27 of a large egg. As with margarine, when trying to reduce your fat intake, opt for one of the many reduced-fat mayonnaises. They tend to have slightly less than half the fat of regular mayonnaise, and they taste good. You will find an abundance of them on your supermarket shelf, since every company worth its vinegar now markets a reduced-fat mayonnaise.

Which of the many unsaturated oils are best to use? You can use a variety, but it makes sense to have a good monounsaturated oil on hand. Choose olive oil (any kind) when you want its distinctive flavor, and canola oil when you do not—canola oil is quite flavorless. Canola oil, if you have not heard of it, comes from the rapeseed plant. Used for centuries in Europe, China, Japan, and India, it has gained favor in recent years in this country because of its very low saturated-fatty-acid content. But remember—unsaturated fats are still fat! Use *any* fat in moderation. A bottle, tub, or jar should last a long time.

OMEGA-3 FATTY ACIDS

Not only are fish relatively low in fat and cholesterol, but they also contain *omega-3 fatty acids* (commonly called fish oils). These are very long-chain, polyunsaturated fatty acids that seem to have cardiovascular benefits. Large population studies have shown that groups of people who eat fish regularly have fewer heart attacks than those which do not, and omega-3 fatty acids are believed in part responsible for this protection.

The omega-3 fatty acids have an antithrombotic effect, which means that they cause blood to take longer to clot. Since most heart attacks ultimately occur when a blood clot forms and becomes lodged in a narrowed coronary artery, a reduced tendency to clot is an obvious advantage. Omega-3 fatty acids can also help lower an extremely elevated serum triglyceride level (the fat in the bloodstream).

Omega-3 fatty acids occur in marine phytoplankton, which are eaten by small fish and work their way up the food chain. All fish and shellfish have some, but cold-water fish have a higher total fat content and more omega-3 fatty acids than fish found in warmer water.

Excellent Sources of Omega-3 Fatty Acids

salmon, trout, mackerel,
sardines, bluefish, herring

Small but significant amounts of omega-3 fatty acids are also found in canola oil (10 percent) and soybean oil (7 percent). Their popular and easier nickname, "fish oils," is therefore a misnomer.

Omega-3 supplements are not a good idea unless your doctor prescribes them for a specific reason. They can be high in calories as well as vitamins A and D, not to mention expensive, and the long-term effects of taking fatty acids in capsule form have not been studied.

To get your omega-3s, eat seafood regularly—at least twice per week. More often is even better. Choose fish that is broiled, grilled, baked, poached, steamed, or microwaved. Avoid fish that is fried or cooked in a sea of butter. Canned fish like tuna is fine, but choose water-packed, not oil. Even if the fish is canned in an unsaturated oil, the total fat content will be very high. When dining on shellfish, pass up rich sauces and butter. Choose boiled lobster with lemon, shrimp cocktail, steamed clams, lightly broiled scallops—you get the idea.

HAVE MORE FIBER

Fiber is the part of plants we do not digest or absorb. Fiber is broadly classified into two categories: water-soluble and insoluble. Many foods, like fruits and vegetables, are good sources of both types.

Water-soluble fiber in particular has been shown in several studies to have a cholesterol-lowering effect. The exact mechanism is unknown. One theory proposes that the fiber binds with bile acids in the intestinal tract, and from there they are excreted. To produce more bile acids, the liver pulls cholesterol from the bloodstream, thereby lowering the blood-cholesterol level. It has also been suggested that eating foods high in water-soluble fiber does not in itself lower the cholesterol level, but prevents one from filling up instead on cholesterol-raising options. In other words, if you are having oatmeal and fruit for breakfast, you are not having bacon, eggs, and butter! Though questions about water-soluble fiber remain, regularly including good sources in your diet is clearly beneficial. Foods high in water-soluble fiber include oatmeal and oat bran, barley, legumes (dried beans, peas, and lentils), and fruits and vegetables (especially apples, figs, and carrots). Note that these foods are also highly nutritious.

Increasing water-soluble fiber in your diet

- Eat hot oatmeal or oat bran (or a mixture) for breakfast. Add raisins, apples, and cinnamon if you like.
- Choose a ready-to-eat breakfast cereal that contains oat bran. Look in the ingredient list for *oat bran, rolled oats,* or *whole oat flour.*
- Sprinkle a teaspoonful of oat bran on your favorite ready-to-eat cereal, on yogurt, and on top of casseroles.
- Choose bread made with oats or oat bran.
- Eat fruit—in cereal, with yogurt, for dessert and snacks.

- Add barley to your favorite homemade soup.
- Eat beans and lentils often: make your own baked beans, three-bean salad, lentil or bean soup, chili, and hummus.

Don't be misled by the myriad products that contain oat bran, but also a lot of fat, salt, or sugar. Oat bran muffins are one example. Most commercially-prepared muffins contain about twelve grams of fat, whether or not they have oat bran (you can make your own muffins at home with much less fat). Oat bran doughnuts and potato chips are other examples of oat bran added to junk foods: being fried, by definition they cannot be considered even remotely heart-healthy.

What about insoluble fiber? Found in wheat bran, whole-wheat flour and bread, as well as many cereals, fruits, and vegetables, this type of fiber has many health benefits of its own, such as preventing constipation and certain other gastrointestinal conditions. A healthy diet will include it in generous amounts.

DIET AND HYPERTENSION

Diet is an important component of the treatment for high blood pressure. Lowering sodium intake, and losing weight if necessary, can bring about significant improvement in blood pressure readings. Some studies suggest that sodium is not the only mineral of concern: adequate amounts of dietary potassium and calcium may also improve blood pressure control. Limiting caffeine and alcohol is also of benefit, since both can raise blood pressure.

If you are trying to lose weight and change your diet to improve your high blood pressure, chapter 9 offers information and recommendations.

The problem with sodium

Many people with hypertension are sodium-sensitive, meaning that excess sodium intake raises blood pressure. Since there is no test to determine sodium-sensitivity, almost everyone with hypertension should restrict dietary sodium. Anyone with a condition that causes fluid retention in the body should also avoid excess sodium, since sodium enhances fluid retention. Cardiac disease falls in this category, since having had a heart attack, congestive heart failure, or heart surgery can all cause the body to retain fluid.

The average American consumes over 4,500 milligrams of sodium per day. This is ten times the amount our bodies require to function. This large amount is due to our reliance on highly-processed foods and the habit of shaking overly-generous amounts of salt on our food. Unlike fresh foods, which contain only small amounts of sodium, highly-processed foods have large amounts of salt added. For examples, pickles, olives, canned and powdered soups, and most fast foods are all heavy on the sodium. Table salt is sodium chloride—40 percent sodium, 60 percent chloride. A level teaspoon of salt is about 2,300 milligrams of sodium. Knowing this, you can easily see how using the salt shaker liberally can add up to a lot of sodium.

The Estimated Minimum Requirement for sodium is extremely small—only 500 milligrams per day. A sensible and frequently advised daily limit for people with high blood pressure or cardiac disease is 2,000 milligrams (two grams). This is the limit we recommend in our Behavioral Medicine Cardiovascular Programs.

A preference for highly-salted food is not innate. Most of us acquire this taste during childhood, eating canned soups, luncheon meats, and other sodium-laden foods. Fortunately, the taste for salt can be reduced by eating less of it. After cutting back on salty foods, craving them for several weeks or months is not unusual. Be patient—after a while, the desire for salt diminishes, accompanied by an enhanced appreciation for the taste of the food, not the salt. Some foods may even begin to taste too salty.

To keep your sodium intake below 2,000 milligrams per day, use mainly fresh (unprocessed) foods. Get in the habit of cooking from scratch much of the time. You may, for example, want to start making your own salad dressings or large batches of soups and sauces to freeze and pull out when you need them.

Take a Moment To . . .

List two dishes you will prepare from scratch this week. (They can be simple!)

_____

_____

When buying prepared foods, read the labels: products with salt or another form of sodium listed among the first five ingredients are generally high in sodium. (Hint: With certain canned foods, like tuna, salmon, and beans, the added salt is mostly in the water. Rinse these foods thoroughly in a strainer, under running water, to remove much of the salt.)

The Food and Drug Administration has established standards for sodium labeling. Any manufacturer labeling its product to attract attention to the sodium content must obey the following guidelines:

Sodium Labeling

Sodium Free	5 mg sodium or less per serving
Very Low Sodium	35 mg sodium or less per serving
Low Sodium	140 mg sodium or less per serving
Reduced Sodium	the usual sodium level is decreased by at least 75 percent
No Salt Added, Unsalted, or Salt Free	the food has been processed without salt (the food for which it is a substitute contains salt)

Try using low-sodium soups, sauces, breads, and condiments. Many low-sodium products work well in cooking, such as low-sodium chicken broth as a base for a stir-fry and canned unsalted tomato sauce for making spaghetti sauce.

Instead of adding salt, be creative with other flavorings. Use herbs and spices—shake on your favorites and experiment with some new ones. Try fresh herbs like dill, basil, and parsley. Use old standbys: garlic, onion, and pepper. Grated fresh ginger root is very appealing on chicken and in stir-fries. Fresh lemon juice and flavored vinegars go well on vegetables, fish, and chicken. Fruit juices make nice marinades.

Take a Moment To . . .

List two new flavorings you will try in the next week:

_____

_____

A patient who has been happily eating a heart-healthy diet for the past year was eagerly describing her latest success in creating a low-fat salad dressing. She paused and reflected on her late mother-in-law's cooking:

She cooked everything in this much butter, and, oh! her pie crusts were so flaky; they were made with lard. Everything she made was delicious, you'd think you were in heaven . . . but of course you might get there faster!

Judith Linsey Palken, M.S., R.D.

SAMPLE

HEART HEALTHY NUTRITION

HEALTH COMMITMENT

Long-Term Goal:

Eat a diet that is heart-healthy

_____

Signature

_____

Witness

Expected Date of Reaching Goal: _____

Readiness to Change	Short-Term Goals	Comments (supports, rewards, etc.)
Never considered change; need information.	1. Review chapter 23 ("Eating for the Health of Your Heart") and highlight suggestions that seem especially pertinent to me. 2. Discuss the benefits of following a heart-healthy diet with my dietitian, doctor, or other health care provider.	
Considered change, but not yet committed.	1. Buy a cookbook that features low-fat recipes. 2. Try three new healthy recipes.	
Desire change; need motivation.	1. Have a heart-healthy dinner with interested friends. Arrange for everyone to bring one dish. 2. Treat myself to a new appliance that will keep my cooking efforts—a food processor or a wok, for example.	

(continued)

Readiness to Change	Short-Term Goals	Comments (supports, rewards, etc.)
Attempting change; need structures, support, and skills.	1. Take the time for my own "supermarket tour." Explore healthful options for cheese, cereal, yogurt, desserts, and other items. Buy and try some of them. 2. By next week I will: —have at least two to three pieces of fruit per day. —be using skim and/or 1% fat milk. —be limiting red meat to a maximum of twice per week.	
Change made; need reinforcement.	1. Dine out, making a conscious effort to order a completely healthful and delicious meal. 2. Prepare a favorite recipe, omitting salt and substituting herbs, spices, or other flavorings.	
Change made; slipping back into old habits, need renewed motivation and support.	1. Keep a thorough food diary for one week. Review it critically and write down ways I can improve my diet. 2. Look back over the healthful recipes I made that were a success. Plan to make two this week.	

436

HEART HEALTHY NUTRITION
HEALTH COMMITMENT

Long-Term Goal: _____

_____

_____

_____
Signature

_____
Witness

Expected Date of Reaching Goal: _____

Short-Term Goals	*Comments (supports, rewards, etc.)*

437

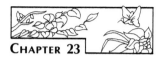

CHAPTER 23

INSTRUCTIONS FOR KEEPING YOUR FOOD RECORD

Keep a food record for three consecutive days. Eat as you normally would. Look up and record the sodium content of everything you eat and drink. Total your sodium intake for each day.

Remember, your long-term goal is to limit your daily sodium intake to no more than 2,000 milligrams.

Note: *The Complete Book of Food Counts* by Corrine T. Netzer (New York: Dell, 1988) lists the amount of sodium in over 8,000 foods.

FOOD RECORD

Name _____

Day and Date _____

Time	Location	Food or Beverage	Amount Eaten	Sodium (milligrams)

439

FOOD RECORD

Name _____

Day and Date _____

Time	Location	Food or Beverage	Amount Eaten	Sodium (milligrams)

FOOD RECORD

Name _____

Day and Date _____

Time	Location	Food or Beverage	Amount Eaten	Sodium (milligrams)

441

FOOD RECORD

Name _____

Day and Date _____

Time	Location	Food or Beverage	Amount Eaten	Sodium (milligrams)

FOOD RECORD

CHAPTER 23

Name _____

Day and Date _____

Time	Location	Food or Beverage	Amount Eaten	Sodium (milligrams)

PART 6

RELAPSE PREVENTION

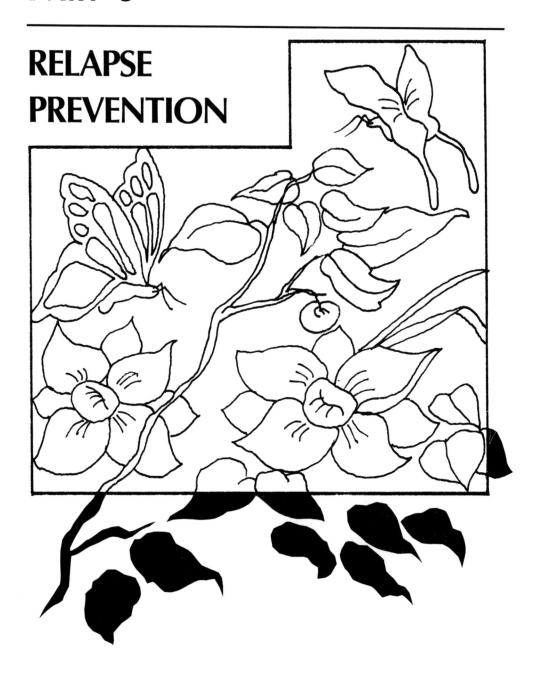

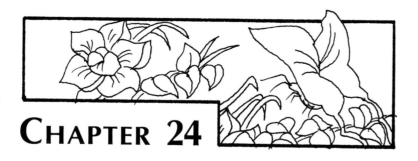

CHAPTER 24

THE END OF THE BEGINNING

Now this is not the end. It is not even the beginning of the end.
But it is, perhaps, the end of the beginning.

Sir Winston Churchill

In this chapter you will explore

- setting new goals for the next three months
- how to maintain the desired or needed changes
- how and why relapse occurs and how to make a plan to get back on track with your goal
- prioritizing your time

Throughout *The Wellness Book*, we have discussed the relationship between thoughts, feelings, behaviors, and health. We have presented many techniques to help you maximize health and minimize the symptoms of illness. You may already have begun to make some healthy changes in your lifestyle. If so, congratulations!

You may have come to the realization that initial behavioral change is in fact possible . . . and perhaps less difficult than you expected. It may have required a reassessment and affirmation of what you value. It certainly required motivation, willpower, self-discipline, and, perhaps, additional support.

And if you have not yet integrated health-enhancing changes into your life, now may be the ideal time to begin. Use finishing *The Wellness Book* as a marker to make a commitment to a healthier life.

Life changes take place over months and years. It took years to acquire your patterns of thoughts, feelings, and behaviors (in many cases detrimental); you cannot expect to eliminate or modify unhealthy behaviors in just a few weeks. Former smokers know that the urge rarely disappears completely and that being smoke-free requires a constant commitment. You need a lifelong and flexible plan to enable you to incorporate new, healthy changes into your life and to maintain these changes.

Having given you information and tools to implement healthy lifestyle changes, we will now focus on maintaining these changes. We will introduce you to techniques which prevent relapses, or the tendency to revert back to a familiar but less healthy lifestyle.

MAKING THE COMMITMENT FOR LONG-LASTING CHANGE

Chapter 3, "Getting Started," introduced in some depth the idea of setting health goals which reflected the mind/body model of health. If you have not yet read chapter 3, you need to do so before reading this chapter. If you have read it, you may want to review it. As you complete this book, return once again to the concept of goal-setting, and make a commitment to the future. If you have achieved the goals you set in chapter 3, you may need to update these goals. If you set goals you were unable to reach, you may need to revise them to be more realistic and attainable. If you did not set goals when you read chapter 3, do so now.

Clarifying what's important/meaningful/valuable to you

Before reevaluating your original goals or setting new ones, first establish or reestablish what is important, meaningful, or valuable to you. Review your responses to the "Ten Loves" exercise (page 19). While reading *The Wellness Book*, you were asked to challenge many of your beliefs, automatic thoughts, and long-standing behaviors. Have your responses to this exercise changed? If so, you may want to do this exercise again.

     Take a Moment To . . .

List below the five things that you discovered or rediscovered you love best.

_____

_____

_____

_____

_____

This list is the basis for reestablishing the specific goals you want to accomplish and the specific behaviors you want to change.

Long-term goals

Long-term goals are your "destination," where you want to be in three, six, twelve months or longer. They are specific, measurable, realistic, positive, and attainable. They should be viewed as a challenge rather than a threat. Now review your list of long-term goals (page 21). Have these changed since you began to read *The Wellness Book*? How? Or were you unable to accomplish them? If so, ask yourself the following questions:

- Does the list reflect things you think are most important, or what other people have told you are most important? You will be far more successful changing behaviors that you want to change than behaviors you feel you should change.
- Were the goals realistic and attainable?
- Were the goals specific and measurable?

Revise and update your long-term goals now, based on the insights you have gained.

Take a Moment To . . .

Set goals you can live with in the coming months and years.

Long-Term Goals:

1. _____
2. _____
3. _____
4. _____
5. _____

Having reestablished and reprioritized your long-term goals, consider once again the obstacles and supports you have for effecting change and successfully achieving these goals. You may want to review what you previously identified as obstacles and supports (pages 26 and 27).

Take a Moment To . . .

Reassess your obstacles to change. Draw upon your experience after beginning to initiate change.

_____

_____

_____

Reassess your supports for change. Again draw upon your experience after beginning to initiate change.

_____

_____

_____

_____

The Health Commitment—a way to achieve your long-term goal

Throughout *The Wellness Book* we have included Health Commitment forms at the end of most chapters, asking you to identify specific strategies (short-term goals) to accomplish each long-term goal. Now review your Health Commitments and revise and update them as needed. Several blank forms are included at the end of this chapter for this purpose. To review directions on how to write a Health Commitment, see page 21.

WHAT ABOUT LAPSES?

Once you have successfully changed a behavior, adapted a new attitude, or developed a more positive feeling, the challenge then is to maintain those changes. Most people have occasional lapses. We need to expect them and allow them some room in order to avoid feelings of discouragement and loss of self-esteem. A *lapse* is "a slight error . . . a temporary deviation or fall" (*Webster's New Collegiate Dictionary*). We all make slight errors now and again. The point is to see them as single events, not catastrophes, and to make sure you do not allow a momentary deviation to push you toward a relapse or the re-emergence of a bad habit. Lapses often accompany feelings of deprivation or other negative emotional states. Feeling deprived can lead to anxiety or tension, which, if left unresolved, can lead to indulgences that quickly alleviate the anxiety or tension. Unfortunately, most activities that produce immediate gratification—such as the use of alcohol, food, cigarettes, or not exercising—are detrimental to health. Plan well to pace yourself as you go about the process of change, and be sure you have established concrete and helpful action plans that can be put into place quickly in situations that come up.

    The greatest single danger during a lapse is to adopt a "saint or sinner" attitude, an expectation of total success or total failure. One outburst of anger, for example, does not negate an entire self-improvement plan. You can learn from your lapses by observing the sequence of events and urges that lead up to them.

    If you do not exercise for several days, for example, what you need to do is:

- State the problem without negative judgment: "I missed a few days of exercise, but I want to get back on track. I am committed."
- Reinforce your contract on the basis of what you have learned: "If I do not exercise in the morning, I don't do it at all. Therefore, I will recommit myself to exercising in the morning."

PREVENTING RELAPSES

Relapse is a more entrenched return to an unhealthy habit. Relapses often occur in "high-risk" situations, the majority of which, according to Drs. Alan Marlatt and Judith R. Gordon, from the University of Washington, evolve from three categories:

1. Negative emotional states—such as boredom, anger, anxiety, frustration, depression—account for 35 percent of relapses.
2. Interpersonal conflicts—perhaps with a spouse, friend, boss—account for about 16 percent.
3. Social pressure accounts for another 20 percent of relapses. Social pressure can be as subtle as a bad example set by someone you know, or as overt as someone actively trying to persuade you to do something you know is wrong for you.

To avoid relapses, start by identifying your high-risk situations. When do they occur? Who is involved? If you know that your brother, for example, will make fun of you jogging, you can be prepared to minimize the negative effects of his ridicule.

 Take a Moment To . . .

List four or five personal high-risk situations that might set you up for a lapse. Be specific. Include names and places.

_____

_____

_____

_____

_____

WHAT TO DO NOW

After identifying your high-risk situations, try these strategies to minimize the chance that a lapse will become more entrenched.

- Watch for the cues. Most habits are paired with certain situations or settings. By controlling these conditioned stimuli, you can lessen the risk. If you know that you and your mother always argue at breakfast, you might eat breakfast separately. You will probably enjoy breakfast more and start the day in better spirits as well.

- Do something else. An alternate activity which can distract you works well in some high-risk situations, especially when the substitute is something you enjoy, like going to a movie, gardening, running.

- Get help. Reach out for social support from friends. Join a group or club to reinforce behavioral change. Studies show that social support, in fact, is one of the keys to long-term success.

- Watch what you are thinking. Your thoughts influence feelings and behavior. Learn to recognize negative thoughts like "I'll never in a million years be able to do this" and replace them with affirmations: "I can do it. I'm ready to take care of myself."

- Outlast the urge. Instead of identifying with the urge and putting yourself behind it—"I really want that piece of chocolate cake!"—become a detached observer—"Ah, there's the old chocolate-cake urge again." If you distance yourself and resist giving in to it, the urge subsides over time.

- Elicit the relaxation response daily. It is your doorway to change. In times of increased stress, releasing physical tension and anxiety is particularly important.

- Balance your lifestyle. Balance can be defined as the equilibrium between external demands ("shoulds") and positive internal satisfactions ("wants"). If shoulds outweigh wants, our life is not in balance. Many of us need to program some free time for balance in an overly crowded schedule.

- Review the stress busters you identified on page 241. Use these resources to buster those situations in which you feel anxiety and tension, and reaffirm your coping capacity.

TAKE TIME! MAKE TIME!

> To choose time is to save time.
> Francis Bacon, "Of Dispatch"

> Time goes, you say? Ah no!
> Alas, Time stays, we go.
> Henry Austin Dobson, "The Paradox of Time"

> We ask for long life, but 'tis deep life, or noble moments that signify. Let the measure of time be spiritual, not mechanical.

> Ralph Waldo Emerson

Dost thou love life? Then do not squander time; for that's
the stuff life is made of.

> Benjamin Franklin, *Poor Richard's Almanac*

Counting time is not so important as making time count.

> James J. Walker

The idea of time is of everlasting fascination. What it is, whether you make it
or take it, and how to use it wisely continues to be talked and written about.

The Wellness Book has challenged you to set long- and short-term goals for
yourself concerning your health. A common lament is "I want to change—but
I do not have the time." Time (or lack thereof) is one of the most commonly
cited deterrents to changing behavior. We repeat Lord Stanley's words, already used to introduce the exercise chapter, because they express so precisely
the facts of the case:

> Those who think they have not time for exercise will sooner or later
> have to find time for illness.
>
> Edward Stanley, 15th Earl of Derby

If we examine time carefully, what is it we are busy being busy at? Why is
it we have no time to take care of ourselves?

Your Time Inventory
(Actual)

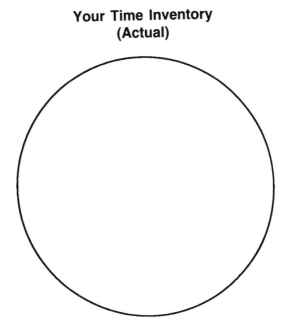

Divide the circle (a time pie) to reflect the major tasks that make up a
typical twenty-four hours for you. Your inventory might include work-related
activities, family responsibilities, self-care activities, recreation, exercise, sleep,
spirituality, community or social obligations.

Look at your circle carefully.

Stop.
Take a breath.
Reflect.

Are you doing the things you want to?
How much time is devoted to fun versus work?
Is everything important?
Could you prioritize?
Do the shoulds outweigh the wants?

Choose.

You have been learning the skills necessary to look at the balance in your life between responsibility to self and others, and to plan your time out of choice, not automatic reaction.

Divide the next time pie into what you consider *ideal* proportions allotted to major tasks of your twenty-four hours. Be sure to allow time for yourself and the health-enhancing behaviors that we have discussed in *The Wellness Book.*

**Your Time Inventory
(Ideal)**

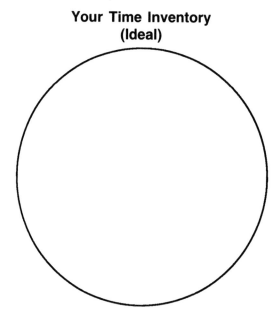

Now that you have given it careful thought—just do it! Take the time, make the time—for yourself.

Cynthia Medich, R.N., M.S.
Sue C. Jacobs, Ph.D.

HEALTH COMMITMENT

Long-Term Goal: _____

_____
Signature

_____
Witness

Expected Date of Reaching Goal: _____

Short-Term Goals

Comments (supports, rewards, etc.)

CHAPTER 24

HEALTH COMMITMENT

Long-Term Goal: _____

_____
Signature

_____
Witness

Expected Date of Reaching Goal: _____

Short-Term Goals

Comments (supports, rewards, etc.)

HEALTH COMMITMENT

Long-Term Goal: _____

_____

_____

_____
Signature

_____
Witness

Expected Date of Reaching Goal: _____

Short-Term Goals

Comments (supports, rewards, etc.)

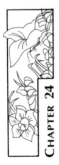

CHAPTER 24

HEALTH COMMITMENT

Long-Term Goal: _____

_____

_____   Signature

_____   Witness

Expected Date of Reaching Goal: _____

Short-Term Goals	*Comments (support, rewards, etc.)*

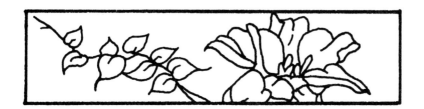

EPILOGUE

SOMETHING TO THINK ABOUT AS WE SAY GOOD-BYE

We have presented you with a vast array of information in *The Wellness Book,* all of which is compatible with the therapies of modern medicine. You have been introduced to the essentials of a healthy lifestyle, including the relaxation response, nutrition, exercise, and stress management. You have learned that thoughts, attitudes, feelings, and behavior are interrelated and that all can affect your health. You have also learned that successfully effecting change requires clarity of purpose, a commitment to yourself, and a realistic plan.

We have challenged you in many ways. Challenged you to think about your behaviors, thoughts, feelings, and attitudes, as well as how they affect your health. Challenged you to ask yourself if you are really doing the things that are important, meaningful, and valuable to you. Challenged you to be creative, flexible, and willing to try new approaches. Challenged you to become stress-hardy. It is not a challenge we take lightly, and so, in addition to teaching you what and how to change, we have incorporated a great deal of information on supports you can muster as you go through this process.

When change is viewed as a challenge and not a threat, success is more likely. Simply accept the challenge, and meet it. Go about it without prejudgment. When you identify the behaviors, thoughts, or attitudes you wish to change, do so without evaluating old patterns as good or bad. Just do it—no goods, bads, or indifferents. If you lapse in your intent, simply return to the plan outlined in your Health Commitment. Again the absence of prejudgment is important. Consider the wisdom of Anne Wilson Schaef's perception, in her book *Meditations for Women Who Do Too Much:* "Recovery is a process, not an event."

Try to see your changes in lifestyle as spurring you to learn and grow. You may experience the world differently, and often the differences will be surprising and unexpected. Your goals may change slightly, and that is fine.

> I don't want to get to the end of my life and find that I just lived the length of it. I want to have lived the width of it as well.
> Dianne Ackerman, in *Meditations for Women Who Do Too Much*

Do not be unduly vigilant about suggested changes. Record them as something you would like to do—as healthy pleasures—and initiate them in the total context of your health and well-being. Make the changes within the perspective of your entire life, and respect the new balance that will follow. Also remember that the changes you will be making are part of a larger process that will evolve and grow with time.

Finally, learn to take an overview of your experiences and changes. Many benefits are not immediately obvious. Often life is shaped by a series of unpredictable events. Consider the lessons in this ancient Zen teaching story about an old Chinese farmer.

> There was once an old farmer who had a mare. One day the mare broke through the fence and ran away. "Now you have no horse to pull your plow at planting time," the neighbors said. "What bad luck this is."
>
> "Good luck, bad luck," replied the farmer. "Who knows?"
>
> The next week the mare returned, bringing with her two wild stallions. "With three horses you are now a rich man," the neighbors said. "What good fortune this is."
>
> "Good fortune, bad fortune," the farmer said. "Who knows?"
>
> That afternoon the farmer's only son tried to tame one of the stallions, but he was thrown and broke a leg. "Now you have no one to help you with planting," the neighbors said. "What bad luck this is."
>
> "Good luck, bad luck," the farmer said. "Who knows?"
>
> The next day the emperor's soldiers rode into town and conscripted the eldest son in every family, but the farmer's son was left behind because of his broken leg. "Yours is the only eldest son in the province who has not been taken from his family," the neighbors said. "What good fortune this is . . ."

As you have learned in *The Wellness Book,* each of life's events can be seen as a challenge, but also as an opportunity. You may not have asked for this opportunity, but it is here nonetheless. How you view it is fundamentally important. Each time you are challenged by change, choose carefully how you want to respond. Stop, Breathe, Reflect, then Choose. Even setbacks can become occasions for remembering and using the skills you have learned. And finally, even the symptoms or illness that brought you to *The Wellness Book* may prove in the long run to have been a catalyst for change and growth that can significantly enrich your life.

Eileen M. Stuart, R.N., M.S.
Herbert Benson, M.D.

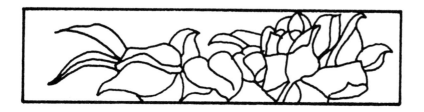

REFERENCES AND SUGGESTED READINGS

CITATIONS WITH AN ASTERISK (*) ARE SUGGESTED READING MATERIAL.

Chapter 2: The Mind/Body Model of Health and Illness

Beecher, H. K. "The Powerful Placebo." *Journal of the American Medical Association* 159 (1955): 1602–06.

Benson, H. *The Mind/Body Effect.* New York: Simon and Schuster, 1979.

————, and M. Epstein. "The Placebo Effect: A Neglected Asset in the Care of Patients." *Journal of the American Medical Association* 232 (1975): 1225–27.

Dawber, T. R. *The Framingham Study: The Epidemiology of Atherosclerotic Disease.* Cambridge, Mass.: Harvard University Press, 1980.

Engel, G. L. "The Need for a New Medical Model: A Challenge for Biomedicine." *Science* 196 (1977): 129–36.

————. "The Predictive Value of Psychological Variables for Disease and Death." *Annals of Internal Medicine* 85 (1976): 673–74.

Goldman, L., and E. F. Cook. "Decline in Ischemic Heart Disease Mortality Rates: An Analysis of the Comparative Effects of Medical Intervention and Changes in Lifestyle." *Annals of Internal Medicine* 101 (1984): 825–36.

Horowitz, R., C. Viscoli, L. Berkman, R. M. Donaldson, S. M. Horowitz, C. J. Murray, D. F. Ransohoff, and J. Sindelar. "Treatment Adherence and Risk of Death After a Myocardial Infarction." *Lancet* 336 (1990): 542–45.

Ornstein, R., and D. Sobel. *The Healing Brain.* New York: Simon & Schuster, 1987.

Pennebaker, J. W. *The Psychology of Physical Symptoms.* New York: Springer Verlag, 1982.

U.S. Department of Health, Education, and Welfare. *Healthy People: The Surgeon General's Report on Health Promotion and Disease Prevention.* Washington, D.C.: U.S. Government Printing Office, DHEW Publication No. 7 79–55071, 1979.

Wolf, S. "Effects of Suggestion and Conditioning on the Action of Chemical Agents in Human Subjects." *Journal of Clinical Investigation* 29 (1950): 100–109.

Chapter 3: Getting Started

DiClemente, C. C., and J. O. Prochaska. "Self-Change and Therapy Change of

Smoking Behavior: A Comparison of Processes of Change in Cessation and Maintenance." *Addictive Behaviors* 7 (1982): 133–42.

Guzetta, C. E., and B. M. Dossey. *Cardiovascular Nursing: Bodymind Tapestry*. Princeton, N. J.: C. V. Mosby Company, 1984.

Simon, S. B. *Meeting Yourself Halfway: 31 Value Clarification Strategies for Daily Living*. Niles, Ill.: Argus Communications, 1974.

———, L. W. Howe, and H. Kirschenbaum. *Value Clarification: A Handbook of Practical Strategies for Teachers and Students*. New York: Hart Publishing Company, 1972.

Strack, F., L. L. Martin, and S. Stepper. "Inhibiting and Facilitating Conditions of the Human Smile: A Nonobtrusive Test of Facial Feedback Hypothesis." *Journal of Personality and Social Psychology* 54 (1988): 768–77.

U.S. Department of Health, Education, and Welfare. *Healthy People: The Surgeon General's Report on Health Promotion and Disease Prevention*. Washington, D.C.: U.S. Government Printing Office, DHEW Publication No. 7 79-55071, 1979.

Chapter 4: The Relaxation Response

Ballentine, R., A. Hymes, and S. Rama. *Science of Breath: A Practical Guide*. Honesdale, Penn.: Himalayan International Institute of Yoga Science and Philosophy Publishers, 1979.

*Benson, H. *The Relaxation Response*. New York: William Morrow, 1975.

*———. *The Mind/Body Effect*. New York: Simon & Schuster, 1979.

*———. *Beyond the Relaxation Response*. New York: Times Books, 1984.

*———. *Your Maximum Mind*. New York: Times Books, 1987.

*Borysenko, J. *Minding the Body, Mending the Mind*. Reading, Mass.: Addison-Wesley, 1987.

Goleman, D. *Meditative Mind: Varieties of Meditative Experience*. Los Angeles: Jeremy P. Tarcher, 1988.

*Hanh, T. N. *The Miracle of Mindfulness: A Manual on Meditation*. Boston: Beacon Press, 1976.

———. [Commentary] *The Sutra on the Full Awareness of Breathing*. Berkeley, Calif.: Parallax Press, 1988.

Kass, J. D., R. Friedman, J. Leserman, P. C. Zuttermeister, and H. Benson. "Health Outcomes and a New Index of Spiritual Experience." *Journal for the Scientific Study of Religion*. 30 (1991): 203–11.

*Kabat-Zinn, J. *Full Catastrophe Living: Using the Wisdom of Your Body and Mind to Face Stress, Pain and Illness*. New York: Delacorte Press, 1990.

LeShan, L. *How to Meditate*. New York: Bantam, 1974.

*Levine, S. *A Gradual Awakening*. Garden City, N.Y.: Anchor Books, 1979.

*Loehr, J., and J. Migdow. *Take a Deep Breath*. New York: Villard Books, 1986.

*Nuernberger, P. *Freedom From Stress: A Holistic Approach*. Honesdale, Penn.: Himalayan International Institute of Yoga Science and Philosophy Publishers, 1983.

Woolfolk, R. L., and P. M. Lehrer, eds. *Principles and Practice of Stress Management*. New York: Guilford Press, 1984.

Chapter 5: Eliciting the Relaxation Response

*Achterberg, J. *Imagery in Healing*. Boston: New Science Library, 1985.

Assagioli, R. *Psychosynthesis*. New York: Viking Press, 1965.

Benson, H. *The Relaxation Response*. New York: William Morrow, 1975.

———. *The Mind/Body Effect*. New York: Simon & Schuster, 1979.

———. *Beyond the Relaxation Response*. New York: Times Books, 1984.

———. *Your Maximum Mind*. New York: Times Books, 1987.

Borysenko, J. *Minding the Body, Mending the Mind*. Reading, Mass.: Addison-Wesley, 1987.

Chidvilasananda, Swami. *Kindle My Heart*. South Fallsburg, N.Y.: SYDA Foundation, 1989.

Campbell, J. *The Power of the Myth*. New York: Doubleday, 1988.

*Dossey, L. *Space, Time and Medicine*. Boulder, Colo.: Shambhala Press, 1982.

Fanning, P. *Visualization for Change*. Oakland, Calif.: New Harbinger Publications, 1988.

*Gawain, S. *Creative Visualization*. New York: Bantam, 1978.

Hanh, T. N. *The Miracle of Mindfulness: A Manual on Meditation*. Boston: Beacon Press, 1976.

———. *Peace in Every Step: The Path of Mindfulness in Everyday Life*. New York: Bantam, 1976.

*Levine, S. *A Gradual Awakening*. Garden City, N.Y.: Anchor Books, 1979.

Pelletier, K. *Mind as Healer, Mind as Slayer*. New York: Dell Publishing, 1977.

*Rossman, M. *Healing Yourself*. New York: Walker & Co., 1987; New York: Pocket Books, 1990.

Sujata. *Beginning to See*. Berkeley, Calif.: Celestial Arts Publishing, 1989.

Chapter 6: Tuning In to Your Body, Tuning Up Your Mind

*Bell, L., and E. Seyfer. *Gentle Yoga*. Berkeley, Calif.: Celestial Arts, 1987.

Dayananda, Swami, and J. Vunderink, eds. *Hatha Yoga for Meditators*. South Fallsburg, N.Y.: SYDA Foundation, 1981.

Eckman, P., R. Levenson, and W. Friesen. "Autonomic Nervous Systems Activity Distinguishes Among Emotions." *Science* 221 (1983): 1208–10.

Gubser, N. J. *The Nunamiut Eskimos: Hunter of Caribou*. New Haven, Conn.: Yale University Press, 1965.

Jacobson, E. *Progressive Relaxation*. 2d ed. Chicago: University of Chicago Press, 1938.

Laird, J. D. "Self-Attribution of Emotion: The Effects of Expressive Behavior on the Quality of Emotional Experience." *Journal of Personality and Social Psychology* 29 (1974): 475–86.

———, J. J. Wagener, M. Halal, and M. Szegda. "Remembering What You Feel: Effects of Emotion on Memory." *Journal of Personality and Social Psychology* 42 (1982): 646–57.

Lowen, A. *Bioenergetics*. New York: Penguin Books, 1976.

Nelson, R. K. *Hunters of the Northern Ice*. Chicago: University of Chicago Press, 1969.

*Nuernberger, P. *Freedom from Stress: A Holistic Approach*. Honesdale, Penn.: Himalayan International Institute of Yoga Science and Philosophy, 1983.

Piaget, J., and B. Inhelder. *The Psychology of the Child*. Translated by H. Weaver. New York: Basic Books, 1969.

Sirota, A. D., G. E. Schwartz, and J. L. Kristeller. "Facial Muscle Activity During Induced Mood States: Differential Growth and Carry-over of Elated Versus Depressed Patterns." *Psychophysiology* 24 (1987): 691–99.

*Tobias M., and M. Stewart. *Stretch and Relax*. Los Angeles: Body Press, 1985.

Whatmore, G. B., and R. M. Ellis. "Some Neurophysiologic Aspects of Depressed States." *Archives of General Psychiatry* I (1959): 70–80.

Chapter 7: Move Into Health

American College of Sports Medicine. *Guidelines for Exercise Testing and Prescription*. Philadelphia: Lea & Febiger, 1986.

American Heart Association. *Exercise and Your Heart*. Dallas: American Heart Association, 1984.

*Bailey, C. *Fit or Fat*. Boston: Houghton Mifflin, 1978.

Blair, S., H. Kohl, R. Paffenbarger, D. Clark, K. Cooper, L. Gibbons. "Physical Fitness and All Cause Mortality: A Prospective Study of Healthy Men and Women." *Journal of the American Medical Association* 262 (1989): 2395–2401.

Blumenthal, J., R. Williams, T. Needels, A. Wallace. "Psychological Changes Accompanying Aerobic Exercise in Healthy Middle Aged Adults." *Psychosomatic Medicine* 44 (1982): 529–36.

Borg, G. "Perceived Exertion: A Note on History and Methods." *Medicine and Science in Sports* 5 (1973): 90–93.

Bortz, W. "Use It or Lose It." *Runners World* 25 (1990): 55–58.

———. "Disuse and Aging." *Journal of the American Medical Association* 248 (1982): 1203–06.

Brehm, B. "Elevation of Metabolic Rate Following Exercise: Implications for Weight Loss." *Sports Medicine* 6 (1988): 72–78.

Cady, L., P. Thomas, R. Karwasky. "Program for Increasing Health and Physical Fitness of Fire Fighters." *Journal of Occupational Medicine* 27 (1985): 110–14.

*Cooper, K. *Aerobics*. New York: Bantam, 1969.

*Getchell, B. *Fitness Book*. Indianapolis: Benchmark Press, 1987.

Health Information Library. *Fitness*. Daly City, Calif.: PAS Publishing, 1983.

Jordan, P. "Seven Key Ingredients to the Fitness Recipe." *Personal Fitness and Weight Loss* (Spring 1990): 59–61.

Kannel, W., and P. Sorlie. "Some Health Benefits of Physical Activity. The Framingham Study." *Archives of Internal Medicine* 139 (1979): 857–61.

Kobasa, S., S. Maddi, M. Puccetti, and M. Zola. "Effectiveness of Hardiness, Exercise and Social Support as Resources Against Illness." *Journal of Psychosomatic Research* 29 (1985): 505–33.

Leon, A., J. Connett, D. Jacobs, and R. Rauramaa. "Leisure-Time Physical Activity Levels and Risk of Coronary Heart Disease and Death: The Multiple Risk Factor Intervention Trial." *Journal of the American Medical Association* 258 (1987): 2388–95.

Morris, J. N., M. G. Everitt, R. Pollard, S. P. Chave, and A. M. Semmence. "Vigorous Exercise in Leisure Time: Protection Against Coronary Heart Disease." *Lancet* ii (1980): 1207–10.

Paffenbarger, R. "Contributions of Epidemiology to Exercise, Science and Cardiovascular Health." *Medicine and Science in Sports and Exercise* 20 (1988): 426–38.

Pollack, M., and V. Froelicher. "Position Stand of the American College of Sports Medicine: The Recommended Quantity and Quality of Exercise for Developing and Maintaining Cardiorespiratory and Muscular Fitness in Healthy Adults." *Journal of Cardiopulmonary Rehabilitation* 10 (1990): 235–45.

Rippe, J. M., A. Ward, J. Porcari, and P. Freedson. "Walking for Health and Fitness." *Journal of the American Medical Association* 259 (1988): 2720–24.

*Rippe, J. M., and A. Ward. *Dr. James M. Rippe's Complete Book of Fitness Walking.* New York: Prentice-Hall Press, 1989.

Schatz, M. "Yoga Relief for Arthritis." *Yoga Journal* 11 (1985): 29–34.

————. "Living With Your Lower Back." *Yoga Journal* 10 (1984): 36–45.

Chapter 8: Nutrition for Good Health

Dietary Guidelines for Americans, 3d ed., 1990. Washington, D.C.: U.S. Department of Agriculture and the U.S. Department of Health and Human Services, 1990.

Foreyt, J. P., et al., eds. *Review of Behavior Therapy.* Vol II. New York: Guilford Press (in press).

Kris-Etherton, P. M., D. Krummel, M. E. Russell, D. Dreon, S. MacKey, J. Borchers, and P. D. Wood. "The Effect of Diet on Plasma Lipids, Lipoproteins, and Coronary Heart Disease." *Journal of the American Dietetic Association* 88 (1988): 1373–1400.

Leonard T. K., R. R. Watson, and M. E. Mohs. "The Effects of Caffeine on Various Body Systems: A Review." *Journal of the American Dietetic Association* 87 (1987): 1048–53.

Pennington, J. A. T. *Bowes & Church's Food Values of Portions Commonly Used.* Philadelphia: J. B. Lippincott, 1989.

Shils, M. E., and V. R. Young. *Modern Nutrition in Health and Disease.* Philadelphia: Lea & Febiger, 1988.

U.S. Department of Health and Human Services. *The Surgeon General's Report on Nutrition and Health.* U.S. Government Printing Office, Washington, D.C.: Publication No. 88–50210, 1988.

Chapter 9: A Sensible Approach to Weight Loss

Council on Scientific Affairs, American Medical Association. "Treatment of Obesity in Adults." *Journal of the American Medical Association* 260 (1988): 2547–51.

Dietary Guidelines for Americans, 3d ed., 1990. Washington, D.C.: U.S. Department of Agriculture and the U.S. Department of Health and Human Services, 1990.

Pi-Sunyer, F. X. "Effect of the Composition of the Diet on Energy Intake." *Nutrition Reviews* 48 (1990): 94–105.

Rock, C. L., and A. M. Coulston. "Weight-Control Approaches: A Review by the California Dietetic Association." *Journal of the American Dietetic Association* 88 (1988): 44–48.

Van Itallie, T. B. "Bad News and Good News About Obesity." *New England Journal of Medicine* 314 (1986): 239–40.

Chapter 10: Managing Stress

*Benson, H. *Mind/Body Effect*. New York: Simon and Schuster, 1979.

*Borysenko, J. *Minding the Body, Mending the Mind*. Reading, Mass.: Addison-Wesley, 1987.

*Farquhar, J. W. *The American Way of Life Need Not Be Hazardous To Your Health*. New York: Norton, 1978.

Friedman, M., and R. H. Rosenman. *Type A Behavior and Your Heart*. New York: Alfred A. Knopf, 1974.

Goldberger, L., and S. Breznitz. *Handbook of Stress*. New York: Free Press, 1982.

Greiff, B. "Who Heals the Healers." Keynote address, Massachusetts Health Council Conference, "Stress in the Workplace: How Can We Cope?" Boston, May 5, 1981.

*Kabat-Zinn, J. *Full Catastrophe Living: Using the Wisdom of Your Body and Mind to Face Stress, Pain and Illness*. New York: Delacorte Press, 1990.

Kobasa, S. C., S. R. Maddi, and M. C. Pucretti. "Personality and Exercise as Buffers in the Stress-Illness Relationship." *Journal of Behavioral Medicine*, 5 (1982): 391–404.

Kobasa, S. C., S. R. Maddi, and S. Kahn. "Hardiness and Health: A Prospective Study." *Journal of Personality and Social Psychology* 42 (1982): 168–77.

*Pelletier, K. *Mind as Healer, Mind as Slayer*. New York: Delacorte Press, 1977.

*Selye, H. *The Stress of Life*. New York: McGraw-Hill, 1956.

Vaillant, G. E., and C. Vaillant. "Natural History of Male Psychological Health, XII: A 45-year Study of Predictors of Successful Aging at Age 65." *American Journal of Psychiatry* 147 (1990): 31–37.

*Williams, R. *The Trusting Heart*. New York: Times Books, 1989.

Woolfolk, R. L., and P. M. Lehrer, eds. *Principles and Practice of Stress Management*. New York: Guilford Press, 1984.

Yerkes, R. M., and J. D. Dodson. "The Relation of Strength of Stimulus to Rapidity of Habit-Formation." *Journal of Comparative Neurology and Psychology* 18 (1908): 459–82.

Chapter 11: How Thoughts Affect Health

Beck, A. *Cognitive Therapy and the Emotional Disorders*. New York: International Universities Press, 1976.

Burns, D. D. *The Feeling Good Handbook: Using the New Mood Therapy in Everyday Life*. New York: William Morrow, 1989.

*Carson, R. D. *Never Get a Tattoo,* New York: Harper & Row, 1990.

*_____. *Taming Your Gremlin.* New York: Harper & Row, 1983.

Davis, M., E. Eshelman, and M. McKay. *The Relaxation and Stress Reduction Workbook.* 3rd ed. Oakland, Calif.: New Harbinger Publications, 1988.

Ellis, A., and R. Greiger. *Handbook of Rational Emotive Therapy.* New York: Springer, 1977.

*Fulghum, R. *All I Really Need to Know I Learned in Kindergarten: Uncommon Thoughts on Common Things.* New York: Villard Books, 1986.

*Lazarus, A. A. *Behavior Therapy and Beyond.* New York: McGraw-Hill, 1972.

Meichenbaum, D. *Cognitive Behavior Modification: An Integrative Approach.* New York: Plenum Press, 1977.

_____. *Stress Inoculation Training.* New York: Pergamon Press, 1985.

Rimm, D. C., and J. C. Masters. *Behavior Therapy: Techniques and Empirical Findings.* Orlando, Fla.: Academic Press, 1979.

*Winn, D. *The Manipulated Mind.* London: Octagon Press, 1983.

Chapter 12: Feelings, Moods, and Attitudes

*Borysenko, J. *Guilt Is the Teacher, Love Is the Lesson.* New York: Warner Books, 1990.

Bower, S. A., and G. Bower. *Asserting Yourself: A Practical Guide for Positive Change.* Reading, Mass.: Addison-Wesley, 1976.

Burns, D. D. *The Feeling Good Handbook: Using the New Mood Therapy in Everyday Life.* New York: William Morrow, 1989.

Friedman, H. S., and M. R. DiMatteo. *Health Psychology.* Englewood Cliffs, N.J.: Prentice Hall, 1989.

Friedman, M., and D. Ulmer. *Treating Type A Behavior and Your Heart.* New York: Knopf, 1984.

*Jeffers, S. *Feel the Fear and Do It Anyway.* San Diego, Calif.: Harcourt, Brace, Jovanovich, 1987.

*Lerner, H. G. *The Dance of Anger: A Woman's Guide to Changing the Patterns of Intimate Relationships.* New York: Harper & Row, 1985.

Maddi, S. R., and S. Kobasa. *The Hardy Executive: Health under Stress.* Chicago: Dorsey Professional Books, 1984.

*McKay, M., and P. Fanning. *Self-Esteem: A Proven Program of Cognitive Techniques for Assessing, Improving and Maintaining Your Self-esteem.* Oakland, Calif.: New Harbinger Publications, 1987.

Peterson, C., M. E. Seligman, and G. E. Vaillant. "Pessimistic Explanatory Style Is a Risk Factor for Physical Illness: A Thirty-Five-Year Longitudinal Study." *Journal of Personality and Social Psychology* 55:1 (1988): 23–27.

Tubesing, N., and D. Tubesing, eds. *Structured Exercises in Stress Management.* Volume II. Duluth, Minn.: Whole Person Press, 1990.

Vaillant, G. E., and C. Vaillant. "Natural History of Male Psychological Health, XII: A 45-Year Study of Predictors of Successful Aging at Age 65." *American Journal of Psychiatry* 147 (1990): 31–37.

Williams R. *The Trusting Heart.* New York: Times Books, 1989.

Chapter 13: Coping and Problem-Solving

Benson, H. *Your Maximum Mind*. New York: Times Books, 1987.

Frankl, V. *Man's Search for Meaning*. Boston: Beacon Press, 1963.

Jeffers, S., *Feel The Fear and Do It Anyway*. San Diego, Calif.: Harcourt, Brace, Jovanovich, 1987.

Kobasa, S. C., S. R. Maddi, and S. Kahn. "Hardiness and Health: A Prospective Study." *Journal of Personality and Social Psychology* 42 (1982): 168–77.

Lazarus, R. S., and S. Folkman. *Stress, Appraisal and Coping*. New York: Springer Publishing Company, 1984.

*Lynch, J. J. *The Broken Heart: The Medical Consequences of Loneliness*. New York: Basic Books, 1977.

*Meichenbaum, D. *Cognitive Behavior Modification: An Integrative Approach*. New York: Plenum Press, 1977.

Orth-Gomer, K., A. L. Unden, and M. E. Edwards. "Social Isolation and Mortality in Ischemic Heart Disease: A Ten-Year Follow-up Study of 150 Middle-aged Men." *Acta Medica Scandinavica* 224 (1988): 205–15.

*Pennebaker, J. W., J. K. Kiecolt-Glaser, and R. Glaser. "Disclosure of Traumas and Immune Function: Health Implications for Psychotherapy." *Journal of Consulting and Clinical Psychology* 56 (1988): 239–45.

Ray, M., and R. Myers, *Creativity in Business*. New York: Doubleday, 1986.

Spiegel, D., J. R. Bloom, H. C. Kraemer, and E. Gottheil. "Effect of Psychosocial Treatment on Survival of Patients with Metastatic Breast Cancer." *Lancet* ii (1989): 888–91.

Chapter 14: Communicating

*Blanchard, K., and S. Johnson. *The One Minute Manager*. New York: Berkley Books, 1983.

*Blanchard, K., and R. Lorber. *Putting the One Minute Manager to Work*. New York: Berkley Books, 1985.

Burns, D. D. *The Feeling Good Handbook: Using the New Mood Therapy in Everyday Life*. New York: William Morrow, 1989.

*Fisher, R., and W. Ury. *Getting to Yes: Negotiating Agreement Without Giving In*. New York: Penguin Books, 1983.

*Tannen, D. *You Just Don't Understand: Women and Men in Conversation*. New York: William Morrow, 1990.

Chapter 15: Jest 'n' Joy

*Barry, D. *Dave Barry's Guide to Marriage and/or Sex*. Emmaus, Penn.: Rodale Press, 1987. Also, all other works by Dave Barry.

Berk, L. S., S. A. Tan, W. F. Fry, B. J. Napier, J. W. Lee, R. W. Hubbard, J. E. Lewis, and W. C. Eby. "Neuroendocrine and Stress Hormone Changes During Mirthful Laughter." *American Journal of the Medical Sciences* 298 (1989): 390–96.

*Bombeck, E. *Family—The Ties That Bind . . . And Gag!* New York: Fawcett Press, 1987. Also, all other works by Erma Bombeck.

*Brilliant, A. *I May Not Be Totally Perfect, But Parts of Me Are Excellent.* Santa Barbara, Calif.: Woodbridge Press, 1988.

Cogan, R., D. Cogan, W. Waltz, and M. McCue. "Effects of Laughter and Relaxation on Discomfort Thresholds." *Journal of Behavioral Medicine* 10 (1987): 139–44.

Cohen, M. "Caring for Ourselves Can Be Funny Business." *Holistic Nursing Practice* 4 (1990): 1–11.

*Cousins, N. *Anatomy of an Illness.* New York: W. W. Norton, 1979.

Ekman, P., R. W. Levenson, and W. V. Friesen. "Autonomic Nervous System Activity Distinguishes Among Emotions." *Science* 221 (1983): 1208–10.

*The Humor Project—a clearinghouse for theory, research, and practical ideas related to humor—publishes *Laughing Matters Magazine.* Address: 110 Spring St., Saratoga Springs, N.Y. 12866; or phone (518) 587-8770.

*Klein, A. *The Healing Power of Humor.* Los Angeles: Jeremy P. Tarcher, 1989.

Peterson, C., M. E. Seligman, and G. E. Vaillant. "Pessimistic Explanatory Style Is a Risk Factor for Physical Illness: A Thirty-Five-Year Longitudinal Study." *Journal of Personality and Social Psychology* 55 (1988): 23–27.

Poland, W. S. "The Gift of Laughter: On the Development of a Sense of Humor in Clinical Analysis." *Psychoanalytic Quarterly* 59 (1990): 197–225.

Vaillant, G. E. *Adaptation to Life.* Boston: Little, Brown, 1977.

Yovetich, N. A., J. A. Dale, and M. A. Hudak. "Benefits of Humor in Reduction of Threat-Induced Anxiety." *Psychological Reports* 66 (1990): 51–58.

Chapter 16: Improving Your Sleep

Bootzin, R. R., M. Engle-Friedman, and L. Hazelwood. "Insomnia." In *Clinical Geropsychology: New Directions in Assessment and Treatment,* edited by P. M. Lewinsohn and L. Teri. New York: Pergamon Press, 1983.

Campbell, S. S., and J. Zulley. "Ultradian Components of Human Sleep/Wake Patterns during Disentrainment." *Experimental Brain Research* Supplement 12 (1985): 234–55.

Hauri, P. *The Sleep Disorders.* Kalamazoo: The Upjohn Company, 1982.

————, and S. Linde. *No More Sleepless Nights.* New York: John Wiley and Sons, 1990.

Jacobs, G. D., and J. F. Lubar. "Spectral Analysis of the Central Nervous System Effects of the Relaxation Response Elicited by Autogenic Training." *Behavioral Medicine* 15 (1989): 125–32.

Jacobs, G., D. Rosenberg, R. Friedman, J. Matheson, G. Peavy, A. Domar, and H. Benson. "Multifactor Behavioral Treatment of Chronic Sleep-Onset Insomnia Using Stimulus Control and the Relaxation Response." (Submitted for publication.)

Lacks, P. *Behavioral Treatment for Persistent Insomnia.* New York: Pergamon Press, 1987.

Lichstein, K. L., and S. M. Fischer. "Insomnia." In *Handbook of Clinical Behavior Therapy With Adults,* edited by M. Hersen and A. S. Bellack. New York: Plenum Publishing, 1985.

Lichstein, K. L., and T. L. Rosenthal. "Insomniacs' Perceptions of Cognitive Versus Somatic Determinants of Sleep Disturbance." *Journal of Abnormal Psychology* 89 (1980): 105–07.

Reynolds, C. F. "The Implications of Sleep Disturbance Epidemiology." *Journal of the American Medical Association* 262 (1989): 1514.

Sewitch, D. "Slow Wave Sleep Deficiency Insomnia: A Problem in Thermo-Down Regulation at Sleep Onset." *Psychophysiology* 24 (1987): 200–15.

Stampi, C. "Ultrashort Sleep/Wake Patterns and Sustained Performance." In *Sleep and Alertness: Chronobiological, Behavioral and Medical Aspects of Napping,* edited by D. Dinges and R. Broughton. New York: Raven Press, 1989.

Stepanski, E., F. Zorick, T. Roehrs, D. Young, and T. Roth. "Daytime Alertness in Patients With Chronic Insomnia Compared With Asymptomatic Control Subjects." *Sleep* 11 (1988): 54–60.

Sugerman, J., J. Stern, and J. Walsh. "Daytime Alertness in Subjective and Objective Insomnia: Some Preliminary Findings." *Biological Psychiatry* 20 (1985): 741–50.

Chapter 17: Infertility and Women's Health

*Collins, J., and T. Rowe. "Age of the Female Partner Is a Prognostic Factor in Prolonged Unexplained Infertility: A Multicenter Study." *Fertility and Sterility* 52 (1989): 15–20.

*Domar, A. D., and M. Seibel. "Emotional Aspects of Infertility." In *Infertility: A Comprehensive Text,* edited by M. Seibel. Norwalk, Conn.: Appleton and Lange, 1990.

*Domar, A. D., et al. "The Mind/Body Program for Infertility: A New Behavioral Treatment Approach for Women With Infertility." *Fertility and Sterility* 53 (1990): 246–49.

Frisch, M., and G. Rapoport. *Getting Pregnant.* Tuscon: Body Press, 1987.

*Germaine, L., and R. Freedman. "Behavioral Treatment of Menopausal Hot Flashes: Evaluation of Objective Methods." *Journal of Consulting and Clinical Psychology* 52 (1984): 1072–79.

Glazer, E. *The Long-Awaited Stork: A Guide to Parenting After Infertility.* Lexington, Mass.: Lexington Books, 1990.

*Greenwood, S. *Menopause Naturally: Preparing for the Second Half of Life.* Volcano, Calif.: Volcano Press, 1989.

Harkness, C. *The Infertility Book: A Comprehensive Medical and Emotional Guide.* San Francisco: Volcano Press, 1987.

Nachtigall, R., and E. Mehren. *Overcoming Infertility.* New York: Doubleday, 1991.

*Omer, H., et al. "Life Stresses and Premature Labor: Real Connection or Artificial Findings?" *Psychosomatic Medicine* 48 (1986): 362–69.

Salzer, L. *Infertility: How Couples Can Cope.* Boston: G. K. Hall, 1986.

Stangel, J. *The New Fertility and Conception.* New York: Plume Books, 1988.

*Sturdee, D. "Hormone Replacement Therapy: Risks and Benefits." *Practitioner* 234 (1990): 471–74.

*Swartzman, L., R. Edelberg, and E. Kemmann. "Impact of Stress on Objectively Recorded Menopausal Hot Flushes and on Flush Report Bias." *Health Psychology* 9 (1990): 529–45.

Wells, J., et al. "Presurgical Anxiety and Postsurgical Pain and Adjustment: Effects of a Stress Inoculation Procedure." *Journal of Consulting and Clinical Psychology* 54 (1986): 831–35.

Chapter 18: Behavioral Medicine and Cancer

Achterberg, J. *Imagery in Healing.* Boston: New Science Library, 1985.

Borysenko, J. *Guilt Is the Teacher, Love Is the Lesson.* New York: Warner Books, 1990.
_____. *Minding the Body, Mending the Mind.* Reading, Mass.: Addison-Wesley, 1987.

Casarjian, R., and N. Reiselle. *The Stress Reducer.* Boston: Sound Discoveries, 1983.

Cella, D. F. "Health Promotion in Oncology: A Cancer Wellness Doctrine." *Journal of Psychosocial Oncology* 8 (1990): 17–31.

*Cunningham, A. J. *Helping Yourself.* Toronto: Ontario Cancer Institute, 1989.

Greer, S., and M. Watson. "Mental Adjustment to Cancer: Its Management and Prognostic Importance." *Cancer Surveys* 6 (1987) 439–53.

LeShan, L. *Cancer as a Turning Point.* New York: Plume Books, 1990.

Locke, S., and D. Colligan. *The Healer Within.* New York and Scarborough, Ont.: Mentor Books, 1987.

Love, S. M., and K. Lindsey. *Dr. Susan Love's Breast Book.* Reading, Mass.: Addison-Wesley, 1990.

Radner, G. *It's Always Something.* New York: Simon & Schuster, 1989.

Rossman, M. L. *Healing Yourself.* New York: Walker and Co., 1987.

Schaef, A. W. *Medications for Women Who Do Too Much.* New York: Harper & Row, 1990.

Siegel, B. *Love, Medicine and Miracles.* New York: Harper & Row, 1986.

Simonton, D. C., S. Matthews-Simonton, and J. Creighton. *Getting Well Again.* Los Angeles: Jeremy P. Tarcher, 1978; New York: Bantam, 1980.

*Spiegel, D., J. R. Bloom, H. C. Kraemer, and E. Gottheil. "Effect of Psychosocial Treatment on Survival of Patients With Metastatic Breast Cancer." *Lancet* ii (1989): 888–91.

Williams, W. *The Power Within.* New York: Harper & Row, 1990.

Chapter 19: Eating Healthfully to Prevent Undernutrition

American Cancer Society. "Unproven Methods of Cancer Management: Macrobiotic Diets for the Treatment of Cancer." *CA—A Cancer Journal for Clinicians* 39 (1989): 248–51.

American Cancer Society. *Cancer Manual,* 8th ed. Boston: American Cancer Society, Massachusetts Division, Inc., 1990.

American Dietetic Association. "Position of the American Dietetic Association: Vegetarian Diets." *Journal of the American Dietetic Association* 88 (1988): 351–55.

Beisel, W. R., R. Edelman, K. Nauss, and R. M. Suskind. "Single-Nutrient Effects on Immunologic Functions." *Journal of the American Medical Association* 245 (1981): 53–58.

Blackburn, G. L., B. S. Maini, B. R. Bistrian, and W. V. McDermott, Jr. "The Effect of Cancer on Nitrogen, Electrolyte, and Mineral Metabolism." *Cancer Research* 37 (1977): 2348–53.

*Brody, J. E. *Jane Brody's Nutrition Book.* New York: W. W. Norton, 1987.

Cahill, G. F., Jr. "Starvation in Man." *New England Journal of Medicine* 282 (1970): 668–75.

Centers for Disease Control. "Revision of the Centers for Disease Control Surveillance Definition for Acquired Immunodeficiency Syndrome." *Morbidity and Mortality Weekly Review* 36 (1987) (1S): 3S–15S.

Chandra, R. K. "Immunodeficiency in Undernutrition and Overnutrition." *Nutrition Review* 39 (1981): 225–31.

_____. "Nutrition, Immunity and Infection: Present Knowledge and Future Directions." *Lancet* i (1983): 688–91.

Cunningham-Rundles, S. "Effects of Nutritional Status on Immunological Function." *American Journal of Clinical Nutrition* 35 (1982): 1202–10.

*Kelly, K. "An Overview of How to Nourish the Cancer Patient by Mouth." *Cancer* 58 (Suppl.) (1986): 1897–1901.

Kotler, D. P., A. R. Tierney, J. Wang, and R. N. Pierson, Jr. "Magnitude of Body-Cell-Mass Depletion and the Timing of Death from Wasting in AIDS." *American Journal of Clinical Nutrition* 50 (1989): 444–47.

Lertzman, M. M., and R. M. Cherniak. "Rehabilitation of Patients With Chronic Obstructive Pulmonary Disease." *American Review of Respiratory Disease* 114 (1976): 1145–65.

Levine, A. S., and G. K. W. Yim. "Neuropeptidergic Regulation of Food Intake." *Federation Proceedings* 43 (1984): 2888–2906.

*Mayer, J. *Dr. Jean Mayer's Diet and Nutrition Guide.* New York: Pharos Books, 1990.

Myrvik, Q. N. "Nutrition and Immunology." In *Modern Nutrition in Health and Disease,* edited by M. E. Shils and V. R. Young. Philadelphia: Lea & Febiger, 1988.

Pietsch, J. B., and J. L. Meakins. "Predicting Infection in Surgical Patients." *Surgical Clinics of North America* 59 (1979): 185–97.

Prasad, A. S., et al. "Hypocupremia Induced by Zinc Therapy in Adults." *Journal of American Medical Association* 240 (1979): 2166–68.

Roe, D. A. *Drug-Induced Nutritional Deficiencies.* Westport, Conn.: AVI Publishing, 1985.

Shils, M. E. "Nutrition and Diet in Cancer." In *Modern Nutrition in Health and Disease,* edited by M. E. Shils and V. R. Young. Philadelphia: Lea & Febiger, 1988.

Office of Technology Assessment, U. S. Congress. *Unconventional Cancer Treatments,* OTA-H-405. Washington, D.C.: U.S. Government Printing Office, September 1990.

U. S. Department of Health and Human Services, Public Health Service, National Institutes of Health National Cancer Institute. "Eating Hints—Recipes and Tips for Better Nutrition During Cancer Treatment." NIH Publication No. 91–2079, Revised April 1990.

Visintainer, M. A., J. R. Volpicelli, and M. E. P. Seligman. "Tumor Rejection in Rats After Inescapable or Escapable Shock." *Science* 216 (1982): 437–39.

Webster, A., L. Stolbach, and R. Friedman. "Personality Characteristics Do Not Identify Patients at Risk for Developing Anticipatory Nausea and Vomiting due to Chemotherapy." Abstract presented at Poster Session, Society of Behavioral Medicine Meeting, Tenth Anniversary Meeting, San Francisco, 1989.

Chapter 20: Psychoneuroimmunology and HIV Disease

Antoni, M., N. Schneiderman, M. Fletcher, D. Goldstein, G. Ironson, and A. Laperriere. "Psychoneuroimmunology and HIV-1." *Journal of Consulting and Clinical Psychology* 58 (1990): 38–49.

Food and Drug Administration. *Eating Defensively: Food Safety Advice for Persons with AIDS* [film]. Rockville, Md.: FDA Office of Public Affairs Communications, (1989).

Frankl, V. *Man's Search for Meaning.* Boston: Beacon Press, 1963.

Kiecolt-Glaser, J. K., and R. Glaser. "Psychological Influences on Immunity." *American Psychologist* 43 (1988): 892–98.

Kiecolt-Glaser, J. K., L. Fisher, P. Ogrocki, J. Stout, C. Speicher, and R. Glaser. "Marital Quality, Marital Disruption, and Immune Function." *Psychosomatic Medicine* 49 (1987): 13–34.

Kiecolt-Glaser, J. K., W. Garner, C. Speicher, G. Penn, and R. Glaser. "Psychological Modifiers of Immunocompetence in Medical Students." *Psychosomatic Medicine* 46 (1984): 7–14.

Kiecolt-Glaser, J. K., R. Glaser, D. Welliger, J. Stout, G. Messick, S. Sheppard, D. Ricker, S. Romisher, W. Briner, G. Bonnell, and R. Donnerberg. "Psychosocial Enhancement of Immunocompetence in a Geriatric Population." *Health Psychology* 4 (1985): 25–41.

Levy, S., J. Lee, M. Lippman, and T. DeAngelo. "Survival Hazards Analysis in First Recurrent Breast Cancer Patients: Seven-Year Follow-up." *Psychosomatic Medicine* 50 (1988): 520–28.

*Pennebaker, J., J. K. Kiecolt-Glaser, and R. Glaser. "Disclosure of Traumas and Immune Function: Health Implications for Psychotherapy." *Journal of Consulting and Clinical Psychology* 56 (1988): 239–45.

Solomon, G. F., L. Temoshok, A. O'Leary, J. Zich. "An Intensive psychoimmunologic Study of Long-Surviving Persons With AIDS." *Annals of the New York Academy of Sciences* 496 (1987): 647–55.

Weiss, J. M., S. K. Sundar, K. J. Becker, and M. A. Cierpial. "Behavioral and Neural Influences on Cellular Immune Responses: Effects of Stress and Interleukin-1." *Journal of Clinical Psychiatry* 50 Suppl. (1989): 43–53.

Chapter 21: Cardiovascular Disease: The Heart of the Matter

Advanced Therapeutics Communications. "Cardiac Risk Factor Questionnaire," from "New Approaches to Cardiovascular Risk Management: A Mandate for the 90's." In *Highlights of the Saddlebrook Symposium: Reducing Cardiovascular Risk Factors in the Hypertensive Patient*. Physicians World Communications, P.O. Box 1505, Secaucus, N.J. 07096–1505, 1988.

Baum, C., D. L. Kennedy, M. B. Forbes, and J. K. Jones. "Drug Use and Expenditures in 1982." *Journal of the American Medical Association* 253 (1985): 382–86.

Blair, S. N., H. W. Kohl, R. S. Paffenbarger, D. G. Clark, K. H. Cooper, and L. W. Gibbons. "Physical Fitness and All-Cause Mortality: A Prospective Study of Healthy Men and Women." *Journal of the American Medical Association* 262 (1989): 2395–2401.

Brown, G., J. J. Albers, L. D. Fisher, S. M. Schaefer, J. T. Lin, C. Kaplan, X. Q. Zhao, B. D. Bisson, V. F. Fitzpatrick, and H. T. Dodge. "Regression of Coronary Artery Disease as a Result of Intensive Lipid-lowering Therapy in Men With High Levels of Apolipoprotein B." *New England Journal of Medicine* 323 (1990): 1289–98.

Burke, G. L., M. Sprafka, A. R. Folsom, L. P. Hahn, R. V. Luepker, and H. Blackburn. "Trends in Serum Cholesterol Levels From 1980 to 1987: The Minnesota Heart Survey." *New England Journal of Medicine* 324 (1991): 941–46.

Casscells, W., C. H. Hennekens, D. Evans, B. Rosener, R. A. DeSilva, B. Lown, J. E. Davies, and M. J. Jesse. "Retirement and Coronary Mortality." *Lancet* i (1980): 1288–89.

Cooper, M. J., and M. M. Aygen. "A Relaxation Technique in the Management of Hypercholesterolemia." *Journal of Human Stress* 5 (1979): 24–27.

Cottington, E. M., K. A. Matthews, E. Talbott, and L. H. Kuller. "Environmental Events Preceding Sudden Death in Women." *Psychosomatic Medicine* 42 (1980): 567–74.

Dawber, T. R. *The Framingham Study: The Epidemiology of Atherosclerotic Disease*. Cambridge: Mass.: Harvard University Press, 1980.

Deanfield, J. E., M. Shea, M. Kensett, et al. "Silent Myocardial Ischemia due to Mental Stress." *Lancet* ii (1984): 1001–5.

DeSilva, R. A. "Psychological Stress and Sudden Cardiac Death." In *Biological and Psychological Factors in Cardiovascular Disease*, edited by T. H. Schmidt, T. M. Dembroski, and G. Blumchen. Berlin: Springer-Verlag, 1986.

Frasure-Smith, N. "In-Hospital Symptoms of Psychological Stress as Predictors of Long-Term Outcome After Acute Myocardial Infarction in Men." *American Journal of Cardiology* 67 (1991): 121–27.

————, and R. Prince. "The Ischemic Heart Disease Life Stress Monitoring Program: Impact on Mortality." *Psychosomatic Medicine* 47 (1985): 431–45.

————. "Long-Term Follow-Up of the Ischemic Heart Disease Life Stress Monitoring Program." *Psychosomatic Medicine* 51 (1989): 485–513.

Friedman, M., and R. Rosenman. *Type A Behavior and Your Heart*. New York: Alfred A. Knopf, 1974.

Friedman, M., C. E. Thoresen, J. J. Gill, L. H. Powell, V. A. Price, B. Brown, L. Thompson, D. D. Rabin, W. S. Breall, et al. "Alteration of Type A Behavior and Its Effect on Cardiac Recurrences in Post Myocardial Infarction Patients: Summary Results of the Recurrent Coronary Prevention Project." *American Heart Journal* 112 (1986): 653–65.

Friedman, M., and D. Ulmer. *Treating Type A Behavior and Your Heart.* New York: Fawcett Crest, 1984.

Friedman, M., L. H. Powell, C. E. Thoresen, D. Ulmer, V. A. Price, J. J. Gill, L. Thompson, D. D. Rabin, B. Brown, W. S. Breall, et al. "Effect of Discontinuance of Type A Behavioral Counseling on Type A Behavior and Cardiac Recurrence Rate of Post Myocardial Infarction Patients." *American Heart Journal* 114 (1987): 483–90.

Grundy, S. M., and A. C. Griffin. "Relationship of Periodic Mental Stress to Serum Lipoprotein and Cholesterol Levels." *Journal of the American Medical Association* 171 (1959): 1794–96.

Haft, J. I. "Role of Blood Platelets in Coronary Artery Disease." *American Journal of Cardiology* 43 (1979): 1197–1206.

House, J. S., K. R. Landis, and D. Umberson. "Social Relationships and Health." *Science* 241 (1988): 540–45.

Jenkins, C. D. "Recent Evidence Supporting Psychologic and Social Risk Factors for Coronary Disease." *New England Journal of Medicine* 294 (1976): 987–94; 1033–38.

Joint National Committee on Detection, Evaluation, and Treatment of High Blood Pressure. "The 1988 Report of the Joint National Committee on Detection, Evaluation, and Treatment of High Blood Pressure." *Archives of Internal Medicine* 148 (1988): 1023–38.

Kobasa, S. "Stressful Life Events, Personality, and Health: An Inquiry Into Hardiness." *Journal of Personality and Social Psychology* 37 (1979): 1–11.

Lee, D. D., V. DeQuattro, J. Allen, S. Kimura, E. Aleman, G. Konugres, and G. Davison. "Behavioral vs. Beta-Blocker Therapy in Patients with Primary Hypertension: Effects on Blood Pressure, Left Ventricular Function and Mass, and the Pressor Surge of Social Stress Anger." *American Heart Journal* 116 (1988): 637–44.

Leserman, J., E. M. Stuart, M. E. Mamish, J. P. Deckro, R. J. Beckman, R. F. Friedman, and H. Benson. "Nonpharmacologic Intervention for Hypertension: Long-Term Follow-Up." *Journal of Cardiopulmonary Rehabilitation* 9 (1989): 316–24.

Lown, B., R. A. DeSilva, P. Reich, and B. S. Murawski. "Psychophysiologic Factors in Sudden Cardiac Death." *American Journal of Psychiatry* 137 (1980): 1325–35.

McKool, K. "Facilitating Smoking Cessation." *Journal of Cardiovascular Nursing* 1 (1987): 28–40.

Medalie, J. H., and U. Goldbourt. "Angina Pectoris Among 10,000 Men, II: Psychosocial and Other Risk Factors as Evidenced by a Multivariate Analysis of a Five-Year Incidence Study." *American Journal of Medicine* 60 (1976): 910–21.

Muller, J. E., G. H. Tofler, and P. H. Stone. "Circadian Variation and Triggers of Onset of Acute Cardiovascular Disease." *Circulation* 79 (1989): 733–43.

Muranaka, M., H. Monou, J. Suzuki, J. D. Lane, N. B. Anderson, C. M. Kuhn, S. M. Schanberg, N. McCown, and R. B. Williams, Jr. "Physiological Responses to

Catecholamine Infusions in Type A and Type B Men." *Health Psychology* 7 Suppl. (1988): 145–63.

National Center for Health Statistics. "Annual Summary of Births, Marriages, Divorces, and Deaths: United States, 1989." *Monthly Vital Statistics Report* 38 (13). Hyattsville, Md.: Public Health Service, 1990.

National Cholesterol Education Program. *Report of the Expert Panel on Detection, Evaluation and Treatment of High Blood Cholesterol in Adults.* United States Department of Health and Human Services; Public Health Service, National Institutes of Health; NIH Pub. No. 89–2925, January 1989.

National Institutes of Health. "Nurses: Help Your Patients Stop Smoking." Public Health Service, USDHHS, NIH Pub. No. 90–2962, 1990.

Ockene, J. K., L. H. Kuller, K. H. Svendsen, and E. Meilahn. "The Relationship of Smoking Cessation to Coronary Heart Disease and Lung Cancer in the Multiple Risk Factor Intervention Trial (MRFIT)." *American Journal of Public Health* 80 (1990): 954–58.

Ornish, D. "Can Life-style Changes Reverse Coronary Atherosclerosis? *Hospital Practice* (1991): 107–14.

———. *Dr. Dean Ornish's Program for Reversing Heart Disease.* New York: Random House, 1990.

———. S. E. Brown, L. W. Scherwitz, J. H. Billings, W. T. Armstrong, T. A. Ports, S. M. McLanahan, R. L. Kirkeeide, R. J. Brand, and K. L. Gould. "Can Lifestyle Changes Reverse Coronary Heart Disease? The Lifestyle Heart Trial." *Lancet* 336 (1990): 129–33.

Orth-Gomer, K., A. L. Unden, and M. E. Edwards. "Social Isolation and Mortality in Ischemic Heart Disease: A Ten-Year Follow-up Study of 150 Middle-aged Men." *Acta Medica Scandinavica* 224 (1988): 205–15.

Osler, W. "The Lumleian Lectures on Angina Pectoris." *Lancet* (1910), March 12: 697–702; March 26: 839–44; April 9: 973–7.

Paffenbarger, R. S., R. T. Hyde, A. L. Wing, and C. Hsieh. "Physical Activity, All-Cause Mortality, and Longevity of College Alumni." *New England Journal of Medicine* 314 (1986): 605–13.

Patel, C., M. G. Marmot, D. J. Terry, M. Carruthers, B. Hunt, and M. Patel. "Trial of Relaxation in Reducing Coronary Risk: Four-Year Follow-up." *British Medical Journal* 290 (1985): 1103–06.

Pennebaker, J. W. *Opening Up the Healing Power of Confiding in Others.* New York: William Morrow, 1990.

Pickering, T. G., G. D. James, C. Boddie, G. A. Harshfield, S. Blank, and J. H. Laragh. "How Common Is White-Coat Hypertension?" *Journal of the American Medical Association* 259 (1988): 225–28.

Reed, D. W., D. McGee, K. Yano, and M. Feinleib. "Social Networks and Coronary Heart Disease Among Japanese Men in Hawaii." *American Journal of Epidemiology* 117 (1983): 38–96.

Rees, W. D., S. G. Lutkins. "Mortality of Bereavement." *British Medical Journal* 4 (1967): 13–16.

Rosenberg, L., J. R. Palmer, and S. Shapiro. "Decline in the Risk of Myocardial Infarction Among Women Who Stop Smoking." *New England Journal of Medicine* 322 (1990): 213–17.

Rosengren, A., L. Wilhelmsen, L. Welin, A. Tsipogianni, A. Teger-Nilsson, and H. Wedel. "Social Influences and Cardiovascular Risk Factors as Determinants of Plasma Fibrinogen Concentration in a General Population Sample of Middle-Aged Men." *British Medical Journal* 300 (1990): 634–38.

Rozanski, A., C. N. Bairey, D. S. Krantz, J. Friedman, K. J. Resser, M. Morell, S. Hilton-Chalfen, L. Hestrin, J. Bietendorf, and D. S. Berman. "Mental Stress and the Induction of Silent Myocardial Ischemia in Patients With Coronary Artery Disease." *New England Journal of Medicine* 318 (1988): 1005–12.

Ruberman, W., E. Weinblatt, J. D. Goldberg, and B. S. Chaudhary. "Psychosocial Influences on Mortality After Myocardial Infarction." *New England Journal of Medicine* 311 (1984): 552–59.

Scherwitz, L., L. Perkins, M. Chesney, and G. Hughes. "Cook-Medley Hostility Scale and Subsets: Relationship to Demographic and Psychosocial Characteristics in Young Adults in the CARDIA Study." *Psychosomatic Medicine* 53 (1991): 36–49.

Schnall, P. L., C. Pieper, J. E. Schwartz, R. A. Karasek, Y. Schlussel, R. B. Devereux, A. Ganau, M. Alderman, K. Warren, and T. G. Pickering. "The Relationship Between 'Job Strain,' Workplace Diastolic Blood Pressure, and Left Ventricular Mass Index: Results of a Case-Control Study." *Journal of the American Medical Association* 263 (1990): 1929–35.

Selwyn, A. P., M. Shea, J. E. Deanfield, R. Wilson, and P. Horlock. "Character of Transient Ischemia in Angina Pectoris." *American Journal of Cardiology* 58 (1986): 21B–25B.

Siegler, I. C., B. L. Peterson, J. C. Barefoot, W. G. Dahlstrom, E. C. Suarez, and R. B. Williams. "Hostility Levels at Age 19 Predict Lipid Risk Profile at Age 42." *Circulation* 82 (1990): III–228.

Suarez, E. C., and R. B. Williams, Jr. "The Relationships Between Dimensions of Hostility and Cardiovascular Reactivity as a Function of Task Characteristics." *Psychosomatic Medicine* 52 (1990): 558–70.

Sytkowski, P. A., W. B. Kannel, and R. B. D'Agostino. "Changes in Risk Factors and the Decline in Mortality From Cardiovascular Disease."*New England Journal of Medicine* 322 (1990): 1635–41.

Unden, A. L., K. Orth-Gomer, and S. Elofsson. "Cardiovascular Effects of Social Support in the Work Place: Twenty-Four-Hour ECG Monitoring of Men and Women." *Psychosomatic Medicine* 53 (1991): 50–60.

United States Department of Health and Human Services, Public Health Service, Office on Smoking and Health. *The Health Consequences of Smoking: Cardiovascular Disease, PHS Pub 84–50204.* Washington, D.C. 1983.

United States Pharmacopoeial Convention, Inc. *About Your High Blood Pressure Medicines,* 3rd ed. Rockville, Md.: The United States Pharmacopoeial Convention, Inc., 1989.

Williams, J., and G. Edwards. "The Death of John Hunter." *Journal of the American Medical Association* 204 (1968): 806–09.

Williams, R. B. *The Trusting Heart.* New York: Times Books, 1989.

Working Group on Physician Behaviors to Reduce Smoking Among Hypertensive Patients. *The Physician's Guide: How to Help Your Hypertensive Patients Stop Smoking.* National High Blood Pressure Education Program, National Heart, Lung and Blood Institute, USDHHS. National Institutes of Health Pub. No. 83–1271. Washington, D.C., 1983.

Chapter 22: Living With Heart Disease and Diabetes: Exercise Can Help

*American Health Foundation. *The Book of Health*. New York: Franklin Watts, 1981.

*Bierman, J., and B. Tookey. *The Diabetics Total Health Book*. Los Angeles: Jeremy P. Tarcher, 1988.

Blair, S. N., H. W. Kohl, R. S. Paffenbarger, D. G. Clark, K. H. Cooper, and L. W. Gibbons. "Physical Fitness and All-Cause Mortality: A Prospective Study of Healthy Men and Women." *Journal of the American Medical Association* 262 (1989): 2395–2401.

Ekoe, J. M. "Overview of Diabetes Mellitus and Exercise. "*Medicine and Science in Sports and Exercise* 21 (1989): 353–55.

Fitness, Health, Nutrition Series. Alexandria, Va.: Time-Life Books, 1988.

*Franz, M. *Diabetes and Exercise: Guidelines for Safe and Enjoyable Activity*. Minneapolis: International Diabetes Center, Inc., 1984.

————. "Exercise and the Management of Diabetes Mellitus." *Journal of the American Dietetic Association* 87 (1987): 872–80.

*Gordon, N. F., and L. W. Gibbons. *The Cooper Clinic Cardiac Rehabilitation Program*. New York: Simon & Schuster, 1990.

Helmrich, S., D. Ragland, R. Leung, and R. Paffenbarger. "Physical Activity and Reduced Occurrence of Non-Insulin-Dependent Diabetes Mellitus." *New England Journal of Medicine* 325 (1991): 147–52.

Horton, E. "Role and Management of Exercise in Diabetes Mellitus." *Diabetes Care* 11 (1988): 201–9.

Kahn, J., and A. Vinike. "Exercise Training in the Diabetic Patient." *Internal Medicine* 9 (1988): 117–25.

Kelemen, M., M. Effron, S. Valenti, K. Stewart. "Exercise Training Combined with Antihypertensive Drug Therapy. Effects on Lipids, Blood Pressure and Left Ventricular Mass." *Journal of the American Medical Association* 263 (1990): 2766–71.

Leon, A., C. Certo, P. Comoss., B. Franklin, V. Froelicher, W. Haskell, H. Hellerstein, W. Marley, M. Pollack, A. Ries, E. Savarajon, L. Smith. "Scientific Evidence of the Value of Cardiac Rehabilitation Services with Emphasis on Patients Following Myocardial Infarction—Section I: Exercise Conditioning Component." *Journal of Cardiopulmonary Rehabilitation* 10 (1990): 79–87.

McHenry, P., M. Ellestad, S. Fletcher, V. Froelicher, H. Hartley, J. Mitchell. "A Special Report: Statement on Exercise." *Circulation* 81 (1990): 396–98.

McMillan, D. "Deterioration of the Microcirculation in Diabetes." *Diabetes* 24 (1975): 944–57.

Oldridge, N. B. "Cardiac Rehabilitation After Myocardial Infarction." *Journal of the American Medical Association* 260 (1988): 945–50.

*Ornish, D. *Dr. Dean Ornish's Program for Reversing Heart Disease.* New York: Random House, 1990.

———, S. E. Brown, L. W. Scherwitz, J. H. Billings, W. T. Armstrong, T. A. Ports, S. M. McLanahan, R. L. Kirkeeide, R. J. Brand, and K. L. Gould. "Can Lifestyle Changes Reverse Coronary Disease?" *Lancet* 336 (1990): 129–33.

*Piscatella, J. C. *Choices for a Healthy Heart.* New York: Workman Publishing, 1987.

Shepherd, R. J. "The Value of Exercise in Ischemic Heart Disease: A Cumulative Analysis." *Journal of Cardiac Rehabilitation* 3 (1983): 294–98.

Thompson, P. D. "The Benefits and Risks of Exercise Training in Patients With Chronic Coronary Artery Disease." *Journal of the American Medical Association* 259 (1988): 1537–40.

Chapter 23: Eating for the Health of Your Heart

An Expert Panel of the National Cholesterol Education Program. "Report of the National Cholesterol Education Program Expert Panel on Detection, Evaluation, and Treatment of High Blood Cholesterol in Adults." *Archives of Internal Medicine* 148 (1988): 36–69.

Food and Nutrition Board of the National Research Council, National Academy of Sciences. "Water and Electrolytes." In *Recommended Dietary Allowances,* 10th ed. Washington, D.C.: National Academy Press, 1989.

Grundy, S. M. "Comparison of Monounsaturated Fatty Acids and Carbohydrates for Lowering Plasma Cholesterol." *New England Journal of Medicine* 314 (1986): 745–48.

Houston, M. C. "Sodium and Hypertension—A Review." *Archives of Internal Medicine* 146 (1986): 179–85.

Kris-Etherton, P. M., D. Krummel, M. E. Russell, D. Dreon, S. MacKey, J. Borchers, and P. D. Wood. "The Effect of Diet on Plasma Lipids, Lipoproteins, and Coronary Heart Disease." *Journal of the American Dietetic Association* 88 (1988): 1373–1400.

LaRosa, J. C., D. Hunninghake, D. Bush, M. H. Criqui, G. S. Getz, A M. Gotto, S. M. Grundy, L. Rakita, R. M. Robertson, M. L. Weisfeldt, and J. I. Cleeman. "The Cholesterol Facts: A Summary of the Evidence Relating Dietary Fats, Serum Cholesterol, and Coronary Heart Disease." *Circulation* 81 (1990): 1721–33.

Leaf, A., and P. C. Weber. "Cardiovascular Effects of n-3 Fatty Acids." *New England Journal of Medicine* 318 (1988): 549–57.

Ornish, D., S. E. Brown, L. W. Scherwitz, J. H. Billings, W. T. Armstrong, T. A. Ports, S. M. McLanahan, R. L. Kirkeeide, R. J. Brand, and K. L. Gould. "Can Lifestyle Changes Reverse Coronary Heart Disease?" *Lancet* 336 (1990): 129–33.

Pennington, J. A. T. *Bowes & Church's Food Values of Portions Commonly Used.* Philadelphia: J. B. Lippincott, 1989.

Van Horn, L. V., K. Liu, D. Parker, L. Emidy, Y. Liao, W. Harn Pan, D. Giumetti, J. Hewitt, and J. Stamler. "Serum Lipid Response to Oat Product Intake With a Fat-Modified Diet." *Journal of the American Dietetic Association* 86 (1986): 759–64.

Chapter 24: The End of the Beginning

Abramson, E. E. "A Review of Behavioral Approaches to Weight Control." *Behavior Research Therapy* 11 (1973): 547–56.

Anderson, R., J. K. Davies, I. Kickbusch, D. McQueen, and J. Turner, eds. *Health Behaviour Research and Health Promotion*. New York: Oxford University Press, 1988.

Bandura, A. "Self-Efficacy: Toward a Unifying Theory of Behavior Change." *Psychological Review* 84 (1977): 191–215.

Brownell, K. D., G. A. Marlatt, E. Lichtenstein, and G. T. Wilson. "Understanding and Preventing Relapse." *American Psychologist* 41 (1986): 765–82.

Foreyt, J. P., R. E. Mitchell, P. T. Garner, M. Gee, L. W. Scott, A. M. Gotto. "Behavioral Treatment of Obesity: Results and Limitations." *Behavior Therapy* 13 (1982): 153–61.

Glynn, T. J., G. M. Boyd, and J. C. Gruman. "Essential Elements of Self-Help/ Minimal Intervention Strategies for Smoking Cessation." *Health Education Quarterly* 17 (1990): 329–45.

Haynes, R. B., D. W. Taylor, and D. L. Sackett, eds. *Compliance in Health Care*. Baltimore: Johns Hopkins University Press, 1979.

Jones, J. "A Proposed Model of Relapse Prevention for Adolescents Who Abuse Alcohol." *Journal of Child Adolescence and Psychiatric Mental Health Nursing* 3 (1990): 139–43.

Marlatt, G. A. "Relapse Prevention: A Self-Control Program for the Treatment of Addictive Behaviors." *Adherence, Compliance and Generalizations in Behavioral Medicine*. Edited by R. B. Stuart. New York: Brunner, 1982.

———. J. Gordon. "Determinants of Relapse: Implications for Maintenance of Behavior Change." In *Behavioral Medicine: Changing Health Lifestyles*. Edited by P. O. Davidson and S. M. Davidson. Elmsford, N.Y.: Pergamon, 1980. 410–52.

———. *Relapse Prevention . . . Maintenance Strategies in the Treatment of Addictive Behavior*. New York: Guilford Press, 1985.

Rose-Colley, M., J. M. Eddy, and E. D. Glover. "Relapse Prevention: Implications for Health Promotion Professionals." *Health-Values* 13 (1989): 8–13.

Shiffman, S. "Coping With Temptations To Smoke." *Journal of Consulting and Clinical Psychology* 52 (1984): 261–67.

Super, D. *Work Values Inventory*. Boston: Houghton Mifflin, 1970.

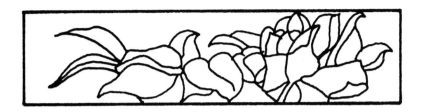

INDEX

Note: *Page numbers in italics refer to illustrations.*